Dermatopathology

Dermatopathology

THIRD EDITION

Edited by

Dirk M. Elston, MD

Professor and Chairman
Department of Dermatology and Dermatologic Surgery
Medical University of South Carolina
Charleston, SC, USA

Tammie Ferringer, MD

Section Head and Fellowship Director of Dermatopathology
Departments of Dermatology and Laboratory Medicine
Geisinger Medical Center
Danville, PA, USA

with

Christine J. Ko, MD
Steven Peckham, MD
Whitney A. High, MD, JD, MEng
David J. DiCaudo, MD
Sunita Bhuta, MD

For additional online content visit http://www.expertconsult.com

ELSEVIER

ELSEVIER

First edition 2009
Second edition 2014

The right of Dirk M. Elston, Tammie Ferringer, Christine J. Ko, Steven Peckham, Whitney A. High, David J. DiCaudo to be identified as authors of this work has been asserted by them in accordance with the Copyright, Designs and Patents Act 1988.

ISBN: 978-0-7020-7280-2
E-ISBN: 978-0-7020-7281-9

Content Strategist: Charlotta Kryhl
Content Development Specialists: Joanne Scott, Kim Benson
Project Manager: Joanna Souch
Design: Ashley Miner
Illustration Manager: Muthukumaran Thangaraj
Marketing Manager: Michele Milano

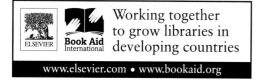

Working together to grow libraries in developing countries

www.elsevier.com • www.bookaid.org

Printed in Poland

Last digit is the print number: 9 8 7 6 5

Contents

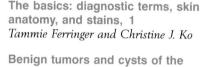
 Indicates additional online material

Online Lectures and Atlas Materials

1. **Author-narrated lectures – 27 presentations with approximately 2000 slides and over 8 hours running time**

2. **Clinical image atlas – with approximately 600 images**

3. **Histopathology atlas – with approximately 400 images**

4. **Infectious disease atlas – with approximately 2500 histopathologic images**

5. **Soft tissue tumor atlas – with approximately 300 histopathologic images**

6. **Lymphoma atlas – with 111 images**

Access the complete contents online at **http://www.expertconsult.com**

Preface

This text is designed to cover the essentials of dermatopathology in a style that is enjoyable and easily understood. **Please note that you are holding only a portion of the book in your hands! Much of it is online in the form of online lectures and extensive digital image atlases. Online material also includes a high-quality clinical image atlas, an extensive infectious disease atlas, a soft tissue tumor atlas, a lymphoma atlas, and more. Be sure to check** out all the online features at http://www.expertconsult.com. For students of dermatopathology, we hope the book and lectures make your way a little easier. For those in practice, we hope the book becomes one of your favorite references and one that you reach for often.

Dirk M. Elston

List of Contributors

With contributions by Patricia Malerich, MD; Lindsay Sewell, MD; Nektarios Lountzis, MD; David Adams, MD; Martie Jewell, MD; Chad Thomas, MD; Sasha Kramer, MD; Eric Hossler, MD; Morgan Wilson, MD; Puja Puri, MD; Michael Conroy, MD; Seth Forman, MD, and Carly Elston.

Monkey pox slides courtesy of Erik Stratman, MD.

Chancroid and granuloma inguinale slides courtesy of Brooke Army Medical Center teaching file.

Lucio phenomenon slide courtesy of David M. Scollard, MD.

Kimura disease slide courtesy of Jim Fitzpatrick, MD.

Peppered moth image courtesy of David Tomlinson, Professor Emeritus Faculty of Life Sciences, University of Manchester.

Sparganum proliferum images courtesy of Richard Bernert, MD.

Contributing authors

Sunita Bhuta, MD
Chief, Head and Neck Pathology
Professor, Pathology and Laboratory Medicine
Director, Transmission Electron Microscopy Laboratory
David Geffen School of Medicine, UCLA
Los Angeles, CA, USA

David J. DiCaudo, MD
Chair, Dermatopathology Division
Associate Professor, Dermatology and Laboratory Medicine/Pathology
Department of Dermatology
Mayo Clinic College of Medicine
Scottsdale, AZ, USA

Dirk M. Elston, MD
Professor and Chairman
Department of Dermatology and Dermatologic Surgery
Medical University of South Carolina
Charleston, SC, USA

Tammie Ferringer, MD
Section Head and Fellowship Director of Dermatopathology
Departments of Dermatology and Laboratory Medicine
Geisinger Medical Center
Danville, PA, USA

Whitney A. High, MD, JD, MEng
Professor, Dermatology and Pathology
Director, Dermatopathology Laboratory (Dermatology)
University of Colorado School of Medicine
Denver, CO, USA

Christine J. Ko, MD
Professor of Dermatology and Pathology
Departments of Dermatology and Pathology
Yale University
New Haven, CT, USA

Steven Peckham, MD
Pathologist/Dermatopathologist
Precision Pathology Services
San Antonio, TX, USA

Acknowledgments

I would like to thank my fellow authors as well as the faculty residents and fellows of the Medical University of South Carolina, the Ackerman Academy of Dermatopathology, the Robert Wood Johnson School of Medicine, Saint Lukes-Roosevelt /Mount Sinai, Palisades Medical Center, China Medical University, Central South University, Peking University, Geisinger Medical Center, Brooke Army Medical Center, and Wilford Hall Medical Center. This book would not have been possible without their support. I would also like to thank my first teachers in dermatopathology: Dean Pearson, Tim Berger, Jim Graham, George Lupton, and Wilma Bergfeld.

John Metcalf and John Maize deserve recognition as true gentlemen and scholars. Special thanks to those who collaborated on projects and made my years at the Ackerman Academy a pleasure. Ed Heilman: You are the ultimate gentleman. Mike Kramer: Your generosity of spirit and commitment to do right are always appreciated. Pat Heller: You are the best of New York wrapped up in one person. Jakki Hopkins: I could not have survived the AAD year without you. Raj Singh: Your work ethic and commitment to education are an example to us all. Jisun Cha and Eun Ji Kwon: The dynamic duo of New Jersey. Ying Guo: Graceful and brilliant. Joan Mones: Passionately devoted to DO education and the Ackerman Academy core team: Elaine Waldo, Elen Blochin, Sau Wong, Jonathan Truong, Geffie Figueroa, and Amy Spizuoco. Mark Jacobsen and Paul Chu were always generous with resources at Port Chester. I would like to thank all of those who contributed to research projects and discussions, especially Viktoryia Kazlouskaya, Alexandra Flamm, Cheng Zhou, Amira Elbendary, Manuel Valdebran, Kruti Parikh, Nathan Cleaver, Filamer Kabigting, Khanh Thieu, Jeffrey Shackelton, Mara Dacso, John R. Griffin, Erick Jacobson-Dunlop, Qiang Xie, Dave Hall, Mary Mcgonagle, Tatyana Groysman, Steve Hammond, Jennifer Lambe, Kalpana Reddy, Sean Stephenson, Elgida Volpicelli, Karen Wu, Munir Idriss, Shengli Chen, Caihong Sun, Liping Zhao, Sherihan Allam, Yanping Bai, Lubna Rizwan, Xiaoqin Wang, Nausheen Yaqoob, Mebratu Ketema Tabor, Raissa Couto, Ying Zhou, Xueling Mei, Lei Zhang, Ying Sun, Shijun Shan, Johanna Sales, Chao Ji, Zhancai Zheng, Yue Zhang, Seniz Ergin, Ruzeng Xue, Shaoshan Cui, Jing Zhang, Kara Melissa Torres, Sarah Velasquez, Yan Yu, Christian Andres, Ciara Maguire, Philip Muller, Carlos Morais, Marc Bodendorf, and Anja Miesel.

The editors and authors would like to thank the editorial and publication team at Elsevier, without whom this work would not have been possible.

Dirk M. Elston

Dedications

This book is dedicated to my wife and best friend Kathy, my children Carly and Nate who make me so proud, and to all of those students of dermatopathology, young and old, who make it such a pleasure to teach.

Dirk M. Elston

This work is dedicated to my daughter Emily who has filled holes in my life that I did not know I had; my husband Jim and mother Judy for their patience, understanding, and support; and to the memory of my father Elzie. None of this would be possible without the incredible guidance and tutelage of Dirk M. Elston and would lack purpose without the curiosity and eagerness of the residents and fellows that go on to become my colleagues and friends.

Tammie Ferringer

To Peter, Dylan, and Owen.

Christine J. Ko

To my Ms, old and new …

Whitney A. High

To my parents, James and Hilda, who have always encouraged me to do my best.

Steven Peckham

To my wife Valerie, our children Matthew and Gianna, and all the dermatology residents, past and present, whom I have had the pleasure to teach.

David J. DiCaudo

The basics: diagnostic terms, skin anatomy, and stains

Tammie Ferringer and Christine J. Ko

Glossary of terms

Acantholysis

- Loss of cell–cell adhesion

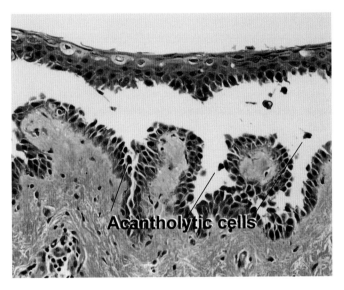

Fig. 1.1 Acantholysis, pemphigus vulgaris

Acanthosis

- Increase in thickness of the epidermis
- Regular (all rete pegs descend to the same level) or irregular (rete pegs descend to different levels in the papillary dermis)

Anaplasia

- Atypical nuclei (abnormal size, shape, staining) and pleomorphism (variation in nuclear characteristics)

Apoptosis (pronounced apohtosis)

- "Programmed cell death"
- "Dead red" keratinocytes with pyknotic nuclei
- Although the term is often applied to any necrotic or dyskeratotic keratinocyte, it is best reserved for physiologic programmed cell death or pathologic processes that produce death through a similar pathway

Arborizing

- Branching, often refers to rete or vasculature

Asteroid body

- Collections of eosinophilic material seen in sporotrichosis
- Also refers to star-shaped intracytoplasmic inclusions seen in giant cells of sarcoidosis or berylliosis or other granulomatous processes

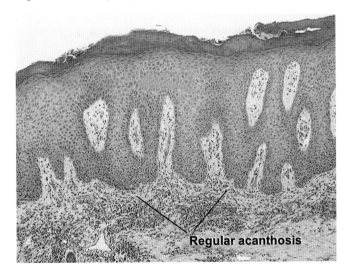

Fig. 1.2 Acanthosis, psoriasis

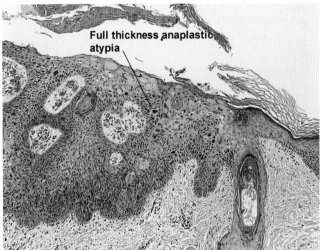

Fig. 1.3 Anaplasia, Bowen disease

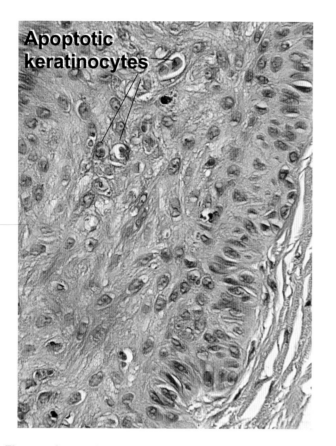

Fig. 1.4 Apoptosis, outer root sheath, catagen follicle

Atrophy

- Decrease in thickness of epidermis

Ballooning degeneration

- Destruction of epidermis by dissolution of cell attachments and intracellular edema

Caterpillar body

- Pale pink linear basement membrane material within epidermis, seen in porphyria cutanea tarda
- Represents degenerated type IV collagen

Civatte/colloid bodies

- Pink, globular remnants of keratinocytes

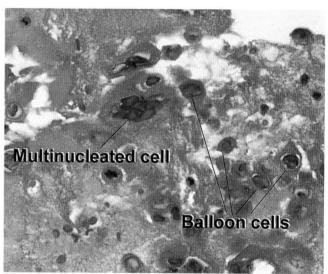

Fig. 1.6 Ballooning degeneration, herpes simplex

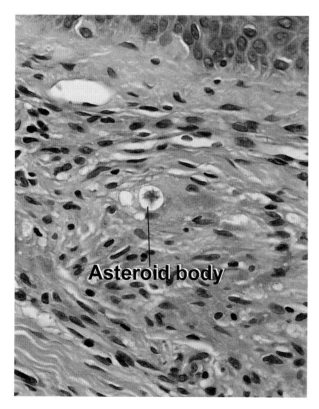

Fig. 1.5 Asteroid body, sarcoidosis

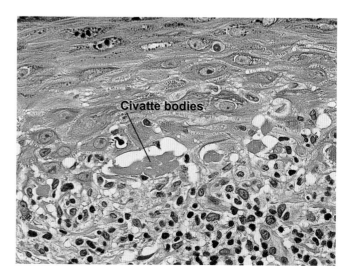

Fig. 1.7 Civatte bodies, lichen planus

Collagen entrapment

- Collagen fibers surrounded by histiocytes/spindle cells (collagen balls)

Cornoid lamellae

- Forty-five–degree angle parakeratosis in a column above a focus with a diminished granular layer and underlying dyskeratotic cells

Corps ronds/grains/dyskeratosis

- Corps ronds = rounded nucleus with halo of pale to pink dyskeratotic cytoplasm
- Grain = dark blue flattened nucleus surrounded by minimal cytoplasm
- Dyskeratosis = abnormal, individual-cell keratinization

Cowdry A body

- Also known as the *Lipschutz body*
- Intranuclear pink inclusions of herpesvirus infection

Cowdry B body

- Intranuclear pink inclusions of adenovirus and poliovirus infection

Crust

- Serum/fluid with inflammatory cells/debris in stratum corneum

Donovan body

- Intracytoplasmic collections of bacteria seen in granuloma inguinale

Dutcher body

- Intracytoplasmic pink masses of immunoglobulin that invaginate into the nucleus of plasma cells and appear to be intranuclear

Effacement

- Loss of normal rete pattern

Eosinophilic spongiosis

- Spongiosis with eosinophils in the epidermis

Epidermolytic hyperkeratosis

- Coarse, irregular hypergranulosis associated with disruption of cell membranes
- Associated with keratin 1 and 10 mutations

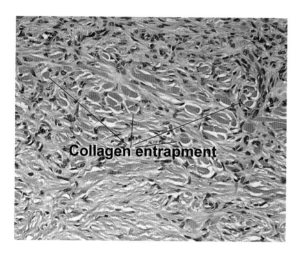

Fig. 1.8 Collagen entrapment, dermatofibroma

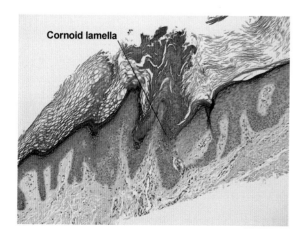

Fig. 1.9 Cornoid lamellae, porokeratosis

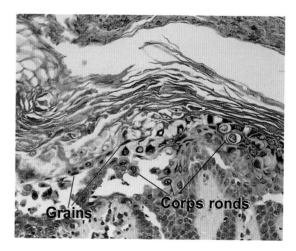

Fig. 1.10 Corps ronds/grains, Darier disease

Epidermotropism

- Lymphocytes in epidermis with relative absence of spongiosis; term usually reserved for mycosis fungoides

Erosion

- Partial thickness loss of epidermis

Exocytosis

- Lymphocytes in the epidermis with associated spongiosis; term usually used when discussing spongiotic dermatitis

Festooning

- Papillary dermis retains an undulating pattern (often used to describe porphyria cutanea tarda)

Flame figure

- Collagen encrusted with major basic protein from eosinophils

Foam cell

- Lipid-laden histiocyte

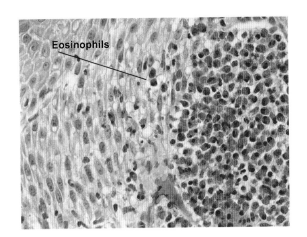

Fig. 1.11 Eosinophilic spongiosis, incontinentia pigmenti

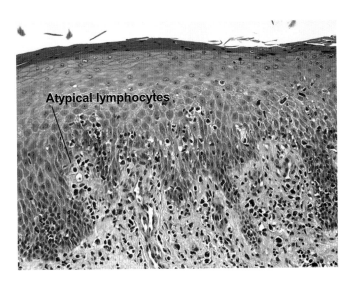

Fig. 1.13 Epidermotropism, mycosis fungoides

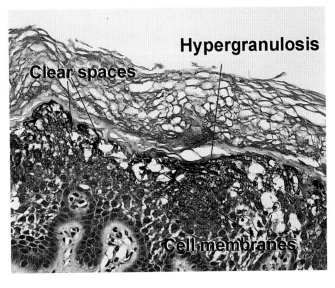

Fig. 1.12 Epidermolytic hyperkeratosis

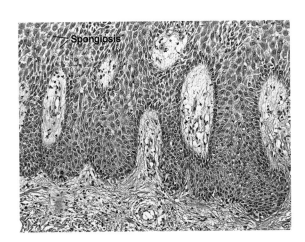

Fig. 1.14 Lymphocyte exocytosis, subacute spongiotic dermatitis

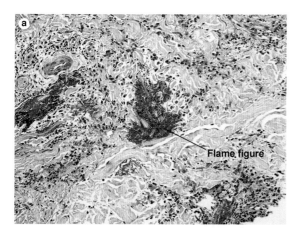

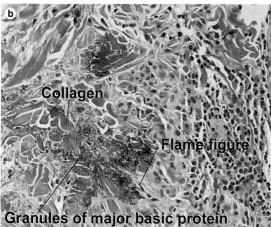

Fig. 1.15 Flame figure, Wells syndrome

Follicular mucinosis

- Alteration of hair sheath anatomy by pools of mucin

Granulomatous

- Composed of granulomas (collections of histiocytes)

Grenz zone

- Uninvolved area of dermis beneath the epidermis or adjacent to a hair follicle (border zone)

Guarnieri body

- Eosinophilic inclusions of smallpox

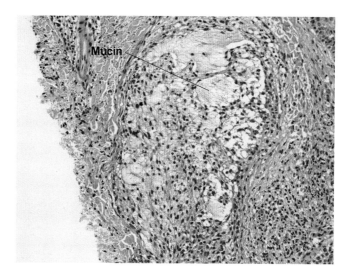

Fig. 1.17 Follicular mucinosis, alopecia mucinosis

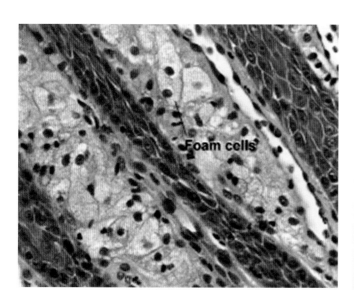

Fig. 1.16 Foam cells, verruciform xanthoma

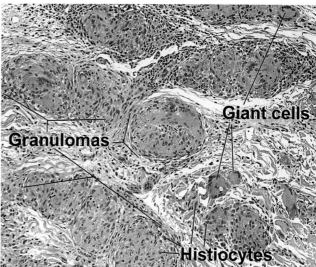

Fig. 1.18 Granulomas, sarcoid

Henderson–Paterson body

• Intracytoplasmic oval, pink inclusions of molluscum infection

Hypergranulosis/hypogranulosis

• Increased/decreased granular layer

Hyperpigmentation/hypopigmentation

• Increased/decreased melanin pigment

Interface

• Generally refers to the dermoepidermal junction

Kamino body

• Dull pink to amphophilic basement membrane material within the epidermis in a Spitz nevus

Karyorrhexis

• Fragmentation of neutrophils (leukocytoclasis). (If neutrophils resemble ants with segmented bodies, then karyorrhexis resembles dismembered ants and scattered ant heads)

Koilocytes

• Keratinocytes with clear cytoplasm and shrunken "raisinlike" pyknotic nuclei

Leishman–Donovan body

• Intracytoplasmic collections of amastigotes in leishmaniasis

Lentiginous epidermal hyperplasia

• Elongated bulbous rete

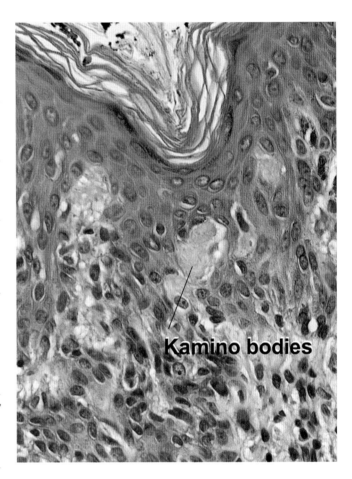

Fig. 1.20 Kamino bodies, Spitz nevus

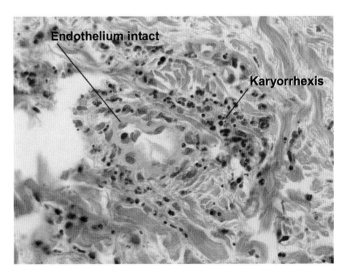

Fig. 1.21 Karyorrhexis, leukocytoclastic vasculitis

Fig. 1.19 Hypergranulosis/hypogranulosis, lichen planus

Lentiginous melanocytic growth pattern

- Proliferation predominantly along the dermoepidermal junction

Leukocytoclasia

- Fragmentation of neutrophils, also referred to as *karyorrhexis*

Lichenoid dermatitis

- Interface dermatitis with destruction of the basal layer and Civatte body formation (Fig. 1.7 and Fig. 1.19)

Lichenoid infiltrate

- A bandlike infiltrate, generally composed predominantly of lymphocytes, located at the dermoepidermal junction

Medlar body

- Brown, round structure resembling overlapping copper pennies
- Divide by septation, resembling a hot-cross bun

Metachromasia

- The property of staining a different color from the stain itself (i.e., the purple color of mast cell granules with the blue stain methylene blue)

Michaelis–Gutman body

- Intracellular and extracellular calcified, concentric circular structures, seen in malakoplakia

Munro microabscess

- Collection of neutrophils in the stratum corneum, as seen in psoriasis

Necrobiosis

- Pale-staining, smudged, necrotic collagen

Negri body

- Inclusions within neurons seen in rabies infection

Orthokeratosis

- Stratum corneum without retained nuclei

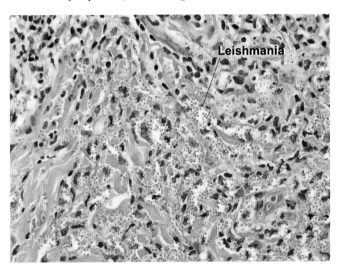

Fig. 1.22 Leishman–Donovan bodies, leishmaniasis

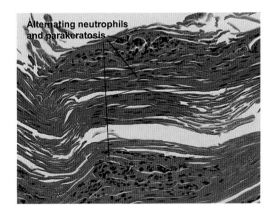

Fig. 1.24 Munro microabscess, psoriasis

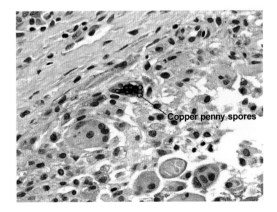

Fig. 1.23 Medlar bodies, chromomycosis

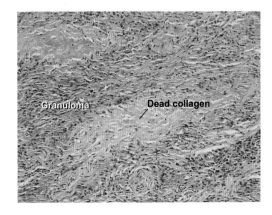

Fig. 1.25 Necrobiosis, necrobiosis lipoidica

Pagetoid cells

- Large cells with abundant cytoplasm within the epidermis

Pagetoid scatter

- Buckshot scatter of atypical cells within the epidermis

Palisading

- Picket fence–like arrangement at the periphery

Papillary mesenchymal body

- Structure that resembles the whorl of plump mesenchymal cells normally present in the hair papilla (seen in trichoblastoma and trichoepithelioma)

Papillomatosis

- Exophytic fingerlike projections

Parakeratosis

- Stratum corneum with retained nuclei

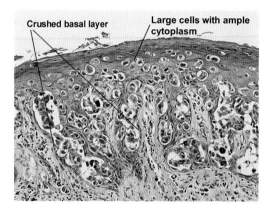

Fig. 1.26 Pagetoid cells and pagetoid scatter, Paget disease

Pigment incontinence

- Melanin within dermal macrophages and free within the dermis

Pleomorphism

- Variation in nuclear size/shape

Psammoma body

- Extracellular laminated, calcified structures seen in meningioma, papillary thyroid carcinoma, and ovarian carcinoma

Pseudoepitheliomatous hyperplasia (PEH)

- Prominent acanthosis of the adnexal epithelium and epidermis, mimics squamous cell carcinoma
- Often associated with trapping of elastic fibers

Pseudohorn cyst

- Keratin-filled cystic structure that is the result of cutting through invaginations of the stratum corneum (similar to a horn cyst, but connects to the surface)

Reticular degeneration

- Destruction of epidermis with cell membranes remaining in a netlike pattern

Reticulated

- Network of interconnecting strands (netlike)

Russell body

- Intracytoplasmic pink collections of immunoglobulins in plasma cells, seen in rhinoscleroma and other conditions with many plasma cells

Schaumann body

- Laminated calcified structure seen in sarcoidosis

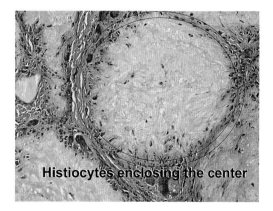

Fig. 1.27 Palisading, gout

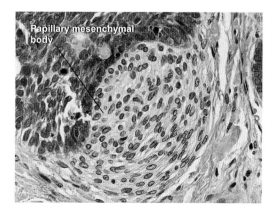

Fig. 1.28 Papillary mesenchymal body, trichoepithelioma

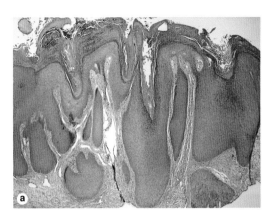 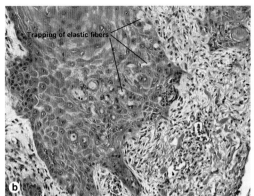

Fig. 1.29 (A) PEH, syringosquamous metaplasia after trauma. **(B)** Elastic fiber trapping in PEH

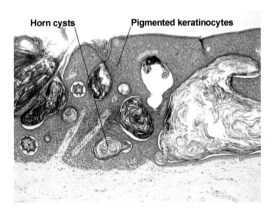

Fig. 1.30 Pseudohorn cyst, seborrheic keratosis

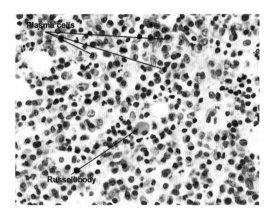

Fig. 1.32 Russell body, rhinoscleroma

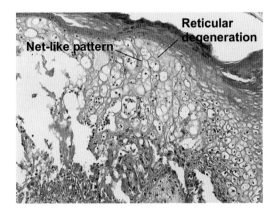

Fig. 1.31 Reticular degeneration, variola

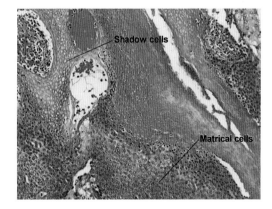

Fig. 1.33 Shadow cells, pilomatricoma

Shadow cells

- Cells with barely visible outlines of nuclei

Spongiform pustule of Kogoj

- Neutrophils in the stratum spinosum, associated with spongiosis at the periphery (typical of psoriasis)

Spongiosis

- Intercellular edema in epidermis with stretching of cell–cell junctions (Fig. 1.14)

Squamotization (or squamatization)

- Loss of cuboidal/columnar basal cells, with deepest layer now being polyhedral, pink squamous cells

Squamous eddies

- Circular whorls of squamous cells

Storiform

- Cartwheel or loosely whorled pattern

Vacuolar change

- Formation of clear spaces within the basal layer

Verocay body

- Structure composed of two nuclear palisades enclosing pink cytoplasmic processes, seen in schwannoma

Villus

- Projection of papillary dermis covered by a layer of epidermal cells into a cavity

Scalp skin

Key Features

- Numerous follicles that extend down into the panniculus
- Associated sebaceous glands, arrector pili muscles

Facial skin

Key Features

- Thin epidermis
- Basket-weave stratum corneum
- Hair follicles and sebaceous glands numerous in the dermis
- *Demodex* mites common
- Eyelid and ear skin have many vellus hair follicles
- In the upper dermis of eyelid skin, skeletal muscle bundles are present
- On the conjunctival surface of the eyelid, stratum corneum and hair follicles are absent, but goblet cells are present

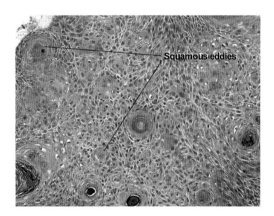

Fig. 1.34 Squamous eddies, irritated seborrheic keratosis

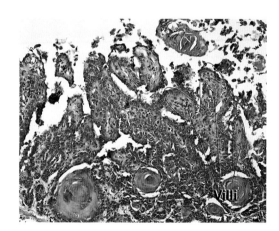

Fig. 1.36 Villi, warty dyskeratoma

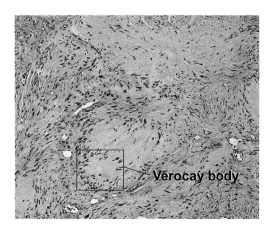

Fig. 1.35 Verocay body, schwannoma

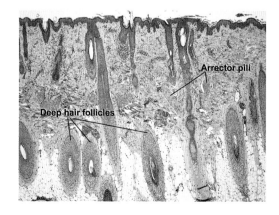

Fig. 1.37 Normal scalp with follicles rooted in the fat

Skin of the trunk

Key Features

- Very thick dermis, especially in skin from the back
- Scattered hair follicles and sebaceous glands
- Projections of fat extend upward to envelop adnexae

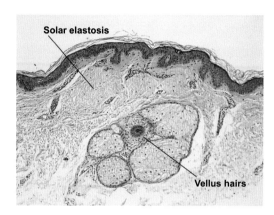

Fig. 1.38 Sun-damaged facial skin

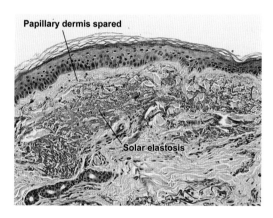

Fig. 1.39 Sun-damaged skin. Solar elastosis spares papillary dermis

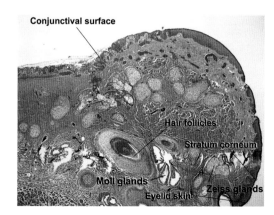

Fig. 1.40 Eyelid

Areolar skin

Key Features

- Slight acanthosis of the epidermis with basilar hyperpigmentation
- Sometimes there is a central invagination of the epidermis that leads to a follicle and sebaceous glands
- Smooth muscle bundles in the mid–deep dermis
- Apocrine glands in the reticular dermis

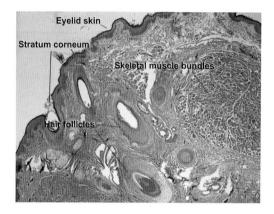

Fig. 1.41 Eyelid

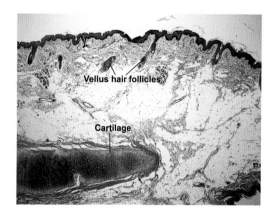

Fig. 1.42 Ear

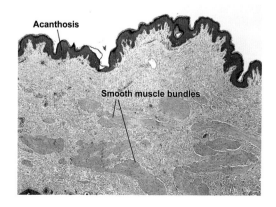

Fig. 1.43 Areolar skin, smooth muscle bundles

Acral skin

Key Features

- Compact eosinophilic stratum corneum
- Slight papillomatosis present on dorsal surfaces

Volar skin

Key Features

- Compact eosinophilic hyperkeratosis with underlying translucent stratum lucidum
- No hair follicles or sebaceous glands
- Eccrine glands numerous
- Meissner and Pacinian corpuscles may be seen

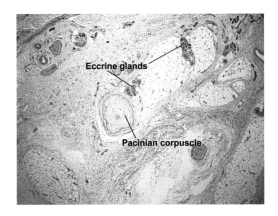

Fig. 1.46 Volar skin, eccrine glands, and Pacinian corpuscle

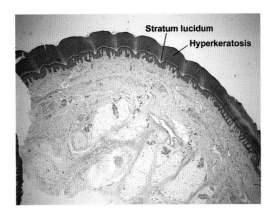

Fig. 1.44 Volar skin, thick stratum corneum, and deep Pacinian corpuscles

Mucosa

Key Features

- Absent granular layer
- Keratinocytes are large and pale (filled with glycogen)
- Dilated vessels in the submucosa
- Smooth muscle bundles may be present

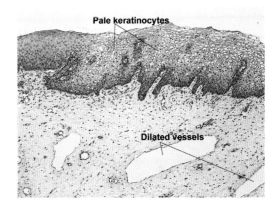

Fig. 1.47 Mucosa

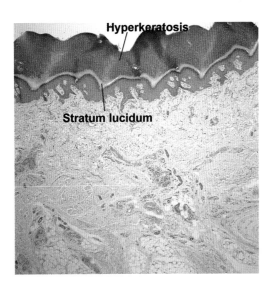

Fig. 1.45 Volar skin, stratum lucidum

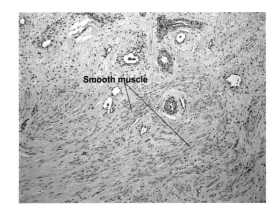

Fig. 1.48 Smooth muscle in submucosa

Nasal turbinate

Key Features

- Erectile tissue with fibrous septa and vascular sinusoids
- Mucous glands

Fetal skin

Key Features

- Stellate and spindled fibroblasts (mesenchyme)
- Densely cellular

Hair anatomy

Infundibulum

Key Features

- From epidermis down to insertion of sebaceous gland
- Intraepidermal portion = acrotrichium
- Keratinizes in the pattern of the normal epidermis with a granular layer (keratohyalin granules)

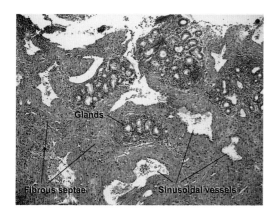

Fig. 1.49 Nasal turbinate mucosa: erectile tissue with mucous glands

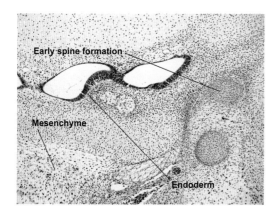

Fig. 1.50 Fetal mesenchyme

Isthmus

Key Features

- From the insertion of the sebaceous gland to the insertion of the arrector pili muscle (bulge)
- Keratin is formed in the absence of a granular layer = trichilemmal keratinization
- The inner root sheath is lost at this level, and the outer root sheath develops an inner corrugated, dense, pink, cornified layer; peripheral palisading of the outer root sheath is seen

Stem

Key Features

- From the insertion of the arrector pili muscle (bulge) to Adamson fringe
- Only present in anagen hairs

Adamson fringe

- The point above which hair cornifies
- Dermatophytes only infect cornified hair above Adamson fringe
- Above Adamson fringe, Huxley layer of the inner root sheath no longer has trichohyalin granules
- Hair tends to retract from the inner root sheath above Adamson fringe
  - The inner root sheath is fused and blue-gray at this level, and trichohyalin granules are not seen
  - The outer root sheath is composed of pink cells with peripheral palisading

Bulb

Key Features

- Below the stem portion of the anagen hair follicle
- From Adamson fringe to the base of the follicle

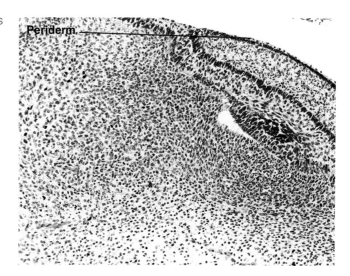

Fig. 1.51 Fetal periderm

- The bulb has three zones: matrix, supramatrix, keratogenous zone
  - Matrix: from base to critical line (widest point of the bulb and papillae)
  - Supramatrix: from critical line to B-fringe (point at which the outer root sheath becomes multilayered and Henle layer no longer has trichohyalin granules)
  - Keratogenous zone: from B-fringe to Adamson fringe
- Layers of the hair follicle that can be seen:
  - Fibrous root sheath
  - Vitreous basement membrane zone
  - Outer root sheath
  - Inner root sheath
    - Henle layer
    - Huxley layer
    - Cuticle of the inner root sheath
  - Hair shaft
    - Cuticle of the hair shaft
    - Cortex
    - Medulla

Anagen hairs have a stem and a bulb, which produces the hair shaft, whereas telogen hairs lack an inferior segment. Telogen hairs are easily recognized in vertical sections, as the club hair and surrounding trichilemmal keratin give the impression of a flamethrower.

Nail anatomy

Key Features

- Nail plate
- Nail bed: between distal edge of lunula and the proximal edge of onychodermal band
- Framing portion: proximal nail fold, lateral nail folds, distal nail fold
- Ensheathing portion: "cuticle," aka eponychium, hyponychium, solehorn, bed horny layer

Cuticle
- "Visible" cuticle (aka eponychium) is the thick keratinous material that borders the proximal nail fold and adheres to the nail plate
- "True" cuticle is located beneath the "visible" portion and is derived from the ventral part of the proximal nail fold
- The true cuticle is generally not seen, but it is sometimes visible as "flakes" of keratinous material parallel to the proximal nail fold

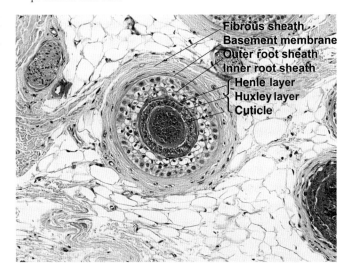

Fig. 1.53 Hair, transverse section

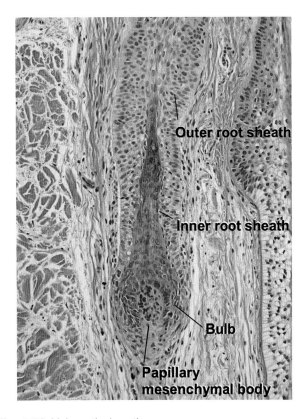

Fig. 1.52 Hair, vertical section

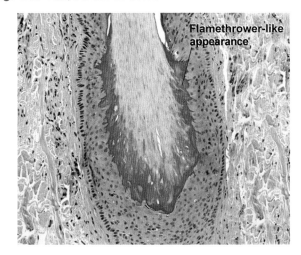

Fig. 1.54 Telogen hair

Hyponychium

- The space, epithelium, and keratinous material ventral to the nail plate

Solehorn

- Subungual white to colorless keratin, extends from the distal nail bed underneath the onychodermal band to below the free, distal edge of the nail plate

Nail matrix

- Proximal part makes the surface of the nail; distal part makes the ventral nail plate

Lunula

- Visible portion of nail matrix
- Anchoring portion (mesenchyme)

Types of keratinization of the nail

Onychokeratinization (no granular layer)

- Hard keratin of nail plate

Onycholemmal keratinization

- Ventral part of proximal nail fold (+ granular layer), bed epithelium (the cuticle, bed horny layer, solehorn) (no granular layer)

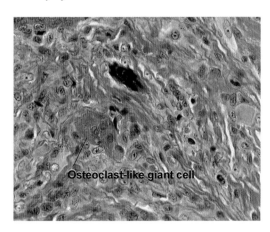

Fig. 1.55 Osteoclast-like giant cell

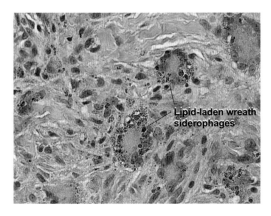

Fig. 1.56 Ringed lipidized siderophage (Touton giant cell with hemosiderin) in dermatofibroma

Epidermoid keratinization

- Dorsal proximal nail fold, lateral folds, hyponychium

Types of inflammatory cells

Dermal dendrocyte

Key Features

- Macrophage-type cells located in the dermis
- Many are factor XIIIa+, some are S100+
- Likely serve as antigen-presenting cells

Giant cell

Key Features

- Cell with multiple nuclei, usually abundant cytoplasm

Types

- Foreign body: nuclei are arranged haphazardly
- Langhans: nuclei are arranged in a horseshoe shape
- Osteoclast-like: nuclei are arranged haphazardly and eccentrically; cytoplasm is deep pink with a scalloped border that molds to adjacent structures
- Touton: nuclei are arranged in a wreath with foamy cytoplasm peripherally
- Ringed siderophage: Touton giant cell with hemosiderin (characteristic of the fibrous histiocytoma type of dermatofibroma)

Histiocyte

Key Features

- Epithelioid cell with a central, round/oval nucleus and surrounding cytoplasm
- Most are derived from a monocyte that takes up residence in tissue
- Functions include phagocytosis and antigen presentation
- Tend to coalesce in tissue with no intervening connective tissue

Langerhans cell

Key Features

- Dendritic cells in epidermis and dermis
- CD1a+, S100+, peanut agglutinin, langerin+
- Nucleus is typically eccentric and may be reniform (kidney shaped)
- Originate in bone marrow and function in presenting antigens to T cells
- Contain Birbeck granules, tennis racket–shaped rod and oval bodies seen on electron microscopy

Lymphocyte

Key Features

- Round, dark nucleus, generally with no visible cytoplasm
- B-cell lymphocytes produce antibodies and are important for humoral immunity

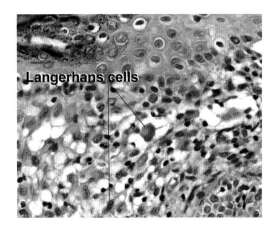

Fig. 1.57 Langerhans cell histiocytosis

- Natural killer (NK) cells are part of the innate immune system
- T-cell lymphocytes mature in the thymus and are important in cell-mediated immunity
- TH1 cells produce interleukin-1 (IL-1), IL-2, IL-12, and interferon-gamma (IFN-γ) and are important for cell-mediated immunity and function in activating macrophages
- TH2 cells produce IL-4, IL-5, and IL-10 and are important for humoral immunity

Mast cell

Key Features

- "Fried-egg" appearance with central round nucleus and surrounding oval, bluish cytoplasm
- Contain metachromatic granules composed of heparin, histamine, tryptase, carboxypeptidase, leukotrienes
- Important in immediate-type hypersensitivity reactions

Neutrophil

Key Features

- Predominant cell in acute infection
- Multilobulated nucleus

Eosinophil

Key Features

- IL-5 induces eosinophil production
- Bilobed nucleus with granular cytoplasm containing major basic protein, eosinophil cationic protein, catalase, and other proteins

Plasma cell

Key Features

- Eccentric nucleus with "clock face"
- Perinuclear pale space corresponding to rough endoplasmic reticulum (described by Hopf)
- Pink cytoplasm

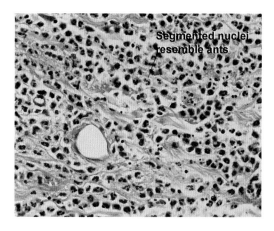

Fig. 1.59 Neutrophils in Sweet syndrome

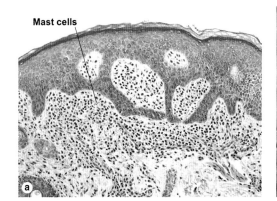

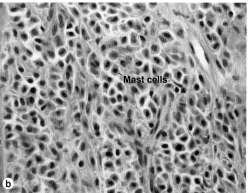

Fig. 1.58 Mastocytoma

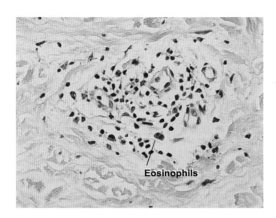

Fig. 1.60 Eosinophils in dermal hypersensitivity response

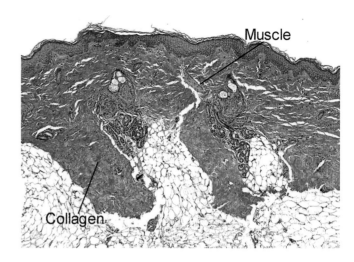

Fig. 1.62 Normal skin with Masson's trichrome

Verhoeff–Van Gieson stain

- Elastic fibers are black
- Examples: absence or reduction in scar, middermal elastolysis, anetoderma, cutis laxa
- Example: distorted fibers in pseudoxanthoma elasticum

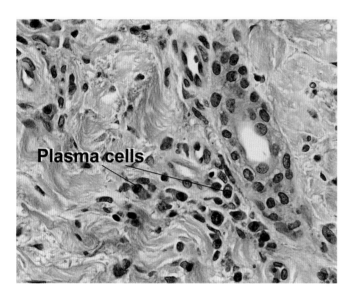

Fig. 1.61 Plasma cells

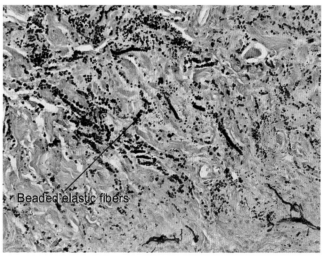

Fig. 1.63 Beaded elastic fibers in elastofibroma dorsi (Verhoeff–Van Gieson)

Histochemical stains

The affinities of various dyes have been exploited as histochemical "special" stains to aid in identification of cell type, mucopolysaccharides, muscle, lipid, iron, melanin, calcium, elastin, collagen, amyloid, and infectious organisms. Hematoxylin and eosin (H&E) is the routine staining choice for microscopic interpretation, resulting in blue nuclei and pink cytoplasm.

Connective tissue stains

Masson trichrome stain

- Differentiates collagen (blue-green) from smooth muscle (red)
- Example: scar versus leiomyoma

Important pitfall: very young collagen can stain red

Mast cell stains

Toluidine blue

- Stains mast cell granules metachromatically (i.e., the dye is blue but the granules stain purple)
- Also stains mucin (see later)

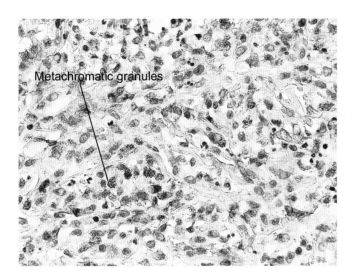

Fig. 1.64 Metachromatic staining of mast cells in urticaria pigmentosa (toluidine blue)

Giemsa

- Stains mast cell granules metachromatically (Fig. 1.82)
- Also stains many types of organisms and myeloid cells (see below)

Leder stain (naphthol ASD chloroacetate esterase)

- Mast cell cytoplasm stains red (not dependent on presence of granules)
- Also stains myeloid cells (example: leukemia cutis)

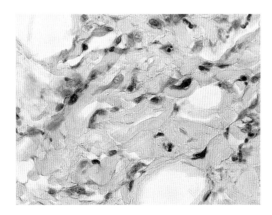

Fig. 1.65 Mast cells in urticaria pigmentosa (Leder)

Carbohydrate stains

PAS (periodic acid–Schiff)

- Stains glycogen, neutral mucopolysaccharides (such as basement membrane), and fungi red
  - Glycogen is diastase labile (i.e., sections exposed to diastase before staining do not stain red with PAS reaction)
    - Useful in clear cell acanthoma, trichilemmoma
  - Fungi and neutral mucopolysaccharides (basement membrane) are diastase resistant (i.e., stain red with PAS after diastase exposure)

- Useful in tinea corporis, tinea versicolor, candida, basement membrane thickening of lupus erythematosus, thickened vessel walls in porphyria
- Acid mucopolysaccharides, such as hyaluronic acid, do not stain with PAS

Alcian blue

- Demonstrates acid mucopolysaccharides by staining them blue

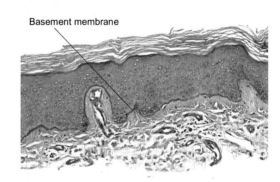

Fig. 1.66 PAS-positive basement membrane

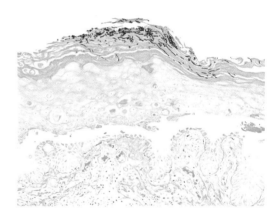

Fig. 1.67 PAS-positive fungi within the stratum corneum of tinea versicolor (PAS with light green counterstain)

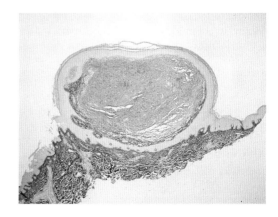

Fig. 1.68 Focal mucinosis with colloidal iron

- In normal skin, most mucin is sulfated acid mucopolysaccharide (heparin, chondroitin, dermatan sulfates). In most pathologic states with increased dermal mucin, the mucin is predominantly nonsulfated hyaluronic acid
  - Nonsulfated acid mucopolysaccharides (hyaluronic acid) stain with Alcian blue at pH 2.5 but not at pH 0.5
  - Examples: follicular mucinosis, granuloma annulare, myxoid cyst, dermal mucin in lupus erythematosus
  - Sulfated acid mucopolysaccharides stain with Alcian blue at both pH 2.5 and pH 0.5
- Alcian blue can be used with and without hyaluronidase to differentiate hyaluronic acid from other mucopolysaccharides

Colloidal iron

- Blue color indicates acid mucopolysaccharides
- As with Alcian blue, hyaluronidase digestion can be combined with colloidal iron to differentiate between hyaluronic acid and other mucosubstances

Toluidine blue

- Similar staining pattern as Alcian blue for acid mucopolysaccharides but metachromatic (reddish purple)
- Technically more complicated than Alcian blue and is used less often
- Metachromatically stains mast cells (see earlier)

Mucicarmine

- Stains acid mucopolysaccharides pink to red
- Stains the mucinous capsule of *Cryptococcus neoformans* pink to red

Amyloid

Congo red

- Amyloid stains brick red and displays "apple green" birefringence with polarized light

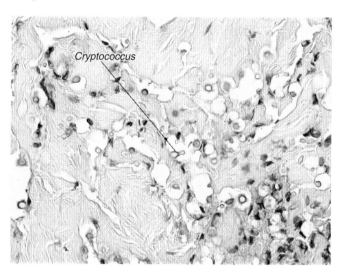

Fig. 1.69 Pink capsule of *Cryptococcus* with mucicarmine

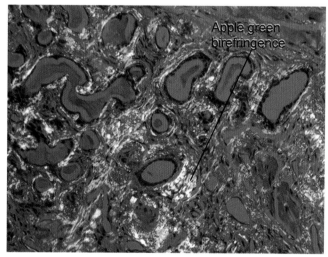

Fig. 1.71 Congo red–stained amyloid in a salivary gland viewed with polarized light

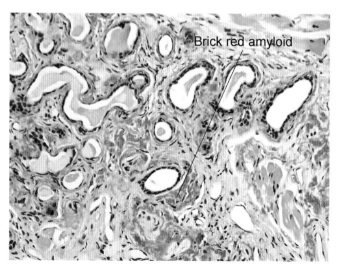

Fig. 1.70 Congo red–stained amyloid in a salivary gland viewed with light microscopy

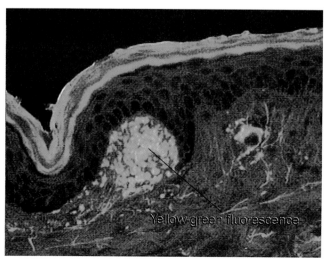

Fig. 1.72 Lichen amyloid with thioflavin T

Thioflavin T

- Sections must be examined with a fluorescent microscope, causing amyloid to have a yellow to yellow-green appearance

Crystal violet

- Metachromatically results in a red-purple color of amyloid

Iron

Prussian blue (Perls stain)

- Ferric ions react to form a deep blue color
- Useful to distinguish melanin from hemosiderin
- Example: hemosiderin in pigmented purpuric dermatosis
- Does not demonstrate iron in intact red blood cells

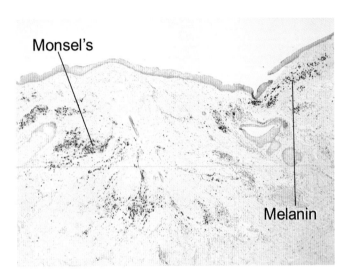

Fig. 1.73 Blue iron deposition from Monsel's (ferric subsulfate) tattoo with Perls iron stain

Melanin

Fontana–Masson

- A silver stain that results in a black precipitate with melanin

Calcium

Von Kossa

- A silver stain that stains calcium salts black
- Examples: pseudoxanthoma elasticum, calcinosis cutis, calciphylaxis

Alizarin red

- Binds directly to calcium ions, resulting in an orange-red color

Lipids

Oil red O

- Requires fresh frozen tissue, as lipid is removed during routine processing

Sudan black

- Requires fresh tissue

Osmium tetroxide

- Requires fresh tissue

Bacteria

Brown–Hopps

- A modification of the Brown–Brenn technique
- Gram-positive organisms stain blue, and gram-negative organisms stain red

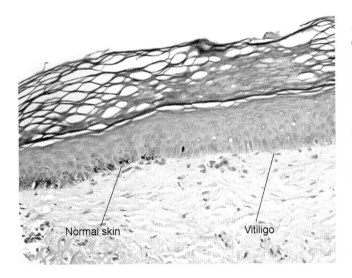

Fig. 1.74 Absence of melanin in vitiligo is contrasted with adjacent normal skin (Fontana–Masson)

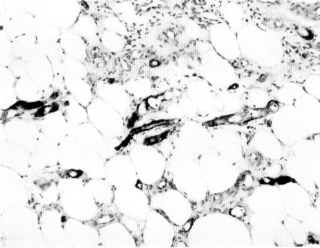

Fig. 1.75 Calcium deposition in the small vessels of the subcutaneous fat in calciphylaxis (Von Kossa)

Fungi

PAS (Periodic acid–Schiff)

• Fungi are PAS positive and diastase resistant (see earlier)

GMS (Grocott's methenamine silver)

• Gray-black reaction with fungal wall
• Also stains *Nocardia* and *Actinomyces*

Mycobacteria

Ziehl–Neelsen acid-fast stain; Fite acid-fast stain; Kinyoun's acid-fast stain

• Mycobacteria appear bright red
• Fite is preferred for "partially acid-fast" organisms such as lepra bacilli, atypical mycobacteria, and *Nocardia*. Fite preserves color due to use of peanut oil before staining and gentle decolorization

Auramine–rhodamine

• Requires a fluorescent microscope
• Mycobacteria fluoresce reddish yellow

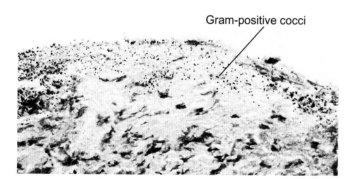

Gram-positive cocci

Fig. 1.76 Gram-positive cocci in an ulcer bed

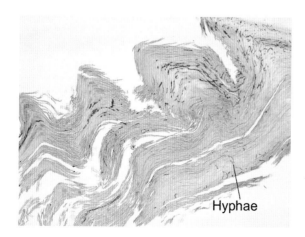

Hyphae

Fig. 1.77 PAS-positive hyphae of onychomycosis

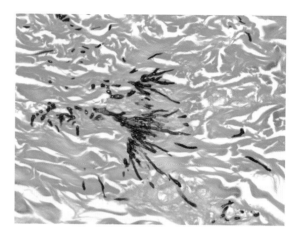

Fig. 1.78 *Aspergillus* with GMS

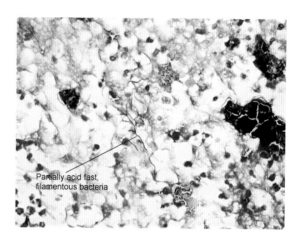

Partially acid fast, filamentous bacteria

Fig. 1.79 *Nocardia* with Fite stain

Spirochetes

Warthin–Starry (technically more difficult than the others, so sometimes referred to as the "worthless Starry")

Dieterle

Steiner (modified Dieterle stain)

• Silver stains resulting in black spirochetes
• Examples: Lyme disease (around vessels and in dermal papillae), syphilis (in lower epidermis)
• Also stains *Legionella*, *Bartonella*, and Donovan bodies of granuloma inguinale

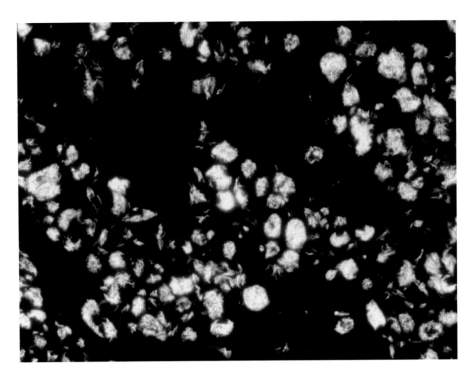

Fig. 1.80 Globi of *Mycobacterium leprae* stained with auramine–rhodamine as viewed with a fluorescent scope

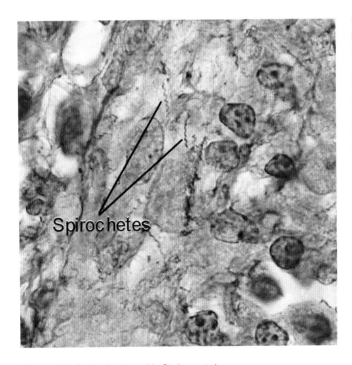

Fig. 1.81 Spirochetes with Steiner stain

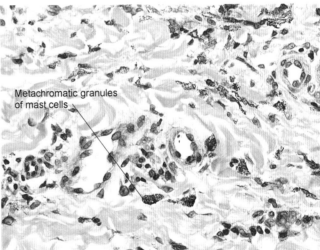

Fig. 1.82 Metachromatic granules within mast cells of urticaria pigmentosa (Giemsa)

Other "special" stains

Giemsa

- Giemsa has many uses, including highlighting myeloid and mast cell granules purplish blue
- Giemsa also stains many types of organisms, including bacteria, *Leishmania*, and *Histoplasma*

Immunohistochemical stains

Histochemical stains are now being supplemented by immunohistochemical techniques in fixed, paraffin-embedded tissue. Antibodies directed toward the antigen of interest are conjugated to peroxidases. Enzyme histochemical reactions for the peroxidase, such as diaminobenzidine method (DAB), are used to visualize the presence of enzyme–antibody–antigen complex fixed to tissue as a stable brown product. 3-amino-9-ethylcarbazole (AEC) can alternatively be used, giving a red reaction, but does not archive as well.

Immunopathologic antibodies are used in dermatopathology to differentiate carcinoma, melanoma, sarcoma, neural neoplasms, and lymphomas. A panel of antibodies is generally recommended rather than a single stain because aberrant staining is common in neoplasms. Independent and internal controls should be assessed to ensure proper reactivity.

Epithelial markers

AE1/AE3

- Cocktail of high- and low-molecular-weight monoclonal cytokeratin antibodies
- Expressed in the epidermis and adnexal epithelium
- Stains all epithelial tumors (squamous cell carcinoma and adnexal tumors) and generally excludes mesenchymal, melanocytic, and hematopoietic tumors
- Also stains epithelioid sarcoma, synovial sarcoma, and mesothelioma

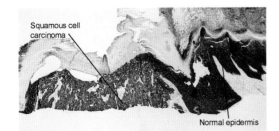

Fig. 1.83 AE1/AE3 positivity of squamous cell carcinoma

CK polyclonal keratin (pankeratin)

- Polyclonal cocktail that offers greater sensitivity than AE1/AE3

p63/p40

- Expressed in basal and spinous cells of the epidermis, germinative cells of sebaceous glands, and myoepithelial cells of the sweat glands

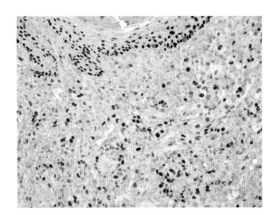

Fig. 1.84 p63 in spindle cell squamous cell carcinoma

- Lack of reactivity in metastatic carcinoma assists in differentiation from primary cutaneous adnexal neoplasms
- Useful in identification of cutaneous spindle cell squamous cell carcinoma from other spindle cell neoplasms

p40

- Recognizes a region of p63
- Useful in identification of cutaneous spindle cell squamous cell carcinoma from other spindle cell neoplasms

CAM5.2

- CAM5.2 detects low-molecular-weight cytokeratins present in most glandular neoplasms without staining the epidermis or stratified squamous epithelium
- Marks Paget disease and extramammary Paget disease

CK7

- Used in determining the origin of metastatic carcinoma
- In general, a marker of adenocarcinomas that originate above the diaphragm (non-gastrointestinal) (see Table 1.1)
- Marks Paget disease and extramammary Paget disease

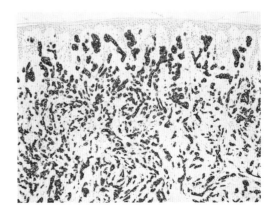

Fig. 1.85 CK7 reactivity of metastatic breast carcinoma

Table 1.1 Metastatic carcinoma of unknown origin

	CK20–	CK20+
CK7+	Breast, lung, mesothelioma	Bladder, pancreatic
CK7–	Hepatocellular, prostate, renal, neuroendocrine, and squamous carcinoma of lung	Colon

CK20

- Marks Merkel cell carcinoma predominantly in a paranuclear pattern and distinguishes from metastatic oat cell carcinoma of the lung that is typically negative
- Used in determining the origin of metastatic carcinoma (see Table 1.1)
- In general, a marker of adenocarcinomas that originate below the diaphragm (gastrointestinal)
- Highlights sparse Merkel cells within the basaloid islands of desmoplastic trichoepithelioma but not basal cell carcinoma

Ber-EP4

- Marks most epithelial cells, but not those undergoing squamous differentiation
- Positive in basal cell carcinoma and negative in squamous cell carcinoma

Epithelial membrane antigen (EMA)

- Highlights normal sebaceous and sweat glands
- Positive in sebaceous carcinoma, Paget and extramammary Paget
- Positive in squamous cell carcinoma but negative in basal cell carcinoma

Carcinoembryonic antigen (CEA)

- Sweat glands are immunoreactive
- Positive in sweat gland neoplasms, Paget, extramammary Paget, and most adenocarcinomas

Adipophilin

- Membrano-vesicular expression in lipid droplets of sebaceous and xanthomatous lesions
- Can help distinguish sebaceous carcinoma from squamous cell carcinoma and basal cell carcinoma

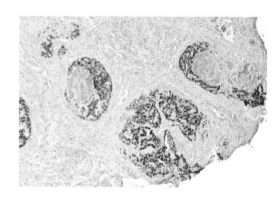

Fig. 1.87 Metastatic colon carcinoma with CDX2

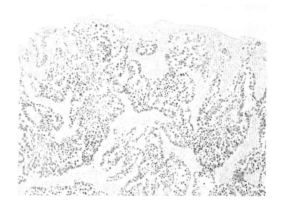

Fig. 1.88 TTF-1 in metastatic adenocarcinoma of the lung

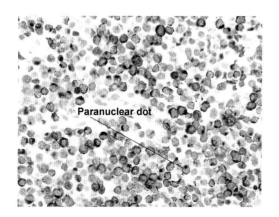

Fig. 1.86 Paranuclear dot with CK20 in Merkel cell carcinoma

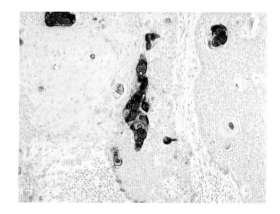

Fig. 1.89 EMA positivity in sebaceous epithelioma

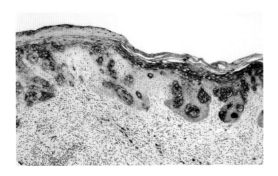

Fig. 1.90 CEA-positive pagetoid cells of Paget disease

Organ-specific markers

CDX2

- Marker of intestinal adenocarcinoma
- Useful for diagnosis of cutaneous metastatic colon adenocarcinoma and extramammary Paget disease associated with an underlying colorectal tumor

PAX-8

- High sensitivity and specificity for renal cell carcinoma metastases and negative in other clear cell tumors of the skin
- Also positive in thyroid and epithelial ovarian neoplasms

Thyroid transcription factor (TTF-1)

- Useful in the small blue cell tumor differential diagnosis
- Reactive in metastatic small cell lung carcinoma and negative in Merkel cell carcinoma

Mesenchymal markers

Desmin (see Table 1.2)

- Positive staining in skeletal and smooth muscle, except vascular smooth muscle
- Negative in myoepithelial cells and focal or weak in myofibroblasts

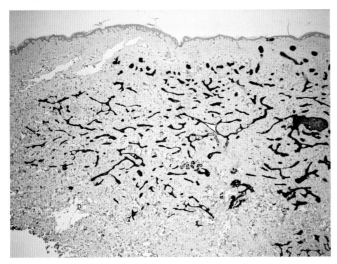

Fig. 1.91 Infiltrating basal cell carcinoma with Ber-EP4

Table 1.2 Muscle markers				
	Smooth muscle	Skeletal muscle	Myofibroblasts	Myoepithelial cells
Desmin	+ except vascular	+	-/+	-
SMA	+	-	+	+

SMA, smooth muscle actin

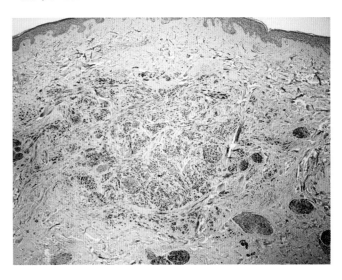

Fig. 1.92 Desmin-positive piloleiomyoma

Smooth muscle actin (SMA) (see Table 1.2)

- Positive in smooth muscle, including vascular smooth muscle
- Also expressed in myofibroblasts and myoepithelial cells
- Negative in skeletal muscle

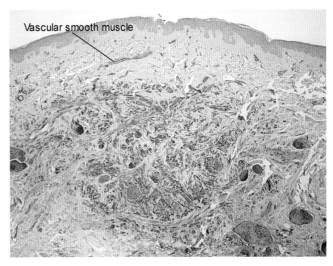

Vascular smooth muscle

Fig. 1.93 Piloleiomyoma with SMA. Note positive staining of normal surrounding vascular smooth muscle in contrast to the absence of reactivity with desmin in Fig. 1.92

CD34

- Marker of vascular endothelium and hematopoietic progenitor cells
- Positive in dermatofibrosarcoma protuberans and negative in dermatofibroma
- Positive in spindle cell lipoma, sclerotic fibroma, solitary fibrous tumor, superficial acral fibromyxoma, pleomorphic fibroma, and pleomorphic hyalinizing angiectatic tumor
- Decreased staining in morphea
- Increased staining in nephrogenic systemic fibrosis
- Stains connective tissue around normal hair follicles
- Typically highlights the stroma of trichoepitheliomas but not basal cell carcinomas
- Positive in tumors with outer root sheath differentiation such as trichilemmoma

Factor XIIIa

- Highlights a population of dermal dendritic cells
- Positive in dermatofibroma and negative in dermatofibrosarcoma protuberans
- Positive in fibrous papule of the face

CD31

- Helpful in confirming vascular origin of tumors
- More specific vascular marker than CD34

D2-40 (podoplanin)

- Lymphatic endothelial marker
- Increases detection of lymphovascular invasion
- Lack of reactivity in metastatic carcinoma assists in differentiation from primary cutaneous adnexal neoplasms

ERG

- Nuclear stain for endothelial cells

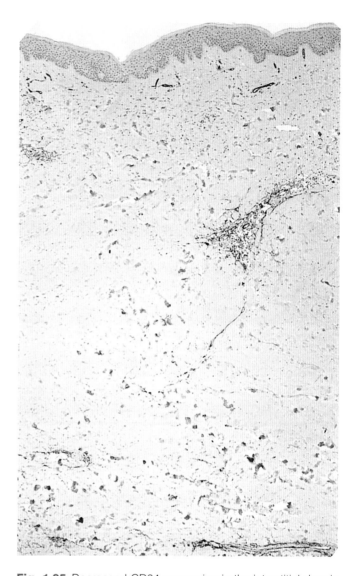

Fig. 1.95 Decreased CD34 expression in the interstitial dermis of morphea

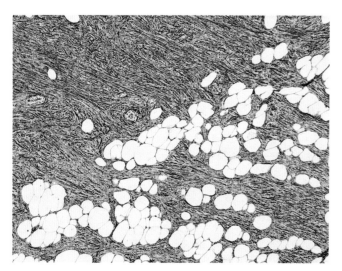

Fig. 1.94 Dermatofibrosarcoma protuberans with CD34

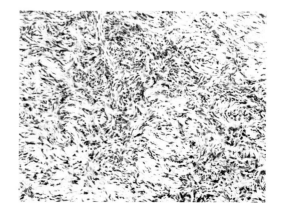

Fig. 1.96 Dermatofibroma with factor XIIIa

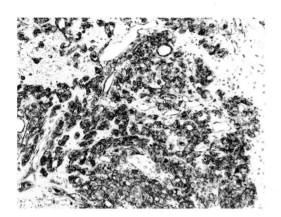

Fig. 1.97 CD31-positive angiosarcoma

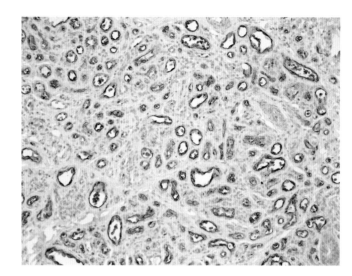

Fig. 1.99 GLUT1 in infantile hemangioma

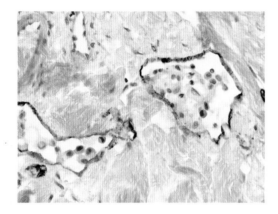

Fig. 1.98 Intralymphatic invasion of melanoma with D2-40 highlighting lymphatics

GLUT1 (glucose transporter)

- Expressed in endothelial cells with blood–tissue barrier function as in placenta
- Positive in infantile hemangiomas (negative in congenital hemangiomas including rapidly-involuting congenital hemangioma [RICH] and non-involuting congenital hemangioma [NICH]) and negative in vascular malformations
- Also stains perineurial cells and perineurioma

Vimentin

- Stains mesenchymal cells, endothelial cells, fibroblasts, melanocytes, lymphocytes, and macrophages, but does not react with keratinocytes or other epithelium
- General marker of sarcomas
- Excludes most carcinomas except rare spindle cell carcinomas

Neuroectodermal markers

S100

- Reactivity is observed for neural crest–derived cells and some mesenchymal lines
- Stains melanocytes, Langerhans cells, sweat glands, nerves, Schwann cells, myoepithelial cells, fat, muscle, and chondrocytes

- Useful in differential diagnosis of spindle cell neoplasms
- Examples: desmoplastic melanoma, Langerhans cell histiocytosis, granular cell tumor, Rosai–Dorfman disease

S100A6 (calcyclin)

- Member of the S100 protein superfamily
- Stains melanocytes, Schwann cells, Langerhans cells, and dermal dendrocytes thus expressed in nevi, particularly those with type C Schwann cell–like features, and some neural and fibrohistiocytic tumors
- Positive in cellular neurothekeoma, whereas S100 is negative
- Reactive in most atypical fibroxanthomas, but is not specific and also stains other entities in the cutaneous spindle cell tumor differential diagnosis
- Has been reported to stain Spitz nevi strongly and diffusely, but spitzoid melanomas have weak or patchy staining in the dermis only

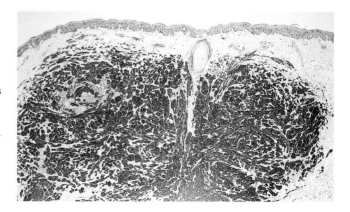

Fig. 1.100 Granular cell tumor with S100

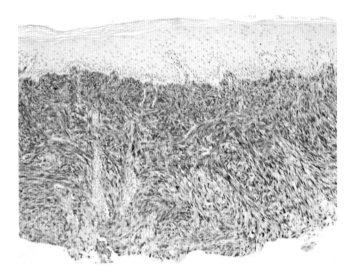

Fig. 1.101 S100A6 in atypical fibroxanthoma

HMB-45

- Premelanosome marker
- Loss of staining of melanocytes with descent into the dermis is a manifestation of loss of premelanosomes. As such, it serves as a marker of normal maturation
- Loss of staining in deep dermal component of most benign nevi, but uniform staining of blue nevi
- Does not stain desmoplastic melanoma reliably

Melan-A and Mart-1

- Two different antibodies that stain the same epitope
- Stain melanocytic lesions
- Do not stain desmoplastic melanoma reliably

p75 (nerve growth factor receptor)

- Early neural crest marker
- Expressed in type C (spindled) melanocytes and Schwann cells
- Sensitive marker for spindle cell and desmoplastic melanoma

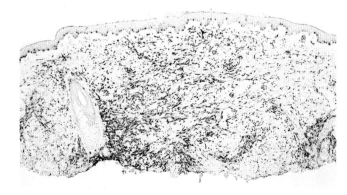

Fig. 1.102 HMB-45–positive staining throughout a blue nevus

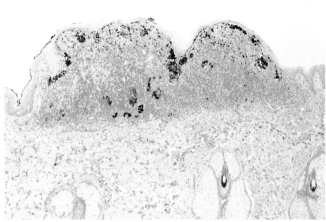

Fig. 1.103 Obscured nevus cells in the lymphocytic infiltrate of halo nevus with Mart-1

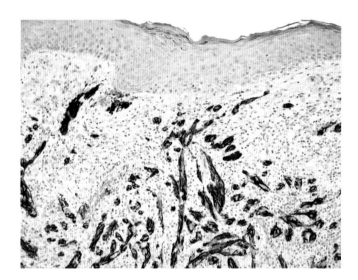

Fig. 1.104 p75 in desmoplastic melanoma

Microphthalmia-associated transcription factor (MITF)

- Essential in development and survival of melanocytes
- Nuclear melanocytic marker
- Positive in cellular neurothekeomas

Sox-10

- Nuclear marker of Schwann cells and melanocytes
- Sensitive marker of melanoma, including conventional, spindled, and desmoplastic types

Neuroendocrine markers

Neuron-specific enolase (NSE)

- Positive in neuroendocrine cells, neurons, and tumors derived from them
- Positive in so many other cell lines that it is sometimes referred to as *nonspecific enolase*

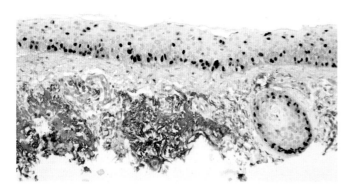

Fig. 1.105 Nuclear reactivity of melanocytes in melanoma in situ with MITF

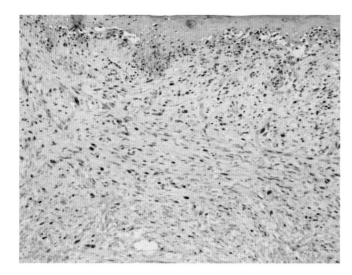

Fig. 1.106 Nuclear reactivity of melanocytes in desmoplastic melanoma with Sox-10

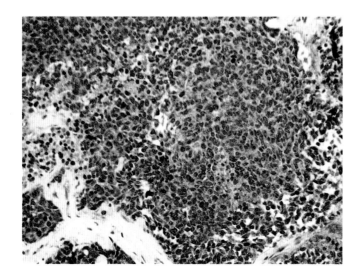

Fig. 1.107 NSE in Merkel cell carcinoma

Chromogranin

• Positive in Merkel cell carcinoma

Synaptophysin

• Positive in Merkel cell carcinoma

Hematopoietic markers

CD1a

• Stains Langerhans cells
• Examples: Langerhans cell histiocytosis

CD3

• Pan-T-cell marker
• Positive in T-cell lymphomas but negative in B-cell lymphomas

CD4

• T-helper lymphocytic marker

CD5

• Pan-T-cell marker like CD3 but aberrant loss in cutaneous T-cell lymphoma (CTCL) is common
• Positive in mantle cell lymphoma and infiltrates of chronic lymphocytic leukemia

CD7

• Immature T-lymphocyte antigen
• Most commonly lost antigen in T-cell lymphoma

CD8

• T-cell cytotoxic/suppressor marker

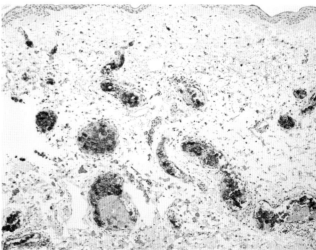

Fig. 1.108 CD20 positivity in intravascular lymphoma using 3-amino-9-ethylcarbazole (AEC) as the enzyme in the enzyme–antibody–antigen complex, resulting in a red product

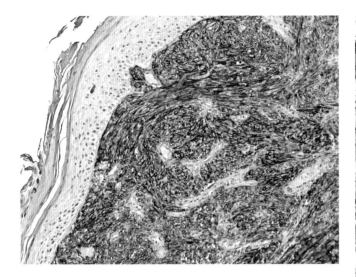

Fig. 1.109 CD10 in atypical fibroxanthoma

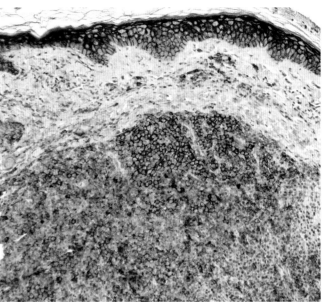

Fig. 1.110 CD138 in plasmacytoma

Table 1.3 Cutaneous B-cell lymphoproliferative disorders

	BCL2	CD10	BCL6	MUM-1
Reactive germinal centers in pseudo B-cell lymphoma	−	+	+	−
PCMZL	+	−	−	−[a]
PCFCL	−[b]	−[c]	+[d]	−
2° CFL	+	+	+	−
PCLBCL-leg	+	−	+/−	+

PCMZL, *Primary cutaneous marginal zone lymphoma;* PCFCL, *primary cutaneous follicle center lymphoma;* 2° CFL, *secondary cutaneous follicular lymphoma;* PCLBCL-leg, *primary cutaneous large B-cell lymphoma, leg type.*
Immunoreactivity refers to the malignant cells in all cases except the reactive germinal center. BCL2 also stains background normal T cells.
[a]*Plasma cells are positive with MUM-1 but the neoplastic B cells are negative in PCMZL.*
[b]*Only 10%–20% of PCFCL are BCL-2 positive.*
[c]*Most PCFCL have a diffuse histologic pattern and are CD10 negative, but cases with a follicular pattern are CD10 positive.*
[d]*The BCL6-positive malignant cells are outside the follicle.*

CD10 (CALLA)

- Common acute lymphoblastic leukemia antigen (CALLA) is an early marker of B-cell differentiation
- Useful in differential diagnosis of B-cell lymphoproliferative disorders (see Table 1.3)
- Positive in periadnexal mesenchymal cells, staining only the stroma of trichoblastomas but the epithelial cells of basal cell carcinoma

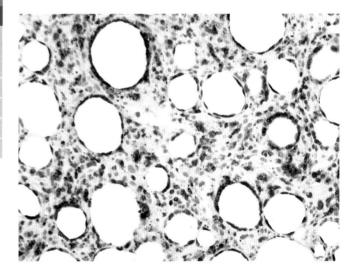

Fig. 1.111 CD3-positive lymphocytes of subcutaneous T-cell lymphoma

- Expressed in most atypical fibroxanthomas but not uncommonly seen in the other tumors in the differential diagnosis of cutaneous spindle cell tumors
- Marker of renal cell carcinoma but also expressed in other cutaneous clear cell lesions including: balloon cell nevi, clear cell hidradenoma, and sebaceous tumors

CD20

- B-cell antigen (often absent in plasma cells)
- Positive in B-cell lymphomas and negative in T-cell lymphomas
- Target for rituximab. Loss correlates with rituximab resistance

CD21

- Follicular dendritic cell marker
- Highlights residual follicle in lymphoma
- CD23 has a similar staining pattern

CD30 (Ki-1, BERH2)

- Originally identified on Reed–Sternberg cells of Hodgkin disease
- Positive in activated lymphocytes of anaplastic large cell lymphoma and lymphomatoid papulosis
- Many positive cells may be seen in scabies nodules and chronic tick bites

CD43 (Leu-22)

- Pan-T-cell marker
- Aberrant coexpression with B-cell marker CD20 is strongly suggestive of B-cell lymphoma

CD45Ra (LCA)

- Leukocyte common antigen (LCA) is a general marker of hematolymphoid differentiation
- LCA is present on all hematopoietic cells and their precursors with the exception of maturing erythroids and megakeratocytes

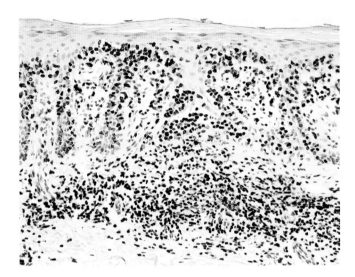

Fig. 1.112 CD4-positive epidermotropic cells of mycosis fungoides

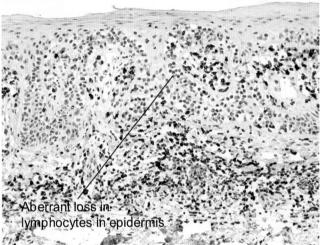

Aberrant loss in lymphocytes in epidermis

Fig. 1.114 Aberrant loss of CD7 in epidermotropic cells of mycosis fungoides (compare with Fig. 1.112)

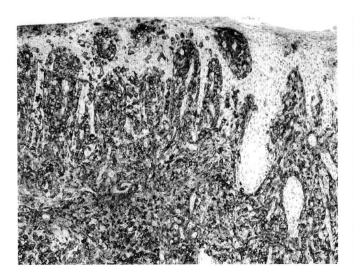

Fig. 1.113 CD30-positive anaplastic large cell lymphoma

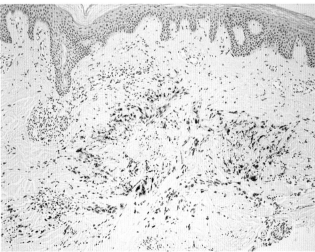

Fig. 1.115 CD68-positive histiocytes of granuloma annulare

CD45Ro (UCHL-1)
- Mature T cells

CD56
- Marker of NK cells and subsets of T cells
- Stains blastic plasmacytoid dendritic cell neoplasm (formerly known as blastic NK/T-cell lymphoma or CD4+/CD56+ hematodermic neoplasm)

CD68 (KP-1)
- Reactive in virtually all monocyte/macrophage cells

CD79a
- Plasma cell and B-cell marker

CD117 (c-Kit)
- Expressed in mast cells and melanocytes
- In nevi and primary melanoma there is a decrease in expression in the dermal component
- Typically lost in metastatic cutaneous melanoma

CD123
- Marker of plasmacytoid dendritic cells
- Clusters of positive cells present in lupus erythematosus
- Positive in blastic plasmacytoid dendritic cell neoplasm

CD138 (syndecan-1)
- Plasma cell marker

CD163
- Reactive in monocytes and macrophages

Langerin (CD207)
- Surrogate marker for presence of Birbeck granules in Langerhans cells

Myeloperoxidase
- Major constituent of granules of neutrophilic myeloid cells
- Marker for acute myeloid leukemia

ALK-1
- Anaplastic lymphoma kinase expressing chromosomal translocation t (2,5)
- Positive in most systemic anaplastic large cell lymphomas and negative in primary cutaneous anaplastic large cell lymphoma
- Those few patients with ALK-1-negative systemic anaplastic large cell lymphoma have a poor prognosis

Kappa/lambda
- Normally expressed in a ratio of two-thirds kappa to one-third lambda

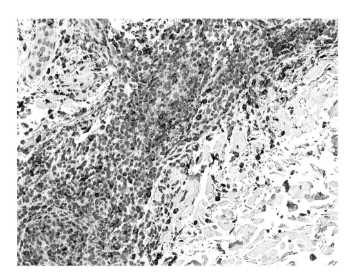

Fig. 1.116 Myeloperoxidase reactivity in leukemia cutis using 3-amino-9-ethylcarbazole (AEC) as the enzyme in the enzyme–antibody–antigen complex, resulting in a red product

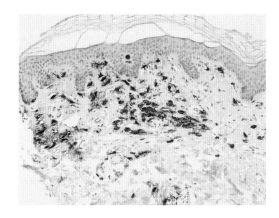

Fig. 1.117 CD117 in urticaria pigmentosa

- Tenfold deviation from this ratio suggests a clonal B-cell proliferation

BCL2
- An oncogene that inhibits apoptosis
- Useful in differential diagnosis of B-cell lymphoproliferative disorders (see Table 1.3)
- Most basal cell carcinomas reveal diffuse BCL2 staining, whereas trichoepitheliomas only show staining of the outermost epithelial layers of the tumor islands

Multiple myeloma oncogene-1 (MUM-1)
- Expressed in plasma cells, activated T cells, and subset of germinal center cells
- Distinguishes primary cutaneous diffuse large B-cell lymphoma, leg type from diffuse follicle center lymphoma (see Table 1.3)

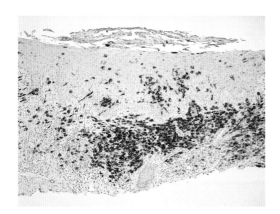

Fig. 1.118 CD1a in Langerhans cell histiocytosis

Table 1.5	Small blue cell tumor				
	S100	Synaptophysin	LCA	TTF-1	CK20
Lymphoma	–	–	+	–/+	–
Merkel cell carcinoma	–/+	+	–	–	+
Malignant melanoma	+	–	–	–	–
Metastatic small cell carcinoma of the lung	–	+/–	–	+	–

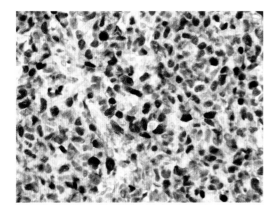

Fig. 1.119 MUM-1 in diffuse large B-cell lymphoma, leg type

Table 1.6	Tumors with intraepidermal buckshot scatter (pagetoid spread)		
	CK7	CEA	S100
Paget disease	+	+	–
Bowen disease	–/+	–	–
Malignant melanoma	–	–	+

Table 1.4	Spindle cell neoplasms			
	AE1/ AE3 and p63	CD10	S100/ Sox-10	Desmin
Squamous cell carcinoma	+	–/+	–	–
Atypical fibroxanthoma	–	+	–	–
Malignant melanoma	–	–/+	+	–
Leiomyosarcoma	–	–/+	–	+

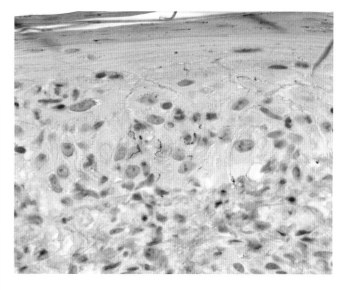

Fig. 1.120 Immunohistochemical identification of *Treponema pallidum* in syphilis

BetaF1

- Identifies αβ T cells

Proliferation markers

Mib-1(Ki-67)

- Nuclear proliferation marker
- Not cell type specific
- Expressed in all active phases of the cell cycle (G1, M, G2, S)

- Pattern and number of reactive melanocytes can be helpful in diagnosing melanocytic lesions

pHH3

- Mitotic marker that only stains cells in the M phase of the cell cycle
- Helps differentiate mitoses from apoptotic or hyperchromatic nuclei

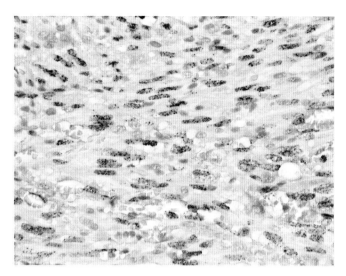

Fig. 1.121 Immunohistochemical identification of HHV8 in Kaposi sarcoma

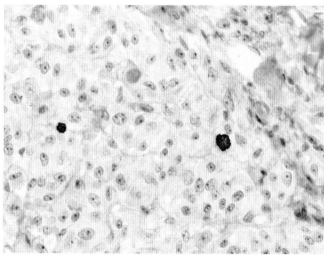

Fig. 1.124 pHH3-positive mitotic figures in malignant melanoma

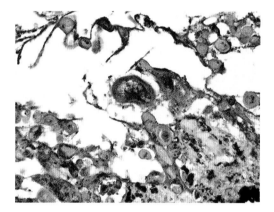

Fig. 1.122 Immunohistochemical identification of VZV in multinucleate giant cell

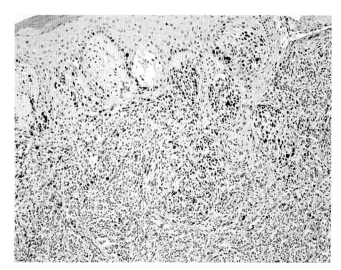

Fig. 1.123 Mib-1 positivity in malignant melanoma. Positive background reactive lymphocytes must be distinguished from Mib-1–positive melanocytes by cytology or double staining technique

Infectious disease markers

Specific immunohistochemical antibodies to viral, bacterial, fungal, and parasitic antigens are available for detection and identification of the causative agents in many infectious diseases including HHV8, HSV, VZV, CMV, EBV, *Bartonella, Rickettsia, Treponema, Borrelia, Aspergillus, Leishmania*, and others.

Transport media

Routine

For most purposes, 10% buffered formalin is the recommended fixative. The length of time for fixation depends on the specimen size: 1–2 hours per millimeter of thickness is required.

Electron microscopy

Glutaraldehyde is the preferred fixative for electron microscopy.

Immunofluorescence

For tissue that is not flash-frozen, Michel's medium (ammonium sulfate) is the preferred transport media for immunofluorescence. Normal saline also performs well.

Further reading

Feller JK, Mahalingam M. c-myc and cutaneous vascular neoplasms. Am J Dermatopathol 2013;35(3):364–9.

Ferringer T. Immunohistochemistry in dermatopathology. Arch Pathol Lab Med 2015;139(1):83–105.

Fuertes L, Santonja C, Kutzner H, et al. Immunohistochemistry in dermatopathology: a review of the most commonly used antibodies (part I). Actas Dermosifiliogr 2013;104(2):99–127.

Fuertes L, Santonja C, Kutzner H, et al. Immunohistochemistry in dermatopathology: a review of the most commonly used antibodies (part II). Actas Dermosifiliogr 2013;104(3):181–203.

Kandalaft PL, Gown AM. Practical Applications in Immunohistochemistry: Carcinomas of Unknown Primary Site. Arch Pathol Lab Med 2016;140(6):508–23.

Molina-Ruiz AM, Cerroni L, Kutzner H, et al. Immunohistochemistry in the diagnosis of cutaneous bacterial infections. Am J Dermatopathol 2015;37(3):179–93.

Molina-Ruiz AM, Santonja C, Rütten A, et al. Immunohistochemistry in the diagnosis of cutaneous viral infections–part I. Cutaneous viral infections by herpesviruses and papillomaviruses. Am J Dermatopathol 2015;37(1):1–14.

Molina-Ruiz AM, Santonja C, Rütten A, et al. Immunohistochemistry in the diagnosis of cutaneous viral infections- part II: cutaneous viral infections by parvoviruses, poxviruses, paramyxoviridae, picornaviridae, retroviruses and filoviruses. Am J Dermatopathol 2015;37(2):93–106.

Naert KA, Trotter MJ. Utilization and utility of immunohistochemistry in dermatopathology. Am J Dermatopathol 2013;35(1):74–7.

Papalas JA, Kulbacki E, Wang E. Anaplastic lymphoma kinase (ALK1) immunohistochemistry in diagnostic dermatopathology; an update. Am J Dermatopathol 2013;35(4):403–8.

Weissinger SE, Keil P, Silvers DN, et al. A diagnostic algorithm to distinguish desmoplastic from spindle cell melanoma. Mod Pathol 2014;27(4):524–34.

Benign tumors and cysts of the epidermis

Dirk M. Elston

🌐 **A clinical image atlas for entities throughout the text can be found in the online content for this book.**

Benign acanthomas

Acanthomas are benign cutaneous neoplasms characterized by an expansion of the epidermis. The acanthoma may be composed of clones of cells that displace or compress the preexisting epidermis. In contrast to the reactive acanthosis seen in inflammatory disorders, the rete ridge pattern is commonly ablated by the neoplastic tissue of an acanthoma.

Seborrheic keratoses

Seborrheic keratoses are acanthomas composed of small polygonal keratinocytes about the size of acrosyringeal keratinocytes (the cells that make up the intraepidermal portion of the eccrine duct). The cells are typically smaller than the cells of the surrounding epidermis, and they are commonly pigmented. Architectural subtypes of seborrheic keratoses include acanthotic, hyperkeratotic, reticulated, and clonal. Any of these subtypes may be pigmented, irritated (spindling of cells and squamous eddy formation), or inflamed (usually lymphoid inflammation). Melanoacanthoma is a distinct subtype of seborrheic keratosis composed of small keratinocytes and dendritic melanocytes.

Seborrheic keratoses produce a characteristic loose lamellar "shredded-wheat" stratum corneum. Exceptions include irritated or inflamed seborrheic keratosis. Instead of the characteristic loose lamellar horn, irritated or inflamed seborrheic keratoses produce a compact, brightly eosinophilic, parakeratotic stratum corneum. Adjacent unaffected areas of the seborrheic keratosis still produce the characteristic loose lamellar stratum corneum, and it is common to see remnants of loose stratum corneum above areas of compact stratum corneum. Melanoacanthomas produce a deeply eosinophilic, compact, parakeratotic stratum corneum, even when they are not irritated or inflamed.

Seborrheic keratoses may express BCL-2, a marker associated with resistance to programmed cell death (apoptosis). Activating point mutations in the gene encoding fibroblast growth factor receptor 3, a tyrosine kinase receptor, are also common in seborrheic keratoses.

Acanthotic seborrheic keratosis

Key Features

- Broad sheets of small polygonal keratinocytes with intervening horn cysts
- Loose lamellar "shredded-wheat" or "onion-skin" keratin
- Commonly pigmented

Acanthotic seborrheic keratoses are composed of broad sheets of cells with intervening horn cysts or pseudohorn cysts. Horn cysts are completely encased within the acanthoma, whereas pseudohorn cysts open to the surface. Like other seborrheic keratoses, they may become irritated or inflamed.

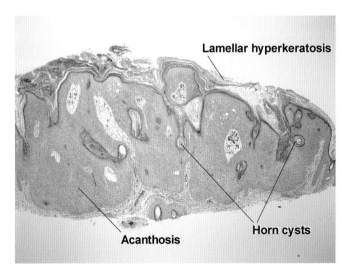

Fig. 2.1 Acanthotic seborrheic keratosis

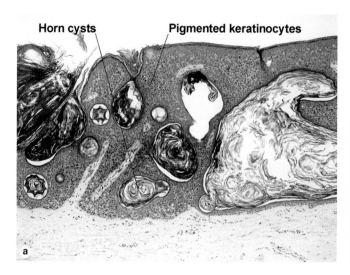

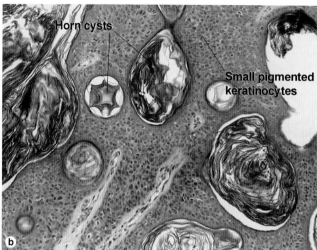

Fig. 2.2 Pigmented acanthotic seborrheic keratosis

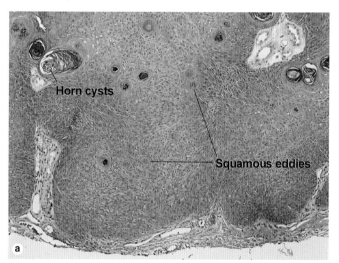

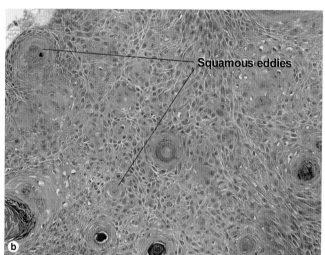

Fig. 2.3 Irritated acanthotic seborrheic keratosis

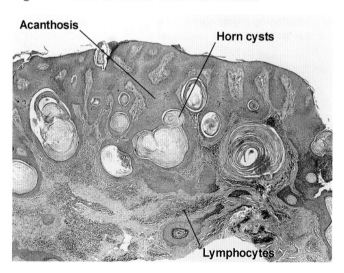

Fig. 2.4 Inflamed acanthotic seborrheic keratosis

Hyperkeratotic seborrheic keratosis

Key Features

- Tall stacks of loose lamellar "shredded-wheat" keratin
- Papillomatosis: hills and dales that may produce a "church-spire" appearance

The tall, stacked stratum corneum is typically much thicker than the epidermis. As in other forms of seborrheic keratosis, the keratin has a loose lamellar "shredded-wheat" appearance unless the lesion has become irritated or inflamed. Papillomatosis is characteristic, but variable in degree. Horn cysts are inconspicuous or absent.

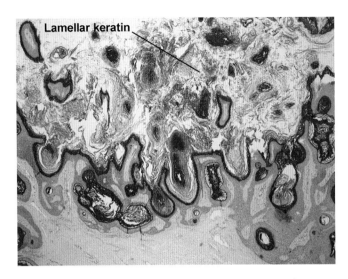

Fig. 2.5 Hyperkeratotic seborrheic keratosis

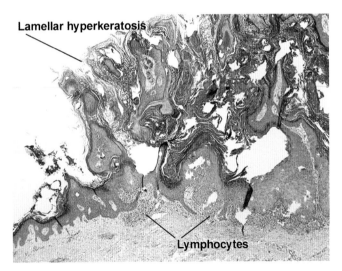

Fig. 2.6 Inflamed hyperkeratotic seborrheic keratosis

Reticulated seborrheic keratosis (adenoid seborrheic keratosis)

Key Features

- Thin, pigmented, interlacing, downward extensions of the epidermis
- Reticular (lacelike) configuration of epidermis interspersed with horn cysts

The lesion is composed of thin, interlacing strands of epidermis, typically two cells thick. These strands are generally pigmented.

Differential Diagnosis

Solar lentigo

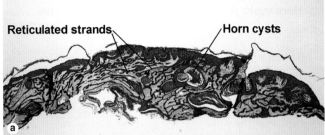

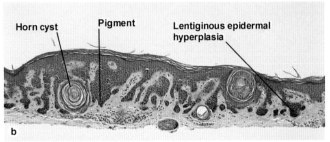

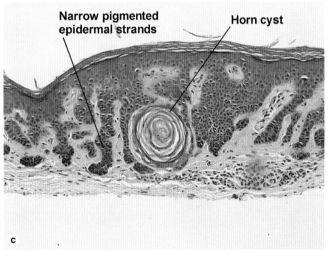

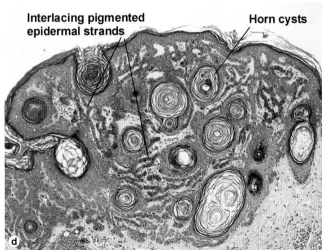

Fig. 2.7 Reticulated seborrheic keratosis. (For the differential diagnosis of Dowling–Degos disease, see Fig. 12.15. For the differential diagnosis of solar lentigo, see Fig. 6.1)

Key Features

- Shares thin, pigmented, interlacing extension of the epidermis
- These are shorter and more bulbous than those in reticulated seborrheic keratosis
- Lacks horn cysts

Clonal seborrheic keratosis

Key Features

- Clonal islands of small keratinocytes within the epidermis
- Bland uniform nuclei
- Absence of duct differentiation within clonal nests

Clonal seborrheic keratosis is characterized by islands of small keratinocytes with uniform bland nuclei. The nests are embedded within the epidermis. Sometimes, the nests are large enough that the normal epidermis is reduced to thin strands separating the large nests. Horn cysts are usually absent. The nests may demonstrate pigment. There may be squamous eddies (irritated seborrheic keratosis), lymphocytes (inflamed seborrheic keratosis), or both. In contrast to Bowen disease, the cells are uniform and atypia is absent. In contrast to hidroacanthoma simplex, no ducts are present within the clones.

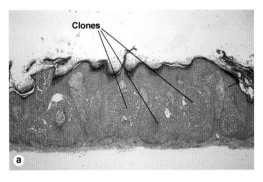

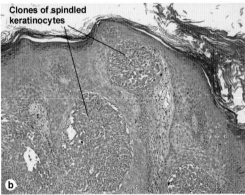

Fig. 2.10 Irritated clonal seborrheic keratosis

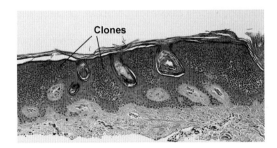

Fig. 2.8 Clonal seborrheic keratosis

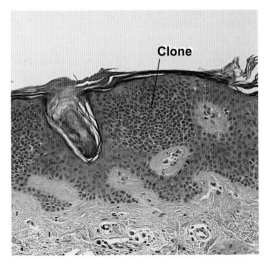

Fig. 2.9 Pigmented clonal seborrheic keratosis

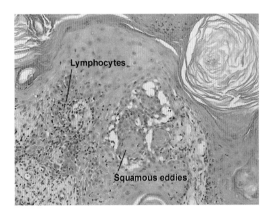

Fig. 2.11 Irritated and inflamed clonal seborrheic keratosis

Differential Diagnosis

Hidroacanthoma simplex

Key Features

- Clonal islands of small keratinocytes similar in appearance to those of clonal seborrheic keratosis
- Ducts present focally within the clonal islands

Bowen's disease

Key Features

- Clonal islands of atypical keratinocytes within the epidermis
- Cells may be anaplastic or glassy and eosinophilic
- Buckshot scatter of cells may be present focally
- Apoptotic keratinocytes commonly scattered within nests
- Overlying stratum corneum becomes compact and parakeratotic where clones touch the surface
- More typical Bowen disease may be present in the adjacent skin

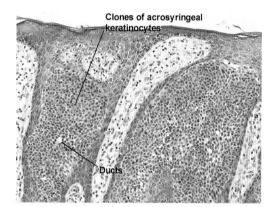

Fig. 2.12 Hidroacanthoma simplex

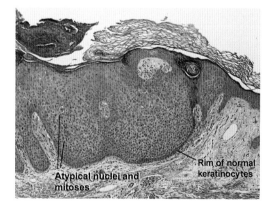

Fig. 2.13 Clonal Bowen disease

Pigmented seborrheic keratosis

Key Features

- Pigment within keratinocytes
- May be acanthotic, hyperkeratotic, reticulated, or clonal
- When clonal, the pigment is restricted to the clonal islands

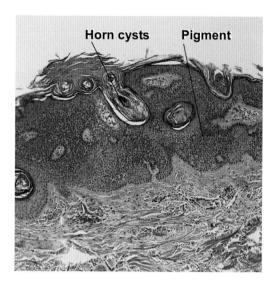

Fig. 2.14 Pigmented seborrheic keratosis

Irritated seborrheic keratosis

Key Features

- Squamous eddies
- Spindled keratinocytes
- Horn cysts common
- Keratin commonly becomes compact, eosinophilic, and parakeratotic
- Keratin often retains a loose lamellar pattern in some areas

Irritated seborrheic keratosis is characterized by the formation of squamous eddies within the epidermis and the presence of spindled keratinocytes. Some areas of the tumor typically still produce a loose lamellar "shredded-wheat" pattern of keratin, and horn cysts composed of loose lamellar keratin are often present. In areas, the keratin becomes compact, eosinophilic, and parakeratotic. A zone of loose lamellar keratin may be seen above the dense eosinophilic keratin. This was produced before the lesion became irritated. It has since been pushed upward.

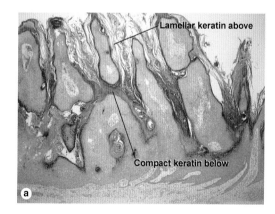

Fig. 2.15 Irritated seborrheic keratosis with prominent squamous eddies

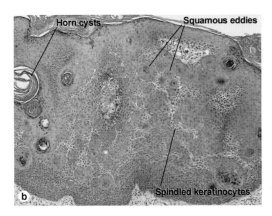

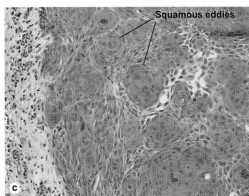

Fig. 2.15, cont'd

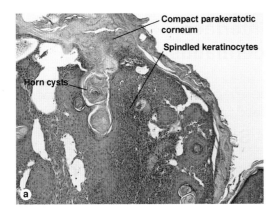

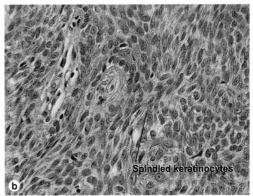

Fig. 2.16 Irritated seborrheic keratosis with prominent spindling of keratinocytes

Inflamed seborrheic keratosis

Key Features

- Lymphocytes and spongiosis
- In areas, the stratum corneum becomes compact, eosinophilic, and parakeratotic
- Loose lamellar keratin is commonly retained in other areas
- Horn cysts are common
- Lichenoid interface dermatitis may be present
- An overlying crust may be present

Inflamed seborrheic keratosis is characterized by lymphocytes and spongiosis within the epidermis or the presence of lichenoid interface dermatitis. Some areas of the tumor typically still produce a loose lamellar "shredded-wheat" pattern of keratin, and horn cysts composed of loose lamellar keratin are often present. As in irritated seborrheic keratoses, a zone of loose lamellar keratin may sometimes be seen above a zone of dense eosinophilic keratin. When clonal, the spongiosis and lymphoid infiltrate are typically restricted to the clonal islands.

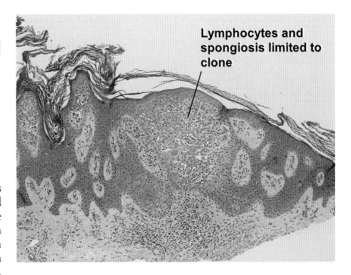

Fig. 2.17 Inflamed seborrheic keratosis with lymphocytes and spongiosis

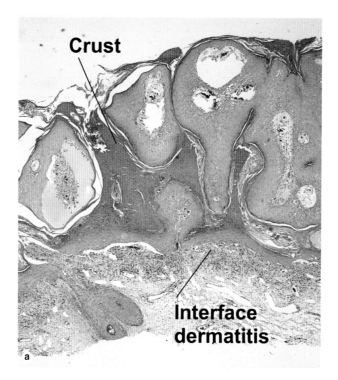

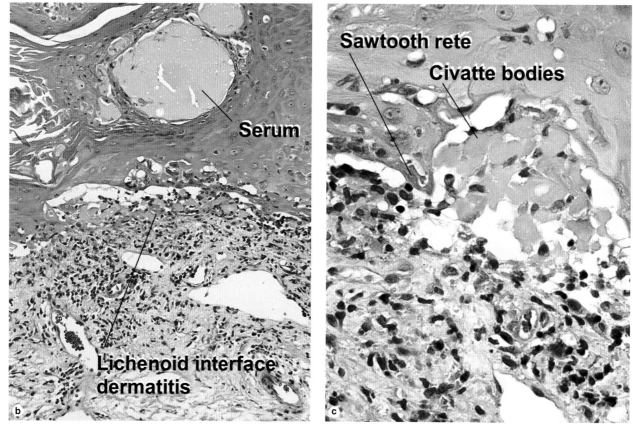

Fig. 2.18 Inflamed seborrheic keratosis with lichenoid interface dermatitis

Melanoacanthoma

Key Features

- Acanthoma composed of both small keratinocytes and pigmented dendritic melanocytes
- Most pigment is within dendrites
- Overlying stratum corneum is almost always compact eosinophilic and parakeratotic

Cutaneous melanoacanthomas are a type of seborrheic keratosis, composed of both small cuboidal keratinocytes and pigmented dendritic melanocytes. Most melanin pigment is contained within the melanocytic dendrites, with little visible pigment within the keratinocytes. Unlike most seborrheic keratoses, horn cysts and loose lamellar horn are typically absent. Instead, the overlying stratum corneum is almost always compact, eosinophilic, and parakeratotic. Cutaneous melanoacanthomas may be clonal. Oral melanoacanthomas are reactive proliferations unrelated to seborrheic keratosis.

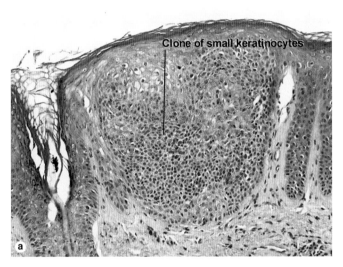

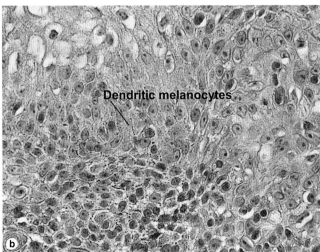

Fig. 2.19 Melanoacanthoma

Clear cell acanthoma (pale cell acanthoma)

Key Features

- Discrete acanthoma with overlying parakeratosis
- Distinct transition between the normal epidermis and the clearer/paler cells in the stratum spinosum
- Peppered with neutrophils

Clear cell acanthomas are recognizable as a clearly defined acanthotic area of the epidermis with ample clear or pale cytoplasm. A thin overlying parakeratotic scale crust is present, and there is a distinct transition between surrounding normal stratum corneum and the parakeratotic stratum corneum, as well as between the normal epidermis and the paler cells comprising the acanthoma. Neutrophils are scattered throughout the lesion. The cells of the acanthoma are deficient in phosphorylase, resulting in an accumulation of glycogen.

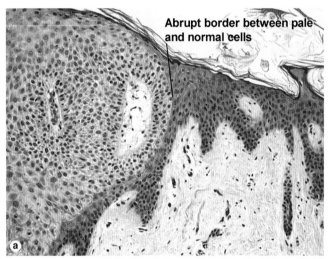

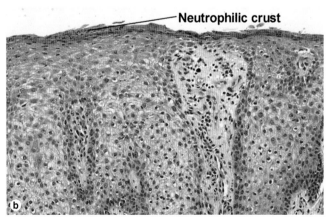

Fig. 2.20 Clear cell acanthoma

Large cell acanthoma

Key Features

- Discrete acanthoma composed of cells with large nuclei
- Overlying lamellar hyperkeratosis is common
- May be pigmented

The rete ridges may be bulbous, or there may be a solid platelike acanthosis. The cells composing the acanthoma have large nuclei, typically twice the size of the nuclei in the surrounding epidermis.

Large cell acanthomas represent a heterogeneous group of lesions. The most common type presents as a slightly hyperkeratotic pigmented patch, resembling a solar lentigo. Other lesions are erythematous. Many appear to represent a histologic variant of solar lentigo, others of Bowen disease. The cells of some lesions have been shown to be aneuploid, and no histologic features predict which lesions demonstrate aneuploid populations. Because of this, many clinicians prefer to destroy any remaining lesion by means of cryotherapy.

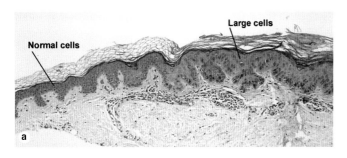

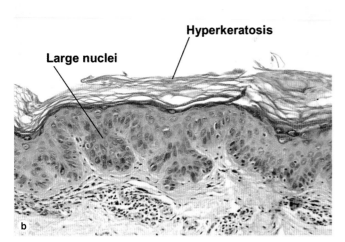

Fig. 2.21 Large cell acanthoma

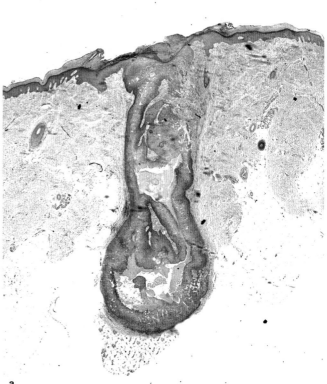

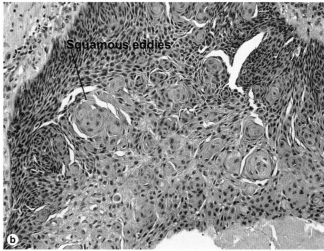

Fig. 2.22 Inverted follicular keratosis

Inverted follicular keratosis (IFK)

Key Features

- Endophytic lesion resembling an expanded hair follicle
- Squamous eddies

The outline of the epithelial column is smooth, with no evidence of jagged invasive growth.

True IFKs are benign follicular proliferations unrelated to human papillomavirus infection. Multiple lesions may be associated with Cowden syndrome. Follicular warts may sometimes have squamous eddies and resemble IFK.

Warty dyskeratoma

Key Features

- Endophytic growth
- Acantholytic dyskeratosis
- Overlying parakeratotic crust may be present

Two types of dyskeratotic cells are noted. Corps ronds are round dyskeratotic cells that stain pale pink to red and may have a wide, clear halo surrounding the nucleus. Grains are flattened basophilic dyskeratotic cells. Either or both may be present. Some lesions are crateriform; others resemble expanded hair follicles.

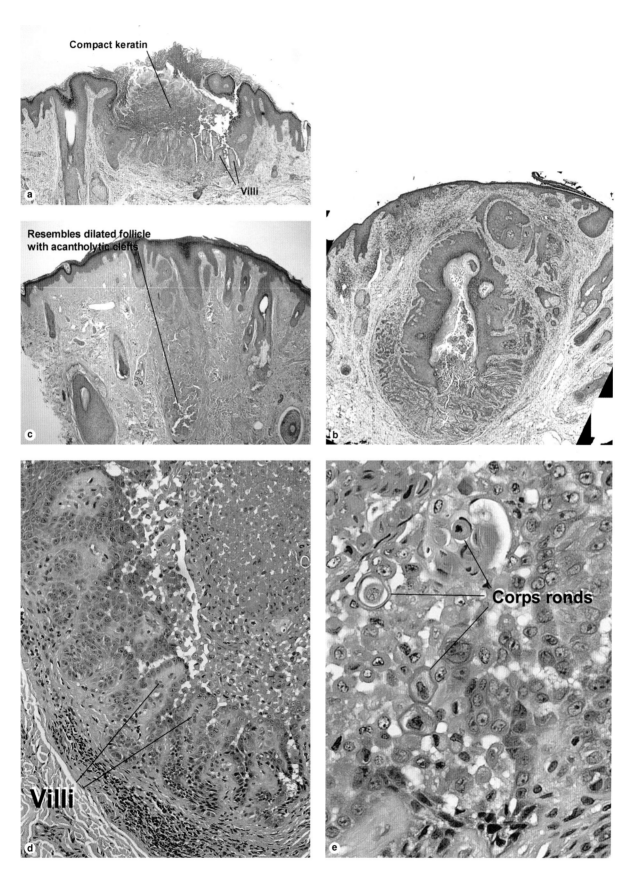

Fig. 2.23 Warty dyskeratoma

Acantholytic acanthoma

Key Features

- Acanthoma composed of bland keratinocytes
- Acantholysis

The appearance resembles the "dilapidated brick wall" of Hailey–Hailey disease.

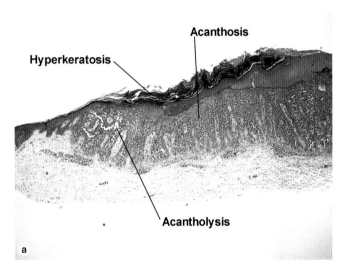

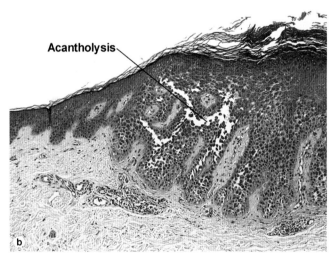

Fig. 2.24 Acantholytic acanthoma

Epidermolytic acanthoma

Key Features

- Often crateriform
- Epidermolytic hyperkeratosis (EHK)

Epidermolytic acanthomas are characterized by EHK. The granular layer is thick and contains irregularly shaped keratohyalin granules, and cytoplasmic borders are indistinct. Clinically, the lesions are solitary discrete acanthomas resembling seborrheic keratoses.

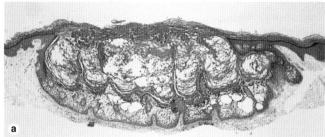

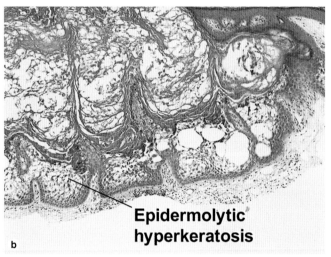

Fig. 2.25 Epidermolytic acanthoma

Epidermal nevi

Key Features

- Discrete acanthomas or hyperkeratotic lesions

Epidermal nevi are typically present at or near birth. Linear epidermal nevi follow Blaschko lines and may represent mosaicism, via postzygotic somatic mutation, lyonization of X chromosomes, or loss of heterozygosity. Patients with multiple epidermal nevi may have associated eye, central nervous, and musculoskeletal abnormalities.

Common epidermal nevus

Key Features

- Resembles seborrheic keratosis

Inflammatory linear verrucous epidermal nevus (ILVEN)

Key Features

- Variable acanthosis
- Stratum corneum with alternating orthokeratosis and parakeratosis
- Parakeratotic areas have no granular layer
- Orthokeratotic areas have a granular layer

The name *inflammatory* linear verrucous epidermal nevus relates to the erythematous clinical appearance of the lesions. Orthokeratosis and parakeratosis alternate from right to left.

Blaschkoid epidermolytic hyperkeratosis (EHK)

Key Features

- Resembles epidermal nevus clinically
- EHK histologically
- Represents mosaicism for keratin 1 and 10 mutations
- Patient can pass on the mutation and have a child with generalized EHK, known as *epidermolytic ichthyosis* (bullous congenial ichthyosiform erythroderma)

Widely separated lesions involving different parts of the body suggest that the mutation occurred in the embryo before gastrulation. In this case, the affected cell line is more likely to contribute to many organ tissues, including the gonads.

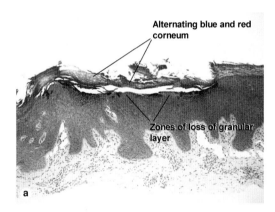

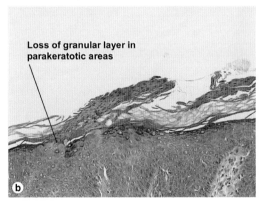

Fig. 2.26 ILVEN

Cysts

Epidermoid cyst (epidermal inclusion cyst, infundibular cyst)

Key Features

- Lining resembles the surface epidermis, but with no adnexal structures
- Loose lamellar "onion-skin" keratin within the cyst

Epidermoid cysts often connect to the surface with a visible punctum. This connection may be visible histologically. In a young cyst, a rete ridge pattern may be present. As tension increases within the cyst, the lining is stretched and the rete pattern disappears. Ruptured cysts demonstrate a neutrophilic infiltrate, histiocytes, and foreign-body giant cells. Flat bits of keratin are noted within giant cells.

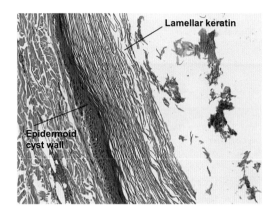

Fig. 2.27 Epidermoid cyst

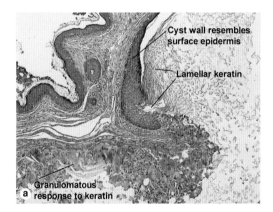

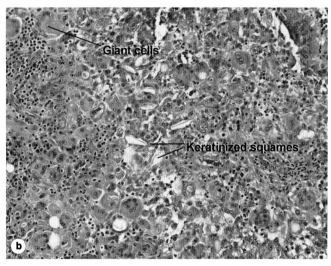

Fig. 2.28 Ruptured and inflamed epidermoid cyst

Epidermoid cyst with pilomatrical differentiation

Key Features

- Areas of ghost cell keratinization as in a pilomatricoma
- Associated with Gardner syndrome

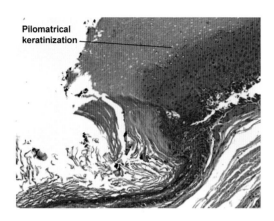

Fig. 2.29 Epidermoid cyst with pilomatrical differentiation

Vellus hair cyst

Key Features

- Wall resembles that of an epidermoid cyst
- Many small vellus hairs within the cyst
- Frequently arise in an eruptive fashion

Eruptive vellus hair cysts may coexist with steatocystomas, and individual cysts may have features of both. Eruptive vellus hair cysts have been reported in association with renal failure and Lowe syndrome (Fanconi-type renal failure, mental retardation, and eye abnormalities).

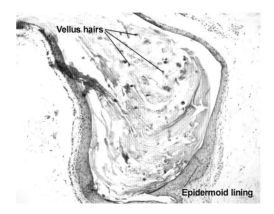

Fig. 2.30 Vellus hair cyst

Dermoid cyst

Key Features

- Wall commonly resembles that of an epidermoid cyst
- Adnexal structures within cyst wall

Adnexal structures within the cyst wall may include terminal hair follicles, sebaceous glands, eccrine glands, and apocrine glands. Terminal hair shafts are commonly noted within the cyst contents. Lamellar keratin is typically present, although some dermoid cysts demonstrate a bright red "shark-tooth" lining similar to that of a steatocystoma. Dermoid cysts occur in embryonic fusion planes and may be associated with underlying skull defects.

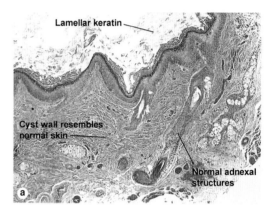

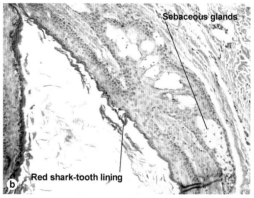

Fig. 2.31 Dermoid cyst

Pilar cyst (trichilemmal cyst, isthmus catagen cyst)

Key Features

- Abrupt keratinization without a granular layer
- Deeply eosinophilic dense keratin
- Focal calcification of contents common
- Typically on scalp
- Often multiple

The abrupt keratinization of pilar cysts resembles that of the outer root sheath (the trichilemma). When the cyst "shells out" during surgery, a single layer of cuboidal epithelium is left behind, resembling a hidrocystoma (see Fig. 2.34).

As the epithelium proliferates, the wall buckles inward, rolling on itself and producing a trabecular or scroll-like appearance ("rolls and scrolls"). A diagnosis of trichilemmal carcinoma should be suspected in tumors with a location other than scalp, recent rapid growth, size greater than 5 cm, infiltrative growth, significant cytologic atypia, and mitotic activity.

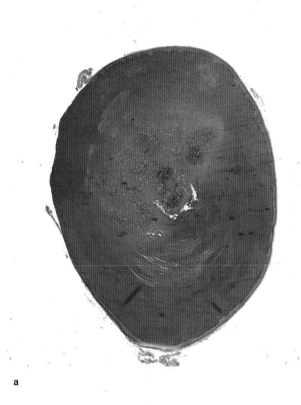

a

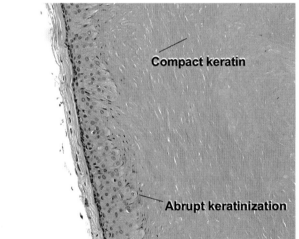

b

Fig. 2.32 Pilar cyst

Proliferating pilar cyst

Key Features

- Rolls and scrolls
- May form small new cysts within the confines of the mother cyst
- Trichilemmal keratinization

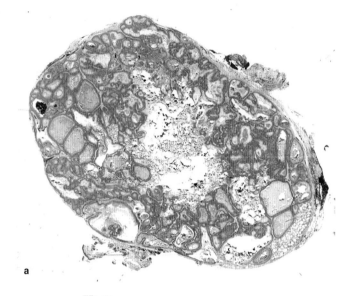

a

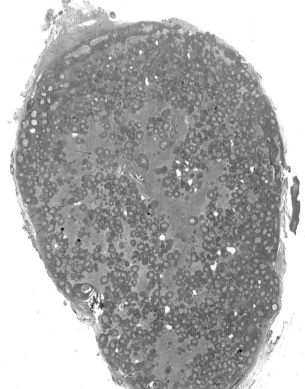

b

Fig. 2.33 Proliferating pilar cyst

continued

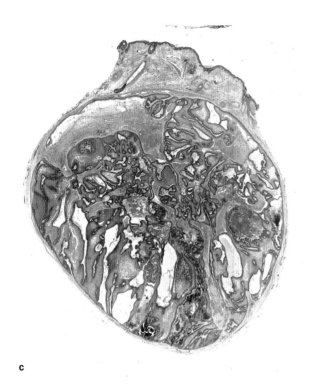

c

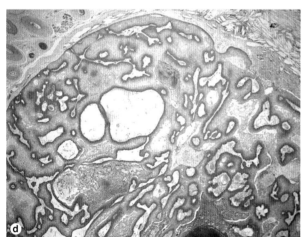

d

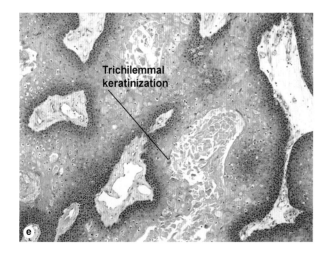

Trichilemmal keratinization

e

Fig. 2.33, cont'd

Differential Diagnosis

Pilomatricoma

Key Features

- Rolls and scrolls
- Ghost cell keratinization, see page 68

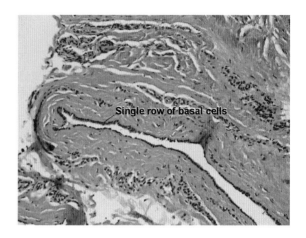

Single row of basal cells

Fig. 2.34 Basal layer left behind when a pilar cyst "shells out"

Branchial cleft cyst

Key Features

- Epidermoid or pseudostratified columnar epithelium
- Lymphoid tissue with germinal centers surrounding the cyst
- Cyst usually appears empty

Branchial cleft cysts are generally found on the lateral part of the neck, anterior to the sternocleidomastoid muscle. They may occur as a result of failure of obliteration of the second branchial cleft in embryonic development. Phylogenetically, the branchial apparatus may be related to gill slits. This analogy is helpful in remembering the typical location on the lateral neck. They are the most common cause of a congenital neck mass, and 2%–3% of cases are bilateral.

Although the classic teaching has been that branchial cleft cysts and bronchogenic cysts are embryologically distinct, cases with overlap in distribution and histology occur. In general, branchial cleft cysts are far more likely to occur on the side of the neck and to demonstrate lymphoid follicles and stratified squamous epithelium. Although smooth muscle may occur, it is rare.

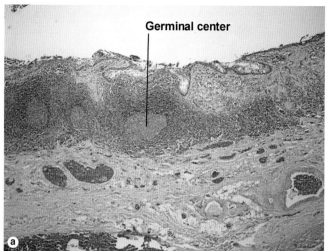

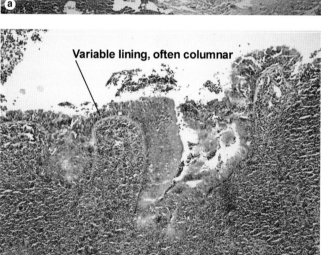

Fig. 2.35 Branchial cleft cyst

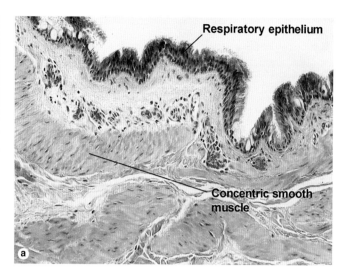

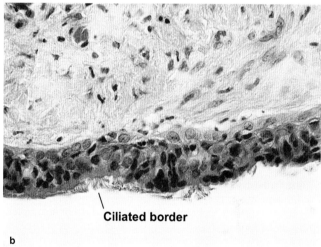

Fig. 2.36 Bronchogenic cyst

Bronchogenic cyst

Key Features

- Ciliated pseudostratified columnar epithelium
- Goblet cells
- May have circumferential smooth muscle around cyst
- May have cartilage

Bronchogenic cysts are typically midline lesions, located in the suprasternal notch. Bronchogenic cysts are thought to result from remnants of the primitive foregut. Although bronchogenic cysts occur predominantly within the chest, *cutaneous* lesions generally present as neck lesions in children.

As compared with branchial cleft cysts, bronchogenic cysts typically lack lymphoid follicles. They typically demonstrate pseudostratified respiratory-type ciliated epithelium, goblet cells, concentric smooth muscle, and cartilage.

Steatocystoma (simple sebaceous duct cyst)

Key Features

- Wavy, eosinophilic, "shark-tooth" cuticle
- Sebaceous glands in cyst wall
- Oily contents, frequently containing vellus hairs

Steatocystomas are commonly inherited, with multiple lesions on the chest. The appearance resembles nodulocystic acne. Solitary lesions are common and sporadic in occurrence. The cyst lining resembles that of the sebaceous duct. Sebaceous glands are common within the cyst wall, but may not be prominent. Some sections lack visible sebaceous glands, but the cyst can still be identified by the characteristic wavy eosinophilic cuticle.

Although dermoid cysts may occasionally demonstrate an identical wavy cuticle, they also commonly demonstrate terminal hair follicles and may have eccrine or apocrine glands within the cyst wall. Grossly, steatocystomas tend to drain oil and collapse when sectioned, whereas dermoid cysts tend to remain rigid because they contain keratin.

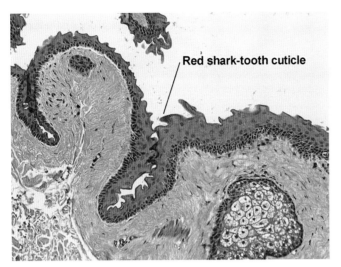

Fig. 2.37 Steatocystoma

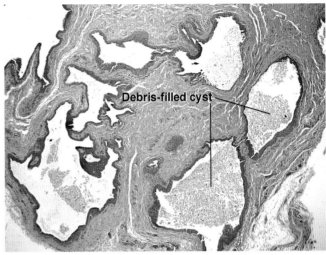

Fig. 2.38 Median raphe cyst

Median raphe cyst

Key Features

- Midline along anogenital raphe
- Debris-filled cyst
- Lining variable
- Surrounding skin has characteristics of genital skin

Median raphe cysts occur in men in a characteristic ventral location from the meatus to the anus. The cyst may first become apparent after intercourse. Median raphe cysts may result from incomplete embryonic fusion of the urethral folds, from ectopic periurethral glands of Littre, or from sequestration of urethral epithelium after closure of the median raphe.

Typically, the cyst is filled with amorphous debris, and the surrounding genital skin is readily identified by the presence of delicate collagen, randomly arranged smooth muscle, many small nerves, and prominent vascularity. Unlike the circumferential smooth muscle of a bronchogenic cyst, the smooth muscle in genital skin has a random, haphazard arrangement throughout the surrounding skin. The cyst wall itself has a highly variable lining. Some areas may appear ciliated, some cuboidal, and some areas may suggest decapitation secretion.

Cutaneous ciliated cyst

Key Features

- Similar to median raphe cysts
- Much less likely to occur on genital skin

Although ciliated cysts typically occur on the legs of women and are thought to relate to Müllerian duct remnants, they are occasionally noted in men. Ciliated cysts are commonly filled with debris, and the appearance of the cyst itself can be indistinguishable from that of a median raphe cyst. Helpful differentiating features are the location, sex of the patient, and characteristics of the surrounding skin. Because ciliated cysts commonly occur on the legs, the skin lacks the typical appearance of genital skin.

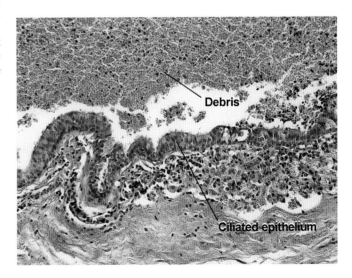

Fig. 2.39 Cutaneous ciliated cyst

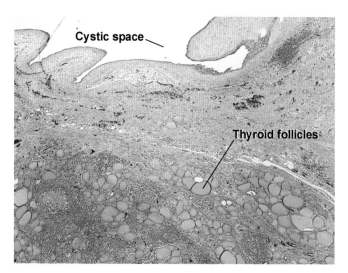

Fig. 2.40 Thyroglossal duct cyst

Thyroglossal duct cyst

Key Features

- Midline of neck
- Typically lined by respiratory-type epithelium
- May be lined by squamous epithelium
- Surrounding thyroid follicles and lymphoid aggregates may be present

Further reading

Abbas O, Wieland CN, Goldberg LJ. Solitary epidermolytic acanthoma: a clinical and histopathological study. J Eur Acad Dermatol Venereol 2011;25(2):175–80.

Argenyi ZB, Huston BM, Argenyi EE, et al. Large-cell acanthoma of the skin. A study by image analysis cytometry and immunohistochemistry. Am J Dermatopathol 1994;16(2):140–4.

Cho S, Chang SE, Choi JH, et al. Clinical and histologic features of 64 cases of steatocystoma multiplex. J Dermatol 2002;29(3):152–6.

Folpe AL, Reisenauer AK, Mentzel T, et al. Proliferating trichilemmal tumors: clinicopathologic evaluation is a guide to biologic behavior. J Cutan Pathol 2003;30(8): 492–8.

Fornatora ML, Reich RF, Haber S, et al. Oral melanoacanthoma: a report of 10 cases, review of the literature, and immunohistochemical analysis for HMB-45 reactivity. Am J Dermatopathol 2003;25(1):12–15.

Goldenberg A, Lee RA, Cohen PR. Acantholytic dyskeratotic acanthoma: case report and review of the literature. Dermatol Pract Concept 2014;4(3):25–30.

Jaworsky C, Murphy GF. Cystic tumors of the neck. J Dermatol Surg Oncol 1989;15(1):21–6.

Kim SH, Choi JH, Sung KJ, et al. Acantholytic acanthoma. J Dermatol 2000;27(2):127–8.

Lyons G, Chamberlain AJ, Kelly JW. Dermoscopic features of clear cell acanthoma: five new cases and a review of existing published cases. Australas J Dermatol 2015;56(3):206–11.

Mehregan DR, Hamzavi F, Brown K. Large cell acanthoma. Int J Dermatol 2003;42(1):36–9.

Romaní J, Barnadas MA, Miralles J, et al. Median raphe cyst of the penis with ciliated cells. J Cutan Pathol 1995;22(4):378–81.

Santos LD, Mendelsohn G. Perineal cutaneous ciliated cyst in a male. Pathology 2004;36(4):369–70.

Sharma R, Verma P, Yadav P, et al. Proliferating trichilemmal tumor of scalp: benign or malignant, a dilemma. J Cutan Aesthet Surg 2012;5(3):213–15.

Vidaurri-de la Cruz H, Tamayo-Sánchez L, Durán-McKinster C, et al. Epidermal nevus syndromes: clinical findings in 35 patients. Pediatr Dermatol 2004;21(4):432–9.

3

Malignant tumors of the epidermis

Dirk M. Elston

Actinic keratosis

Key Features

- Crowding, disorder, and atypia of epidermal keratinocytes
- Arises from the basal layer
- Solar elastosis typically present

Atypical cells commonly surround the follicular infundibulum. In two-dimensional sections, they appear to form a shoulder zone peripheral to the benign follicular epithelium. The overlying stratum corneum may be normal or may have features of a "malignant horn." A malignant horn is a compact, eosinophilic stratum corneum with hyperchromatic bricklike parakeratosis. The brightly eosinophilic zones alternate from left to right with pale, basophilic lamellar keratin originating from adnexal structures (flag sign). Broad-based buds of atypical keratinocytes are commonly seen extending downward from the epidermis. The budding can become complex, and separation from superficially invasive squamous cell carcinoma may sometimes be difficult.

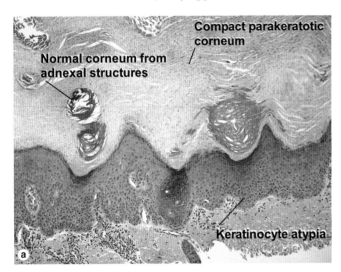

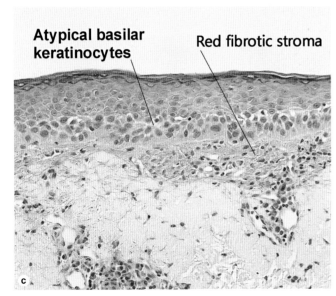

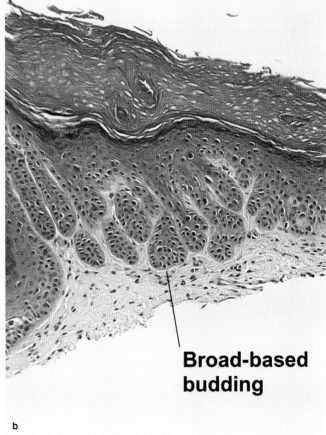

Fig. 3.1 Actinic keratosis

Acantholytic actinic keratosis

Key Features

- Crowding, disorder, and atypia of epidermal keratinocytes
- Acantholysis in areas of atypia
- Overlying "malignant horn" may be present
- Complex epidermal budding may be present

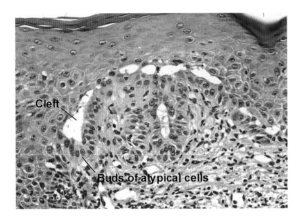

Fig. 3.2 Acantholytic actinic keratosis

Lichenoid actinic keratosis

Key Features

- Crowding, disorder, and atypia of epidermal keratinocytes
- Areas of lichenoid interface dermatitis
- Overlying "malignant horn" may be present

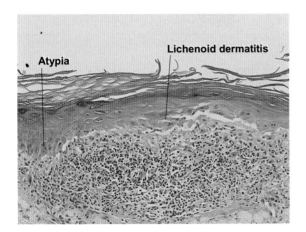

Fig. 3.3 Lichenoid actinic keratosis

Hypertrophic actinic keratosis

Key Features

- Crowding, disorder, and atypia of epidermal keratinocytes
- Prominent overlying "malignant horn"
- Acanthosis, often with complex epidermal budding
- Red, fibrotic stroma often displaces solar elastosis downward

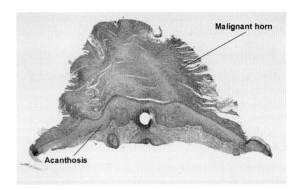

Fig. 3.4 Hypertrophic actinic keratosis

Bowenoid actinic keratosis

Key Features

- Focal, full-thickness atypia

Unlike Bowen disease, bowenoid actinic keratosis never demonstrates anaplastic nuclei, clonal nesting, buckshot intraepidermal scatter of atypical cells, or full-thickness follicular involvement.

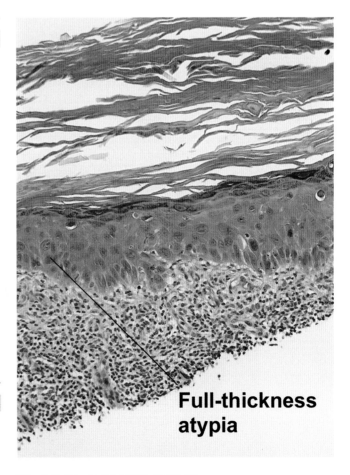

Fig. 3.5 Bowenoid actinic keratosis

Bowen disease

Key Features

- Full-thickness atypia with loss of normal maturation (wind-blown pattern)
- Malignant horn typically present
- Atypical cells may occur in an intraepidermal buckshot or nested pattern
- Full-thickness atypia commonly involves follicles

Bowen disease is a form of squamous cell carcinoma in situ. The malignant cells probably originate in the follicular epithelium. As the malignant cells migrate into the epidermis, they create a buckshot or nested pattern. With time, they involve the full thickness of the epidermis. This is the stage most commonly represented in biopsy specimens. It resembles bowenoid actinic keratosis, except that the cells tend to be more anaplastic with a higher nuclear-to-cytoplasm ratio. Areas with a nested or buckshot pattern may persist. Clear cell change or cells with ample glassy eosinophilic cytoplasm may sometimes be present instead of anaplastic cells. Bowen disease

tends to involve the full thickness of at least some follicles. Some examples show full-thickness involvement of multiple follicles with relative sparing of the overlying epidermis.

Differential Diagnosis

1. Paget disease
2. Melanoma
3. Intraepidermal porocarcinoma
4. Sebaceous carcinoma

The malignant keratinocytes of Bowen disease can keratinize and become part of the stratum corneum. In contrast, the malignant cells of Paget disease or melanoma often "spit out" into the stratum corneum intact. Bowen disease contains glycogen and is periodic acid–Schiff (PAS) positive and diastase sensitive. In contrast, Paget disease contains sialomucin and is PAS positive, diastase resistant. Bowen disease is negative for carcinoembryonic antigen (CEA), whereas Paget stains for CEA. Ducts and sebaceous differentiation distinguish porocarcinoma and sebaceous carcinoma.

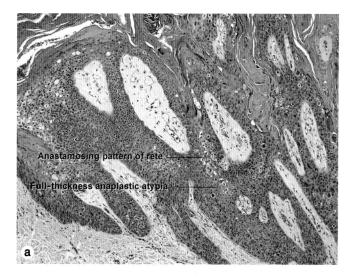

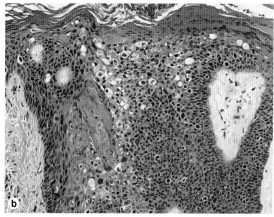

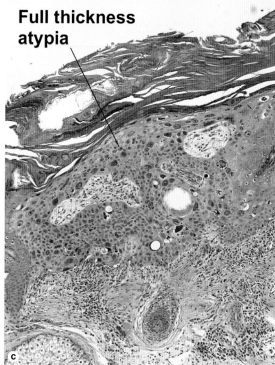

Fig. 3.6 Bowen disease

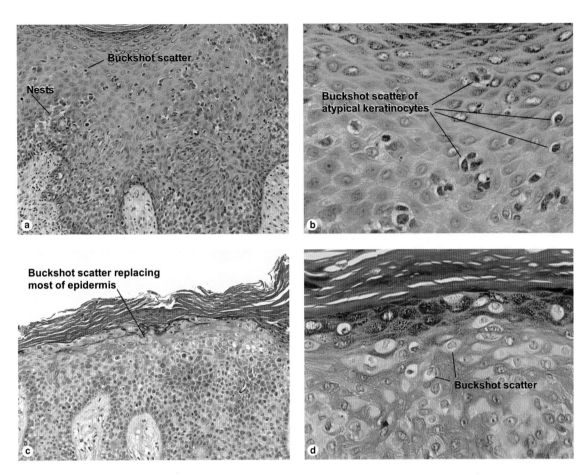

Fig. 3.7 Bowen disease: buckshot scatter of atypical cells

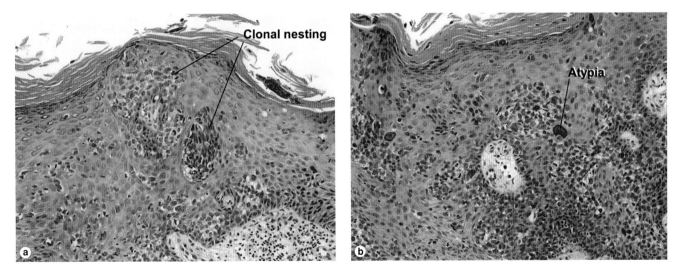

Fig. 3.8 Bowen disease: clonal nesting of atypical cells

continued

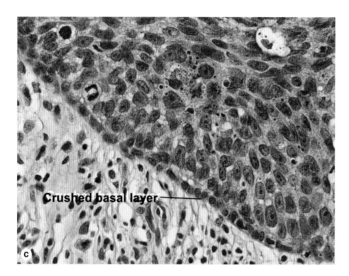

Fig. 3.8, cont'd

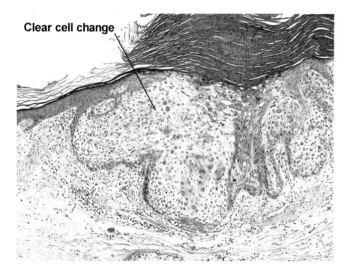

Fig. 3.9 Clear cell change in Bowen disease

Key Features

- Atypical keratinocytes invading the dermis
- Acantholysis may be present
- Desmoplasia may be present

Well-differentiated invasive squamous cell carcinoma closely resembles the surface epidermis in staining characteristics, and keratinization is present. Pseudoepitheliomatous hyperplasia is often noted at the periphery of the tumor, and overlying changes of prurigo nodularis may be present in lesions that have been picked. An adequate biopsy is essential to avoid misdiagnosis.

Nodular lymphoid aggregates are an important clue to the presence of desmoplastic squamous carcinoma. Immunostaining can be used to confirm the presence of atypical squamous cells within the stroma.

Moderately differentiated tumors have a higher nuclear/cytoplastic ratio, but still keratinize. Poorly differentiated tumors are spindled or anaplastic. Keratin immunostaining is typically necessary to confirm the diagnosis of a poorly differentiated tumor.

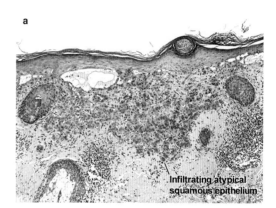

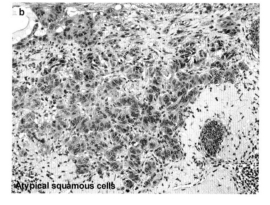

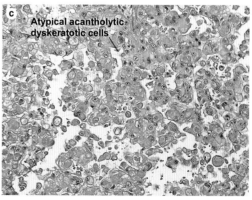

Fig. 3.10 (A and B) Well-differentiated invasive squamous cell carcinoma **(C)** Acantholytic squamous cell carcinoma. **(D and E)** Desmoplastic squamous cell carcinoma (H&E and keratin 903 immunostain)

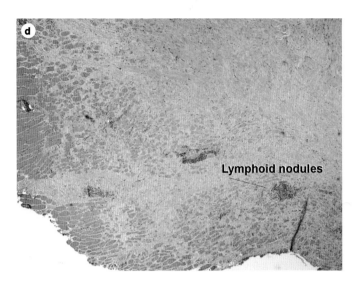

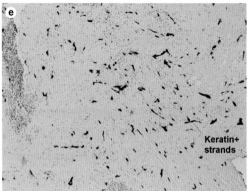

Lymphoid nodules

Keratin+ strands

Fig. 3.10, cont'd

Verrucous carcinoma

Key Features

- Well-differentiated, glassy squamous epithelium
- Rounded border

Whereas most invasive squamous cell carcinomas have a jagged outline, verrucous carcinomas are composed of well-differentiated, glassy eosinophilic keratinocytes and have a blunt, rounded outline. They slowly push into the underlying tissue in a bulldozing fashion.

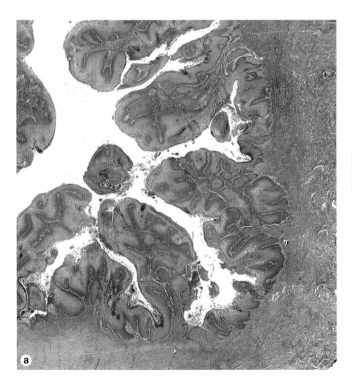

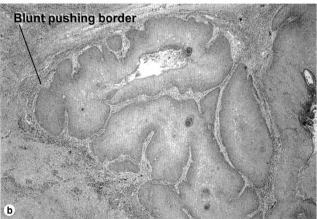

Blunt pushing border

Fig. 3.11 Verrucous carcinoma

Spindled squamous cell carcinoma

Key Features

• Atypical spindle cells abutting the epidermis

Differential Diagnosis

Spindled squamous cell carcinoma can closely resemble other spindle cell neoplasms. The microscopic differential diagnosis for an atypical spindle cell tumor *SLAM*med up against the epidermis includes:
• *S*quamous cell carcinoma (keratin positive)
• *L*eiomyosarcoma (smooth muscle actin and desmin positive)
• *A*typical fibroxanthoma (diagnosis of exclusion)
• *M*elanoma (S100 positive)

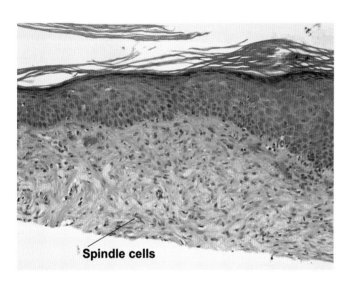

Spindle cells

Fig. 3.12 Spindled squamous cell carcinoma

Keratoacanthoma

Key Features

• Defined by rapid growth and ability to involute spontaneously
• Explosive growth common after biopsy
• Many consider it a form of invasive squamous cell carcinoma capable of regression
• Keratin-filled crater
• Invasive proliferation of glassy, red keratinocytes
• Neutrophil microabscesses common
• Eosinophils common in surrounding infiltrate
• Trapping of elastic fibers common at the periphery of the squamous proliferation
• Hypergranulosis and pseudoepitheliomatous hyperplasia prominent in hair follicles toward the center of early lesions
• Acantholysis is *never* present

Keratoacanthomas grow rapidly and then involute. Unfortunately, they can sometimes be difficult to distinguish from well-differentiated invasive squamous cell carcinomas that will never involute. Perineural extension may be seen in both. Explosive growth after a biopsy is consistent with a diagnosis of keratoacanthoma. In contrast, the presence of acantholysis indicates that the lesion will behave like squamous cell carcinoma. Neutrophilic microabscesses, eosinophils, and elastic trapping are common in keratoacanthoma, but rare in squamous cell carcinoma.

Pseudoepitheliomatous hyperplasia and hypergranulosis in follicles occur in the central portion of early keratoacanthomas, but only at the periphery of squamous cell carcinomas. The defining feature of a keratoacanthoma is its ability to undergo terminal differentiation, a process whereby the tumor keratinizes itself to death.

Table 3.1 Characteristics of keratoacanthoma versus squamous cell carcinoma		
Characteristic	Keratoacanthoma	Squamous cell carcinoma
Pseudoepitheliomatous hyperplasia and hypergranulosis	At center of lesion	At periphery of lesion
Cell type	Large, light-pink, glassy cells	Often large, light-pink, and glassy
Dermal infiltrate	Eosinophils common	Plasma cells common
Gland involvement	Pushes eccrine glands down	Invades eccrine glands
Traps elastic tissue	Commonly	Rarely
Acantholysis	No	Often
Perineural invasion	Yes	Yes
Neutrophilic microabscesses	Commonly	Rarely
Growth	Explosive	Slow
Terminal differentiation	Yes	No

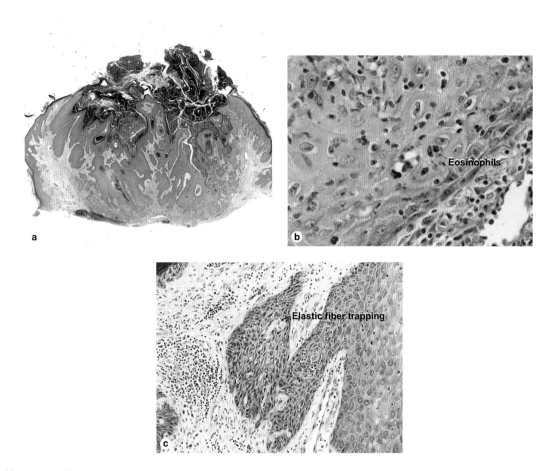

Fig. 3.13 Keratoacanthoma

Regressing keratoacanthoma

Key Features

- Craterlike outline, often with scalloped outline
- Crater filled with keratin
- Proliferative epithelium has involuted to a thin wall resembling the lining of an epidermoid cyst
- Scar peripheral to regressed epithelium

The most striking feature of a regressing keratoacanthoma is the massive keratin within the crater, out of proportion to the thin epithelium that lines the scalloped crater.

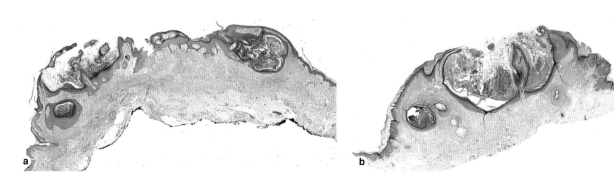

Fig. 3.14 Regressing keratoacanthoma

Basal cell carcinoma (BCC)

Key Features

- Blue islands
- Peripheral palisading
- High nuclear-to-cytoplasmic ratio
- Retraction artifact
- Fibromyxoid stroma

Superficial multifocal BCC

Key Features

- Multifocal blue buds
- Distinctive fibromyxoid stroma displaces solar elastosis downward
- Retraction artifact common

Superficial multifocal BCC grows in a pattern resembling garlands draped from the epidermis. In two-dimensional sections, this gives the appearance of multifocal blue buds. Because the buds are spaced far apart, margin evaluation is based largely on the surrounding tumor stroma. The tumor stroma displaces the reticular dermis and solar elastosis downward. Stroma extending to the margin counts as a positive margin.

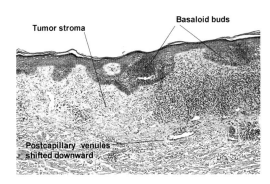

Fig. 3.15 Superficial multifocal basal cell carcinoma

Nodular BCC

Key Features

- Nodular blue islands
- Peripheral palisading
- Retraction artifact
- Distinctive fibromyxoid stroma

Hyperchromatic "monster cells" may be present, but do not affect prognosis.

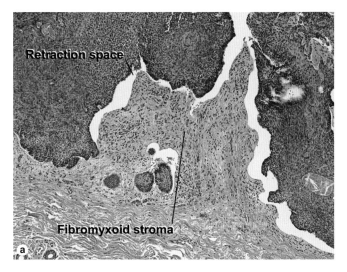

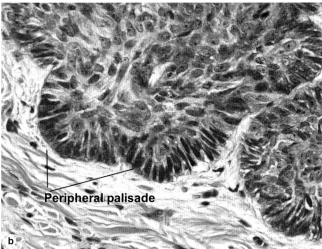

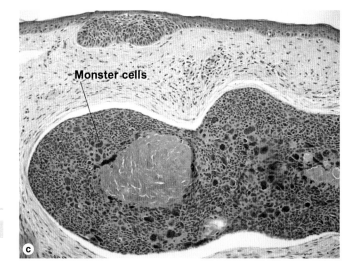

Fig. 3.16 Nodular basal cell carcinoma (Fig. 3.16c demonstrates nodular BCC with monster cells)

Micronodular BCC

- Small blue islands
- Peripheral palisading
- Retraction artifact focally
- Distinctive fibromyxoid stroma surrounds individual islands, but normal dermis is present between islands

Micronodular BCC is characterized by aggressive, wormlike growth into the dermis. In cross-section, the appearance is micronodular. Because of the thick dermal collagen bundles between tumor islands, the tumors are poorly defined clinically, and curettage has a high failure rate.

It should be noted that many ordinary BCCs demonstrate small fingerlike projections that appear as small round balls in cross-section. Only tumor stroma separates the islands, with no thick collagen bundles in between. These tumors do not qualify as micronodular BCC.

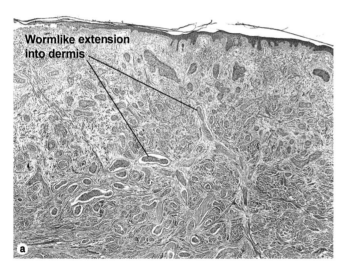

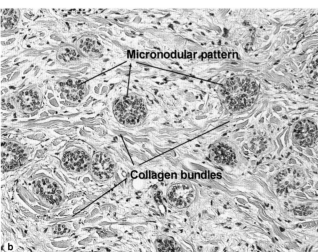

Fig. 3.17 Micronodular basal cell carcinoma

Morpheaform BCC

- Thin infiltrating strands of basaloid cells, usually only two cells thick
- Sclerotic stroma
- Tadpolelike islands with small horn cysts may be present focally

Morpheaform BCC presents clinically as scarlike lesions that gradually expand. Perineural extension is common. It is usually deeply infiltrative by the time the diagnosis is made. The pink sclerotic stroma contains little to no mucin and at first glance may resemble a scar. However, the architecture is not that of a scar. In scars, the collagen has an east/west orientation, whereas blood vessels have a north/south orientation. This is unlike the haphazard structure of the tumor stroma. Occasionally, a superficial biopsy will demonstrate tadpolelike islands with small horn cysts, creating a "paisley-tie" appearance.

1. Morpheaform BCC (older patient with a scarlike lesion)
2. Microcystic adnexal carcinoma (firm plaque on the upper lip, medial cheek, or chin)
3. Desmoplastic trichoepithelioma (doughnutlike firm lesion with central dell on the cheek of a young female)

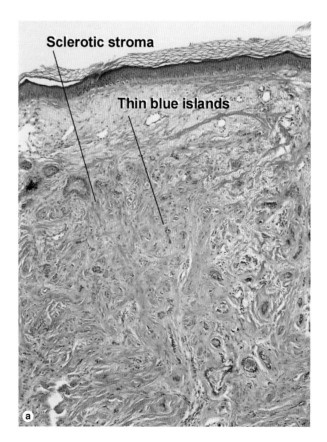

Fig. 3.18 Morpheaform basal cell carcinoma

continued

4. Syringoma (small papules on the lower lids or widely eruptive papules)
5. Eruptive syringomas (chest and back or penis, often skin type VI)

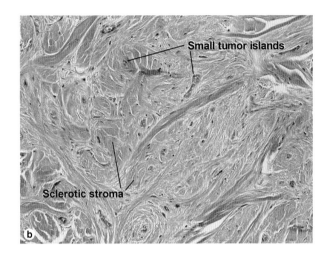

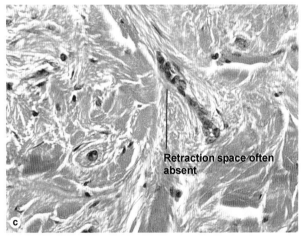

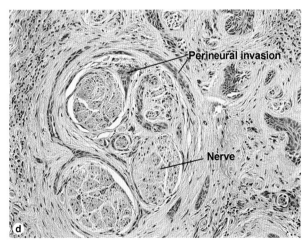

Fig. 3.18, cont'd

Infiltrative BCC

Key Features

- Spiky growth pattern
- Fibroblast-rich stroma with little mucin
- Areas of squamous differentiation common
- Perineural extension common

At first glance, the fibroblast-rich stroma of an infiltrative BCC can resemble the stroma of a trichoepithelioma. Glance again. Trichoepitheliomas never have spiky islands. If you remember that spiky things are likely to hurt you, it may help you to remember that this feature matches with an aggressive form of BCC. Papillary mesenchymal bodies are absent in infiltrative BCC.

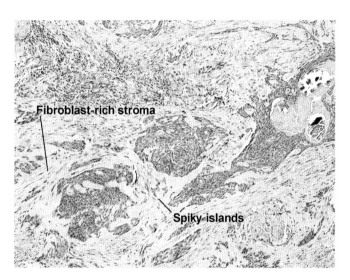

Fig. 3.19 Infiltrative basal cell carcinoma

Infundibulocystic BCC

Key Features

- Radiating pink strands, blue buds
- Horn cysts
- Fibromyxoid stroma

Infundibulocystic BCC differentiates toward the follicular infundibulum. It is characterized by pink strands of squamous epithelium, blue basaloid buds at the tips of the strands, and horn cysts. It closely resembles basaloid follicular hamartoma. The two entities are best distinguished clinically.

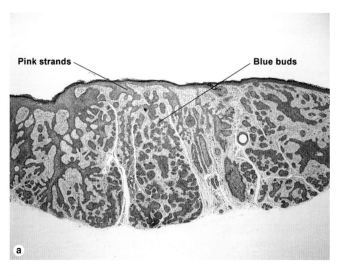

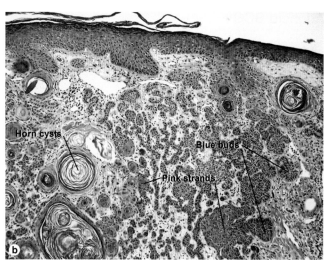

Fig. 3.20 Infundibulocystic basal cell carcinoma

Fibroepithelioma of Pinkus

Key Features

- Anastamosing pink strands, blue buds
- Eccrine ducts often visible within strands
- Ample fibromyxoid stroma

Fibroepithelioma of Pinkus is composed of anastomosing pink epithelial strands embedded in a fibromyxoid stroma. Ducts are often visible within the strands. Blue basaloid buds are present at the tips and periphery of strands.

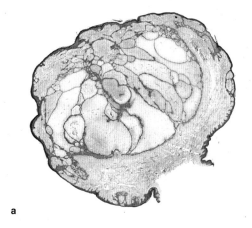

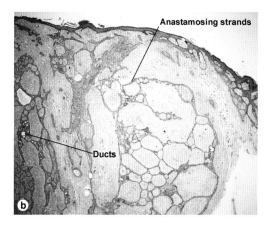

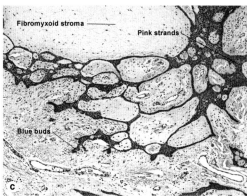

Fig. 3.21 Fibroepithelioma of Pinkus

Adenoid BCC

Key Features

- Blue islands with adenoid pattern (clear spaces in middle of islands)
- Peripheral palisading
- Fibromyxoid stroma
- Retraction artifact

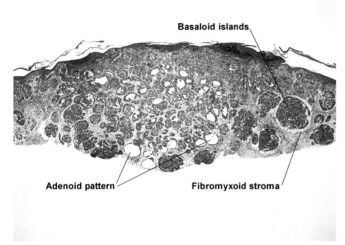

Fig. 3.22 Adenoid basal cell carcinoma

Paget disease

Key Features

- Intraepidermal proliferation of large cells with ample amphophilic cytoplasm
- Tumor cells in buckshot distribution or intraepidermal nests
- Atypical cells crush the basal layer
- Atypical cells may "spit out" into the stratum corneum intact
- CK7+
- CEA+
- S100–
- PAS+, diastase resistant (sialomucin)

Paget disease of the breast represents intraepidermal extension of underlying intraductal carcinoma. Extramammary Paget disease may represent an extension of an underlying adenocarcinoma, but more commonly arises de novo, probably from pluripotent cells or mammarylike glands along milk lines. Sialomucin stains PAS+, diastase resistant, and with Alcian blue and toluidine blue at high (but not low) pH.

Differential Diagnosis

1. Melanoma (S100+, HMB-45+, never crushes basal layer, cells can spit into stratum corneum)
2. Bowen disease (keratin+, CEA–, cells rarely spit into stratum corneum intact)
3. Intraepidermal porocarcinoma (related to acrosyringeal keratinocytes, demonstrates focal duct differentiation, may have adjacent benign hidroacanthoma simplex)

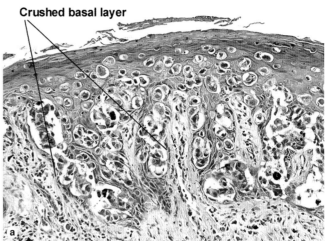

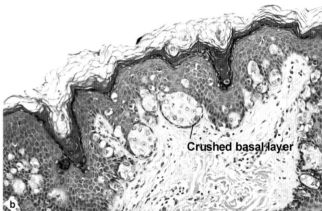

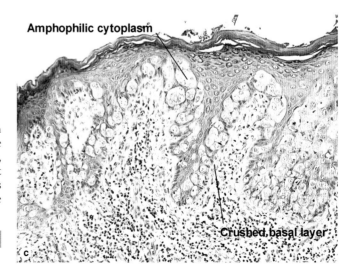

Fig. 3.23 Extramammary Paget disease

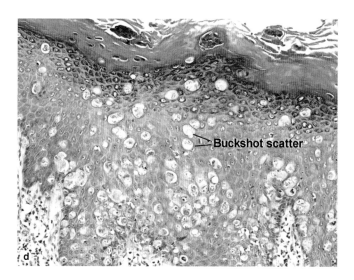

Fig. 3.23, cont'd

Lymphoepithelioma-like carcinoma

Key Features

- At scan, mimics a germinal center or lymphoma
- Central keratin-positive atypical epithelial cells
- Surrounding lymphocytes

Despite the anaplastic character of the cells, the prognosis is generally good. Nasopharyngeal lymphoepithelioma can have a similar appearance, and metastatic disease should be ruled out. Cutaneous lesions are negative for Epstein–Barr virus, unlike the nasopharyngeal counterpart.

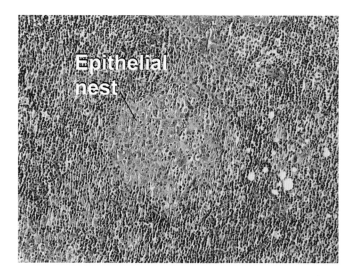

Fig. 3.24 Lymphoepithelioma-like carcinoma

Further reading

Cuevas Gonzalez JC, Gaitan Cepeda LA, Borges Yanez SA, et al. p53 and p16 in oral epithelial dysplasia and oral squamous cell carcinoma: a study of 208 cases. Indian J Pathol Microbiol 2016;59(2):153–8.

Kallam AR, Satyanarayana MA, Aryasomayajula S, et al. Basal cell carcinoma developing from trichoepithelioma: review of three cases. J Clin Diagn Res 2016;10(3):PD17–19.

Mengjun B, Zheng-Qiang W, Tasleem MM. Extramammary Paget's disease of the perianal region: a review of the literature emphasizing management. Dermatol Surg 2013;39(1 Pt 1):69–75.

Pe'er J. Pathology of eyelid tumors. Indian J Ophthalmol 2016;64(3):177–90.

Rudolph R, Zelac DE. Squamous cell carcinoma of the skin. Plast Reconstr Surg 2004;114(6):82e–94.

Suarez MJ, Rivera-Michlig R, Dubovy S, et al. Clinicopathological features of ophthalmic neoplasms arising in the setting of xeroderma pigmentosum. Ocul Oncol Pathol 2015;2(2):112–21.

Pilar and sebaceous neoplasms

Dirk M. Elston

Pilar neoplasms

Pilar neoplasms differentiate toward (resemble) various parts of the normal hair follicle. They are named according to what they resemble. Before reading this chapter, review the discussion of hair anatomy in Chapter 1. Blue pilar tumors differentiate toward elements of the inferior segment of the hair follicle. Red pilar tumors differentiate toward the isthmus and infundibulum. Clear cell tumors differentiate toward the glycogenated outer root sheath.

Pilomatricoma (calcifying epithelioma of Malherbe)

Key Features

- Low-power architecture is a large ball with internal trabeculae (similar in architecture to a proliferating pilar cyst)
- Basophilic cells that resemble those of the hair matrix keratinize to form shadow cells (ghost cells)
- Often calcify
- Giant cell granulomas adjacent to calcifications
- Bone formation common
- Multiple pilomatricomas are associated with myotonic dystrophy

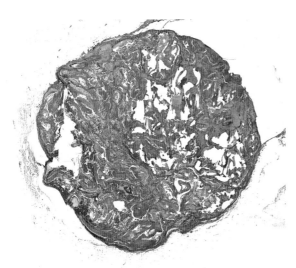

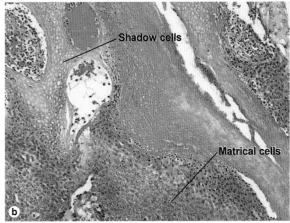

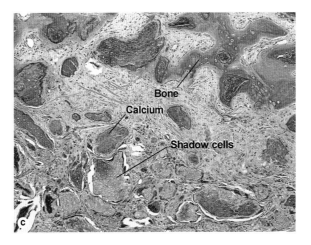

Fig. 4.1 Pilomatricoma

Pilomatrical carcinoma

Key Features

- Rare
- May arise in long-standing pilomatricomas
- Large
- Infiltrative border
- Atypia, mitoses, necrosis

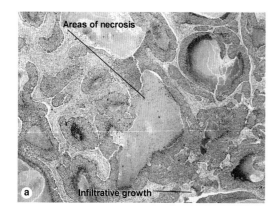

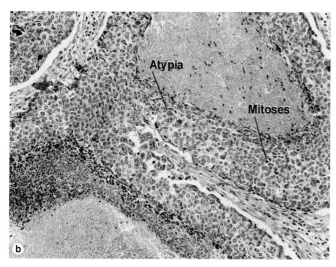

Fig. 4.2 Pilomatrical carcinoma

Trichoblastoma

Key Features

- Family of blue follicular tumors composed of basaloid cells
- Cells resemble those of basal cell carcinoma
- Stroma resembles the normal fibrous sheath of the hair follicle, with concentric collagen and many fibroblasts
- Papillary mesenchymal bodies may be present in the stroma
- Mucin may be present within tumor islands, but never in the stroma
- No retraction artifact

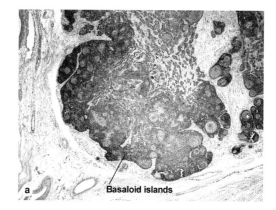

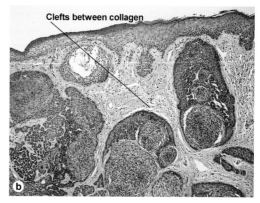

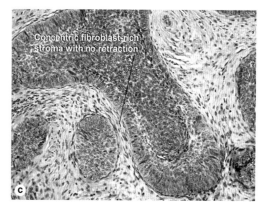

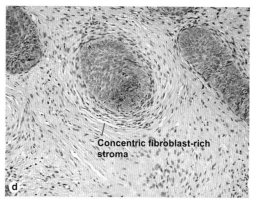

Fig. 4.3 Trichoblastoma

Benign trichoblastomas are large basaloid follicular neoplasms. The tumor islands resemble basal cell carcinoma, but the stroma resembles the normal fibrous sheath of the hair follicle. Trichoepitheliomas and lymphadenomas are distinctive forms of benign trichoblastoma. Trichogerminomas are a type of trichoblastoma with differentiation toward the hair germ. Basal cell carcinoma is the most common malignant counterpart of a benign trichoblastoma. Some trichoblastic carcinomas arising in long-standing trichoblastomas have been very aggressive tumors with metastases.

Trichoepithelioma

Key Features

- Distinctive type of trichoblastoma
- Blue tumor composed of basaloid cells
- At scan, fingerlike projections and cribriform (Swiss-cheese) nodules
- Cells resemble those of basal cell carcinoma
- Stroma resembles the normal fibrous sheath of the hair follicle, with concentric collagen and many fibroblasts (as with any other trichoblastoma)
- Papillary mesenchymal bodies typically prominent
- Mucin may be present within cribriform tumor islands, but never in the stroma
- No retraction artifact

Trichoepitheliomas commonly present as multiple small papules in the nasolabial folds. The multiple type is inherited in an autosomal-dominant fashion. Each papule is composed of basaloid islands in a fibroblast-rich stroma with papillary mesenchymal bodies. Horn cysts and calcification are common. Small clefts may occur between collagen fibers of the tumor stroma, but not between the tumor epithelium and stroma. Papillary mesenchymal bodies are round collections of plump mesenchymal cells resembling those in the follicular papilla.

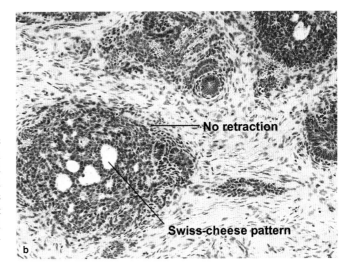

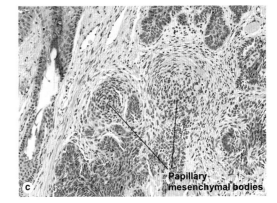

Fig. 4.4 Trichoepithelioma

PEARLS

- Multiple trichoepitheliomas (epithelioma adenoides cysticum) inherited as autosomal-dominant trait
- Brooke–Spiegler syndrome: multiple trichoepitheliomas and cylindromas
- Rombo syndrome: milia, hypotrichosis, trichoepitheliomas, basal cell carcinoma, atrophoderma, vasodilation with cyanosis

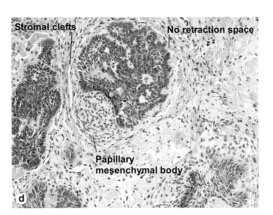

Fig. 4.4, cont'd

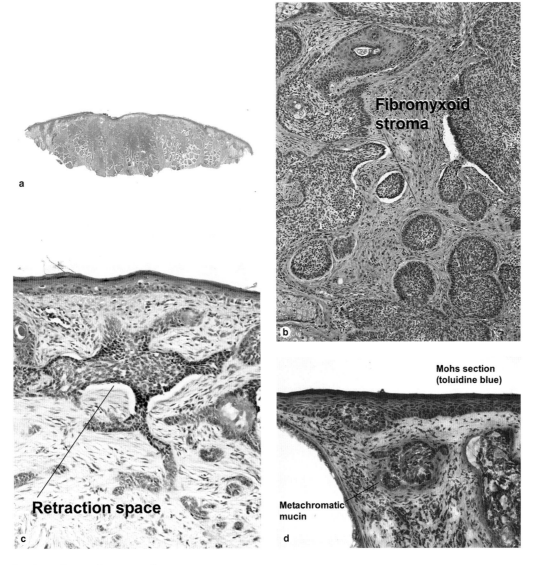

Fig. 4.5 Basal cell carcinoma for comparison

Table 4.1 Characteristics of trichoepithelioma versus basal cell carcinoma

Characteristic	Trichoepithelioma	Basal cell carcinoma
Basaloid cells	Yes	Yes
Peripheral palisading	Yes	Yes
Fingerlike and cribriform	Yes	Sometimes
Stroma	Concentric, fibroblast rich	Myxoid
Mucin	In tumor islands only, none in stroma	Metachromatic mucin in stroma
Papillary mesenchymal bodies	Common	Rare
Horn cysts	Common	Rare
Calcification	Common	Rare
Clefts	Between collagen fibers within stroma	Between epithelium and stroma
CD34 staining	Strong staining in stroma	+/–
BCL-2 staining	Periphery of islands	Strong, diffuse
CK20+ Merkel cells	Present in tumoral islands	Absent in tumoral islands

Desmoplastic trichoepithelioma

Key Features

- Firm doughnut-shaped lesion on a young woman's cheek
- Central dell
- Paisley-tie pattern (tadpole-shaped islands)
- Red desmoplastic stroma
- Calcifications common
- Horn cysts common
- Clefts only within stroma

PEARL

Paisley-tie tumors
- Desmoplastic trichoepithelioma: doughnut-shaped tumor on the cheek of a young female
- Microcystic adnexal carcinoma: firm plaque on the upper lip, medial cheek, or chin
- Morpheaform basal cell carcinoma: scarlike lesion in older patient
- Eruptive syringomas: chest and back or penis, commonly on skin type VI
- Syringomas: small papules on lower lids, very common with Down syndrome and in Asian females

Table 4.2 Characteristics of desmoplastic trichoepithelioma versus morpheaform basal cell carcinoma

Characteristic	Desmoplastic trichoepithelioma	Morpheaform basal cell carcinoma
Paisley-tie pattern	Yes	Sometimes superficially
Stroma	Red, sclerotic	Red, sclerotic
Horn cysts	Common	Occasional
Calcification	Common	Rare
Clefts	Between collagen fibers within stroma	Between epithelium and stroma
Central dell	Yes	No
Age	Younger	Older
Clinical appearance	Firm doughnut	Scarlike

Table 4.3 Characteristics of desmoplastic trichoepithelioma versus microcystic adnexal carcinoma

Characteristic	Desmoplastic trichoepithelioma	Microcystic adnexal carcinoma
Paisley-tie pattern	Yes	Yes
Stroma	Red, sclerotic	Often red, sclerotic
Horn cysts	Common	Common
Calcification	Common	Rare
Lymphoid aggregates	Rare	Typical
Perineural extension	No	Yes
Clinical appearance	Firm doughnut	Plaque on upper lip, cheek, chin
Central dell	Typical	Absent

Table 4.4 Characteristics of desmoplastic trichoepithelioma versus syringoma

Characteristic	Desmoplastic trichoepithelioma	Syringoma
Paisley-tie pattern	Yes	Yes
Stroma	Red, sclerotic	Red, sclerotic
Horn cysts	Common	May occur
Calcification	Common	Rare
Central dell	Typical	Absent
Shape	Broad	Small and round
Clinical appearance	Firm doughnut	Small papules

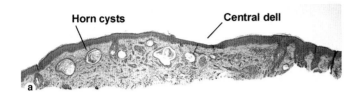

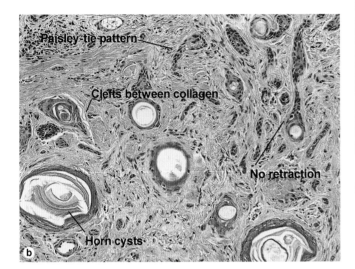

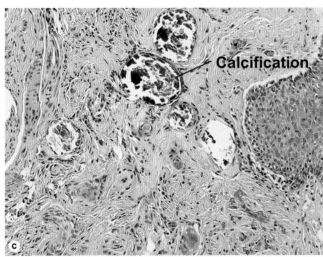

Fig. 4.6 Desmoplastic trichoepithelioma

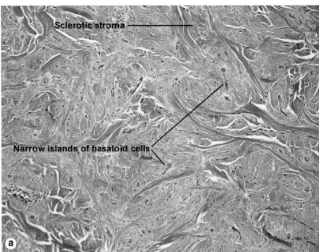

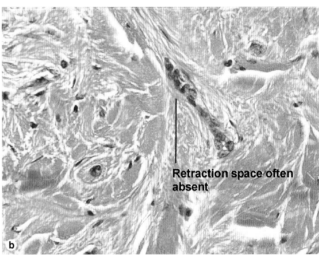

Fig. 4.7 Morpheaform basal cell carcinoma for comparison

Lymphadenoma (adamantinoid trichoblastoma)

Key Features

- Tumor islands with one to two layers of basaloid cells peripherally
- Centers of each island composed of clear cells/ inflammatory cells

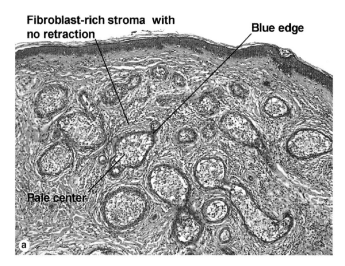

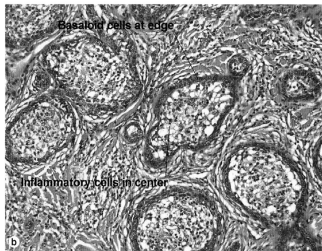

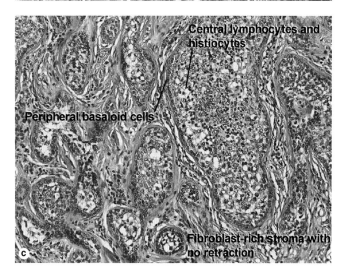

Fig. 4.8 Lymphadenoma

Fibrofolliculoma

Key Features

- Fibrous pink orb or amphophilic fibromucinous orb
- Epithelial strands radiating outward from central follicle-like structure
- No hair fibers

In fibrofolliculomas, the strands of epithelium are not well enough differentiated to form hair fibers. No bulb, inner root sheath, or outer root sheath is present. The strands of epithelium may have an anastomosing pattern. *Trichodiscomas* are simply fibrofolliculomas cut in a plane of section that does not reveal the epithelial strands.

PEARL

Birt–Hogg–Dubé syndrome
- Multiple fibrofolliculomas, "trichodiscomas," and "acrochordons" (all three are probably fibrofolliculomas cut at various angles)
- Chromophobe renal carcinoma, renal oncocytoma, and spontaneous pneumothorax

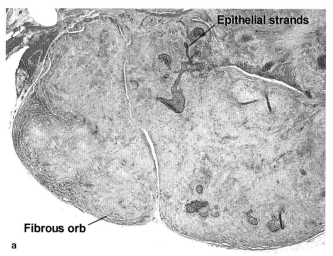

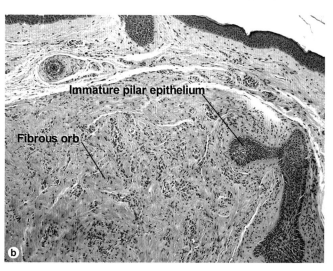

Fig. 4.9 Fibrofolliculoma

Trichofolliculoma

Key Features

- Many small hair follicles emptying into a central large follicular infundibulum (momma and her babies)
- Each small hair follicle has a bulb and root sheath and produces a hair fiber
- Central infundibulum contains many small hair shafts
- Clinically, there is a tuft of hairs protruding from a central pore

Trichofolliculomas demonstrate miniature follicles converging on a central infundibulum (*fingers of fully formed follicles forming follicular fibers*). Some examples are embedded in an eosinophilic fibrous orb of stroma.

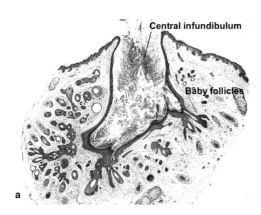

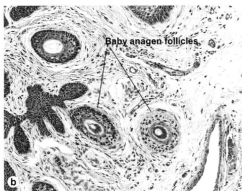

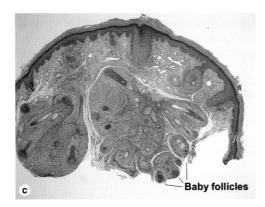

Fig. 4.10 Trichofolliculoma

Trichoadenoma

Key Features

- Multiple red doughnuts in the dermis, each resembling a follicular infundibulum
- Often in pairs resembling eyeglasses or toasted oat cereal

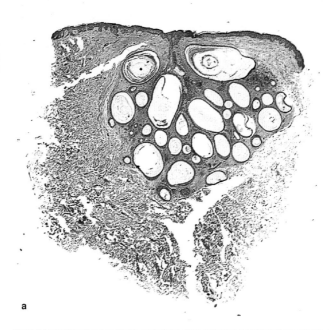

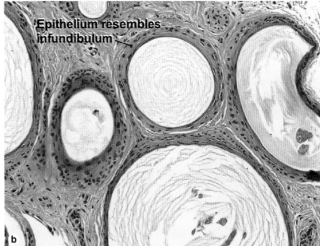

Fig. 4.11 Trichoadenoma

Basaloid follicular hamartoma

Key Features

- Resembles infundibulocystic basal cell carcinoma histologically
- Often multiple with autosomal-dominant inheritance
- Sometimes segmental blaschkoid distribution

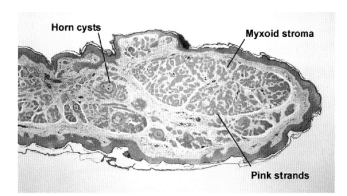

Fig. 4.12 Basaloid follicular hamartoma

Differential Diagnosis

Infundibulocystic basal cell carcinoma can appear identical histologically. The two are best distinguished clinically.

Dilated pore of Winer

Key Features

- Resembles a dilated follicular infundibulum
- Small, radiating, red, fingerlike epithelial projections

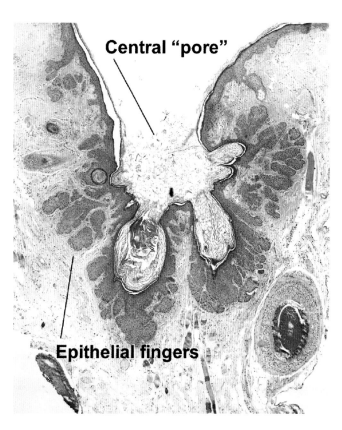

Fig. 4.13 Dilated pore of Winer

Pilar sheath acanthoma

Key Features

- Similar to dilated pore of Winer, but with thick, acanthotic fingers

Pilar sheath acanthoma has been described as a "pore of Winer on steroids"

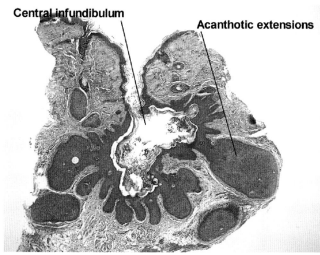

Fig. 4.14 Pilar sheath acanthoma

Trichilemmoma

Key Features

- Often a warty surface
- Smooth lobules of clear glycogenated cells hanging down from the epidermis
- Peripheral palisading
- Outlined by a thick, glassy, eosinophilic "vitreous" basement membrane

Trichilemmomas resemble the glycogenated outer root sheath of the hair follicle. When multiple, they may be a marker for Cowden syndrome.

Differential Diagnosis

Trichilemmomas are composed of lobules of clear glycogenated cells that hang down from the surface epidermis. A clear cell acanthoma is a thickened area of the epidermis. In clear cell acanthoma, a glycogenated pale segment of epidermis is sharply demarcated from the surrounding skin. Neutrophils are noted throughout the lesion and in the overlying crust. There is no thickening of the basement membrane zone.

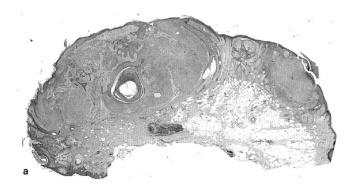

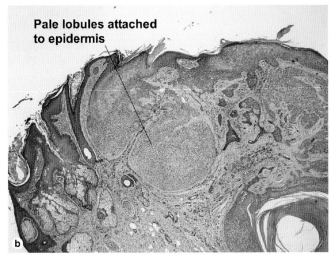

Pale lobules attached
to epidermis

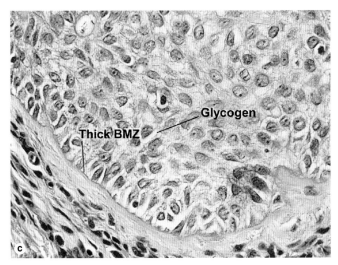

Thick BMZ   Glycogen

Fig. 4.15 Trichilemmoma (*BMZ*, basement membrane zone)

Desmoplastic trichilemmoma

Key Features

- Smooth outline with surrounding glassy basement membrane
- Centrally, broken into jagged islands separated by dense pink stroma

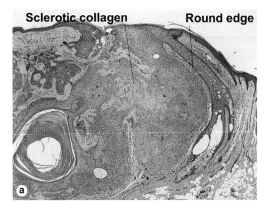

Sclerotic collagen   Round edge

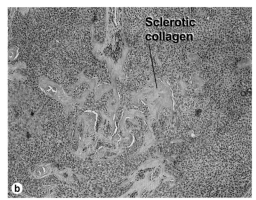

Sclerotic collagen

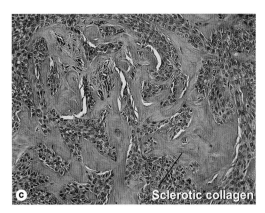

Sclerotic collagen

Fig. 4.16 Desmoplastic trichilemmoma

continued

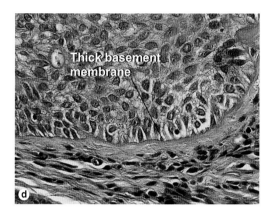

Fig. 4.16, cont'd

Tumor of the follicular infundibulum

Key Features

- Epithelium resembling follicular infundibulum forming garlandlike strands hanging from the epidermis
- Step sections reveal some tumors to be contiguous with adjacent basal cell carcinoma

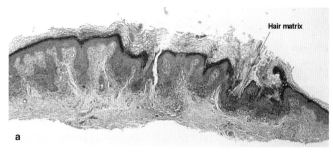

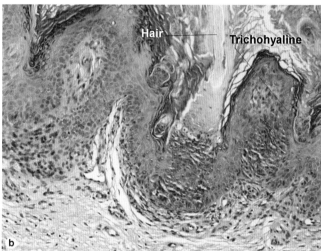

Fig. 4.18 Epidermal panfolliculoma

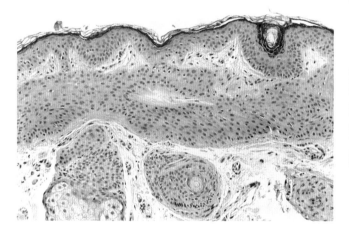

Fig. 4.17 Tumor of the follicular infundibulum

Panfolliculoma

Key Features

- Recapitulates all portions of the hair follicle
- May be cystic or epidermal

Sebaceous neoplasms

Reticulated acanthoma with sebaceous differentiation

Key Features

- The name of the entity pretty much says it all

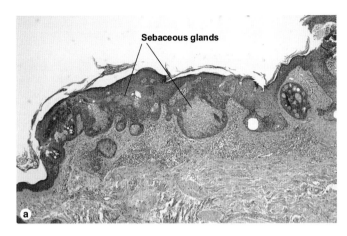

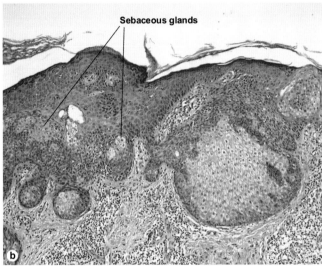

Fig. 4.19 Reticulated acanthoma with sebaceous differentiation

Nevus sebaceus of Jadassohn (organoid nevus)

Postpubertal nevus sebaceus of Jadassohn

Key Features

- "Broad, bald, bumpy, and bubbly"
- Present at birth, becomes cerebriform at puberty
- Dilated apocrine glands in underlying dermis
- Hyperkeratosis, acanthosis, and papillomatosis common
- Secondary tumors, especially syringocystadenoma papilliferum and small trichoblastomas, are common

Postpubertal cerebriform lesions of nevus sebaceus of Jadassohn appear as *broad*, alopecic (*bald*), acanthotic, and papillomatous (*bumpy*) lesions with large sebaceous lobules (*bubbly*) and dilated apocrine glands.

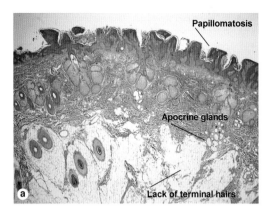

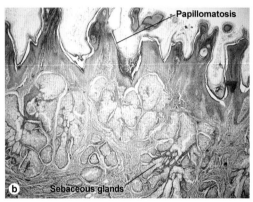

Fig. 4.20 Postpubertal nevus sebaceus of Jadassohn

Prepubertal nevus sebaceus of Jadassohn

Key Features

- "Broad and bald, but not bumpy or bubbly"
- Present at birth, but will not become cerebriform or develop large sebaceous or apocrine elements until puberty
- Primitive epithelial germs resembling fetal hair germs present

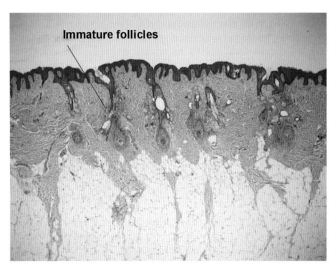

Fig. 4.21 Prepubertal nevus sebaceus of Jadassohn

Sebaceous hyperplasia

Key Features

- Large cluster of sebaceous glands around a patulous follicular opening
- Normal germinative basaloid layer at periphery of lobule

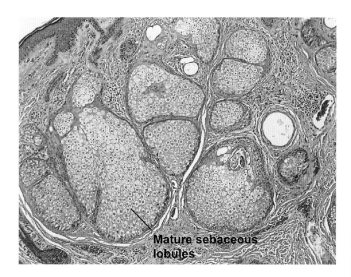

Fig. 4.22 Sebaceous hyperplasia

Sebaceoma

Key Features

- Usually a single blue nodule with red ducts
- Basaloid cells and mature sebocytes in varying proportions
- Some use the term *sebaceous adenoma* for tumors with <50% basaloid cells, and the term *sebaceous epithelioma* for tumors with >50% basaloid cells

Benign sebaceous neoplasms may be markers for the Muir–Torre syndrome (associated with keratoacanthomas and gut carcinoma). The syndrome is allelic to hereditary nonpolyposis colorectal cancer. Gastrointestinal cancers are the most common internal malignancies in the Muir–Torre syndrome (61%), followed by genitourinary tumors (22%). Approximately 15% of female patients with Muir–Torre syndrome develop endometrial cancer. The cancers, although multiple, are usually relatively indolent. Loss of normal nuclear staining for either MSH-2 or MLH-1 but is common in sebaceous neoplasms in patients with no evidence of Muir-Torre syndrome. Patients should be screened by history and not by immunostaining of tumors.

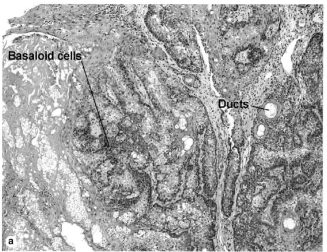

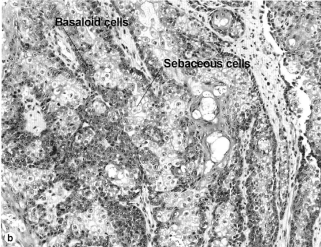

Fig. 4.23 Sebaceous adenoma in Muir–Torre syndrome

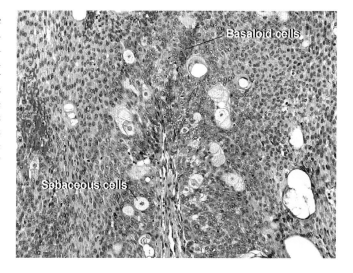

Fig. 4.24 Sebaceous epithelioma

Sebaceous carcinoma

Key Features

- May be predominantly red or blue at scan
- Atypia and mitoses common
- Infiltrative border may be apparent
- Foamy cells with scalloped nuclei
- Atypical cells may extend into the epidermis or conjunctiva in a nested or buckshot pattern

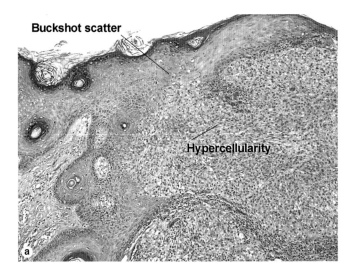
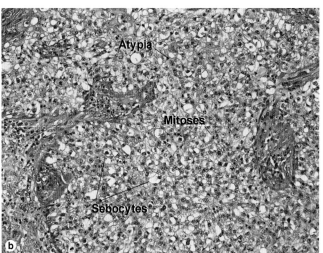
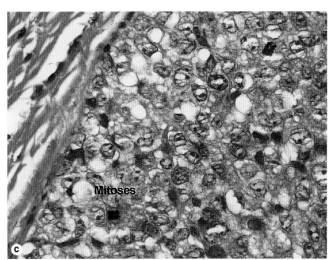

Fig. 4.25 Sebaceous carcinoma

Further reading

Ansai S, Mitsuhashi Y, Kondo S, et al. Immunohistochemical differentiation of extra-ocular sebaceous carcinoma from other skin cancers. J Dermatol 2004;31(12):998–1008.

Morgado B, Agostini P, Rivero A, et al. Extensive and ulcerated malignant proliferating trichilemmal (pilar) tumour, arising from multiple, large, degenerated trichilemmal (pilar) cysts. BMJ Case Rep 2016;2016.

Pereira PR, Odashiro AN, Rodrigues-Reyes AA, et al. Histopathological review of sebaceous carcinoma of the eyelid. J Cutan Pathol 2005;32(7):496–501.

Ponti G, Longo C. Microsatellite instability and mismatch repair protein expression in sebaceous tumors, keratocanthoma, and basal cell carcinomas with sebaceous differentiation in Muir–Torre syndrome. J Am Acad Dermatol 2013;68(3):509–10.

Samaka RM, Alrahabi N. Neuro-folliculo-sebaceous cystic hamartoma is a unique entity. Pol J Pathol 2015;66(1):77–9.

Tebcherani AJ, de Andrade HF Jr, Sotto MN. Diagnostic utility of immunohistochemistry in distinguishing trichoepithelioma and basal cell carcinoma: evaluation using tissue microarray samples. Mod Pathol 2012;25(10):1345–53.

Tellechea O, Cardoso JC, Reis JP, et al. Benign follicular tumors. An Bras Dermatol 2015;90(6):780–96, quiz 797-8.

Welsch MJ, Krunic A, Medenica MM. Birt–Hogg–Dubé Syndrome. Int J Dermatol 2005;44(8):668–73.

CHAPTER 5

Sweat gland neoplasms

Dirk M. Elston

Blue sweat gland tumors differentiate toward the secretory portion of the sweat gland. Red sweat gland tumors differentiate toward the sweat duct. Sweat duct tumors often demonstrate clear cell change. Most sweat gland tumors can show at least focal decapitation secretion, suggesting they are capable of apocrine differentiation.

Cylindroma (turban tumor)

Key Features

- Islands of blue cells with little cytoplasm
- Dark and pale blue nuclei present

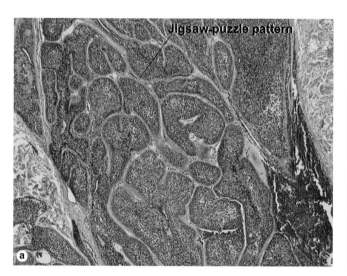

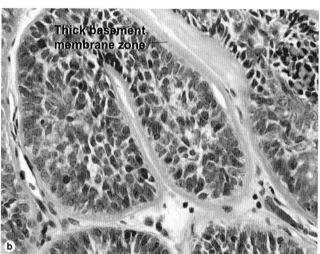

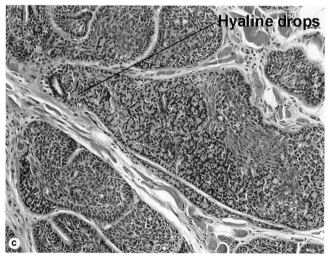

Fig. 5.1 Cylindroma

- Jigsaw-puzzle pattern
- Islands outlined by a deeply eosinophilic basement membrane
- Deeply eosinophilic hyaline droplets may be noted in islands
- Often inherited and multiple on the scalp

Spiradenoma

Key Features

- Larger round islands of blue cells with little cytoplasm
- Dark and pale blue nuclei present
- Islands peppered with black lymphocytes
- Deeply eosinophilic hyaline droplets may be noted in islands
- Usually solitary

Spiradenomas and cylindromas are closely related tumors. Both differentiate toward the secretory portion of the sweat gland. Hybrid tumors occur. Spiradenomas are usually sporadic and solitary, whereas cylindromas are multiple, inherited, and may occur together with trichoepitheliomas. Spiradenomas are inflamed (lymphocytes) and spontaneously tender.

Table 5.1 Characteristics of cylindroma versus spiradenoma

Characteristic	Cylindroma	Spiradenoma
Blue cells with little cytoplasm	Yes	Yes
Dark and pale blue nuclei	Yes	Yes
Peppered with black lymphocytes	No	Yes
Hyaline droplets in nests	Yes	Yes
Jigsaw-puzzle pattern	Yes	No
Deeply eosinophilic basement membrane	Yes	No
Inheritance	Autosomal dominant	Sporadic
Tender	No	Yes

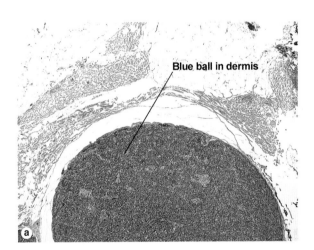

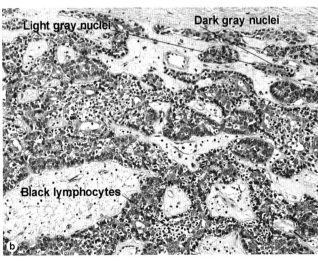

Fig. 5.2 Spiradenoma

PEARL

Tender tumors: BANGLE
- *B*lue rubber bleb nevus
- *A*ngiolipoma
- *N*euroma, neurilemmoma
- *G*lomus tumor
- *L*eiomyoma
- "*E*ccrine" spiradenoma

These tumors are probably tender because they have:
1. Smooth muscle that can contract to cause pain
2. Compressed nerve
3. Inflammation

Spiradenocarcinoma

Key Features

- Rare
- Occurs in long-standing spiradenomas
- Atypia, mitoses, and necrosis

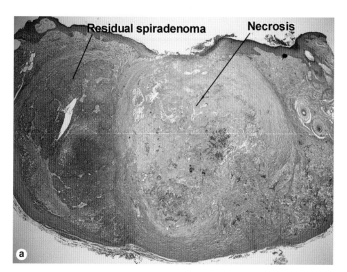

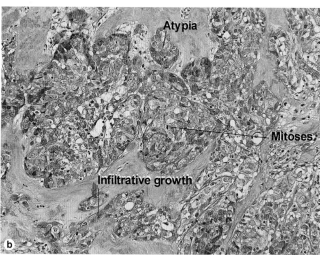

Fig. 5.3 Spiradenocarcinoma

Syringocystadenoma papilliferum

Key Features

- Opens to surface
- Blue papillary fronds extending upward into clear spaces: "fjords and fronds"
- Decapitation secretion
- Plasma cells

Syringocystadenoma papilliform (SPAP) differentiates toward the secretory portion of the sweat gland, and SPAP opens to the surface, which looks as though one could slide into it. Plasma cells are typically present in the mesenchymal core of each frond. Clinically, they appear as raised warty plaques on the head or neck. One third of cases occur within nevus sebaceus.

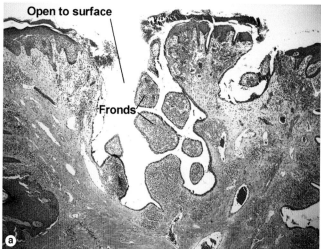

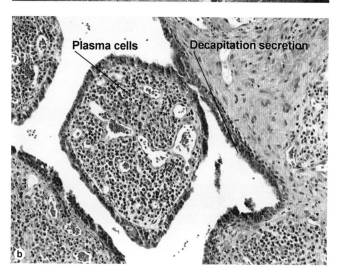

Fig. 5.4 Syringocystadenoma papilliferum

Hidradenoma papilliferum

Key Features

- Blue dermal nodule with branching cystic spaces
- Papillary fronds
- Decapitation secretion

Hidradenoma papilliferum (HPAP) usually presents clinically as a vulvar dermal nodule, but occasionally presents on a breast, eyelid, or ear. Histologically, *H*PAP is a mazelike dermal nodule, which looks as though one could *h*ide in it. The arborizing pattern of blue fronds demonstrates decapitation secretion. Like SPAP, it differentiates toward the secretory segment.

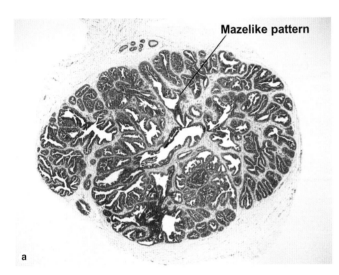

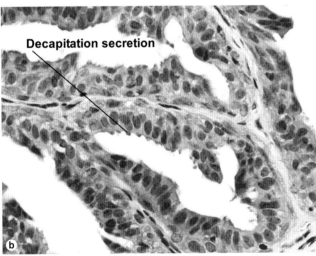

Fig. 5.5 Hidradenoma papilliferum

Papillary digital carcinoma (aggressive digital papillary adenocarcinoma)

Key Features

- Blue tumor nodules with cystic change
- Little to no visible cytoplasm
- Papillary fronds
- Atypia, mitoses, and necrosis variable
- Typically involves the hand
- Many patients are young
- Even bland tumors can metastasize

There can be significant histologic similarities to HPAP. All digital papillary tumors should be considered carcinomas.

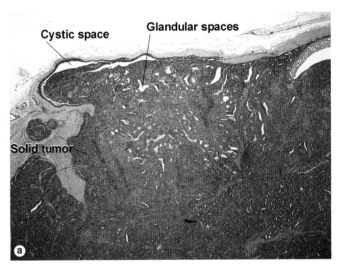

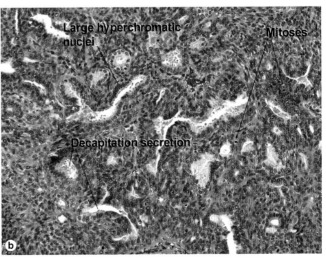

Fig. 5.6 Papillary digital carcinoma

Mucinous carcinoma

Key Features

- Islands of blue cells surrounded by mucin ("blue islands floating in a sea of snot")
- Primary cutaneous mucinous carcinoma and metastatic mucinous carcinoma look identical

Mucinous carcinoma can be primary in the skin or can be metastatic from a primary cancer of the breast or gastrointestinal tract. Imaging studies may be required

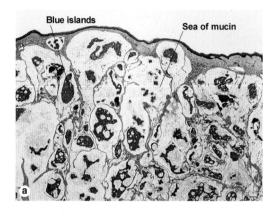

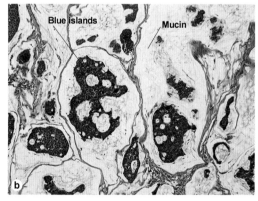

Fig. 5.7 Mucinous carcinoma

Syringoma

Key Features

- Paisley-tie pattern of tadpole-shaped ducts
- Ample pink cytoplasm
- Dense red sclerotic stroma
- Tumor is small and round

Syrinx refers to a pipe or duct. Syringomas usually appear as small papules on the eyelids. They are especially common in Asian women and in children with Down syndrome. Eruptive syringomas typically occur on the chest, back, or penis of a dark-skinned patient. Eruptive syringomas appear as small hyperpigmented papules with no tendency to coalesce.

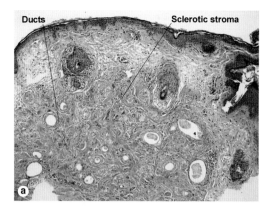

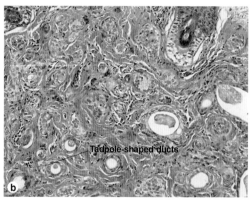

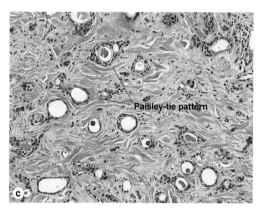

Fig. 5.8 Syringoma

Clear cell syringoma

Key Features

- Paisley-tie pattern of tadpole-shaped ducts
- Clear cells containing abundant glycogen
- Dense red sclerotic stroma
- Tumor is small and round
- Associated with diabetes mellitus

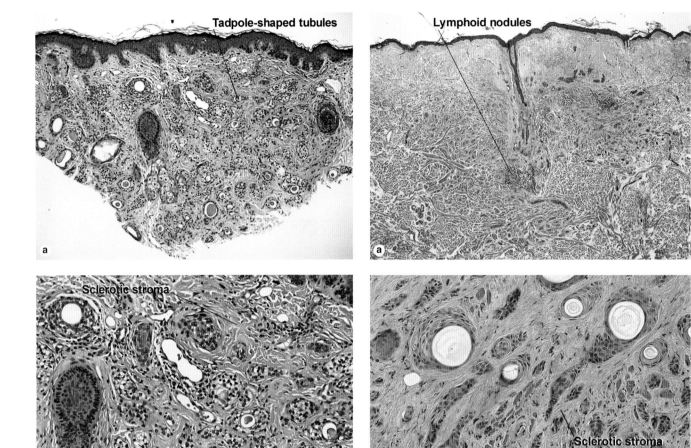

Fig. 5.9 Clear cell syringoma

Microcystic adnexal carcinoma

Key Features

- Biphasic pattern (sweat duct–like and pilar)
- Paisley-tie, tadpole-shaped ducts with ample pink cytoplasm and horn cysts
- Basaloid nests with pilar differentiation common
- Dense pink to red sclerotic stroma
- Deeply invasive
- Lymphoid aggregates
- Perineural extension

Microcystic adnexal carcinoma (MAC) typically presents as a firm plaque on the upper lip, medial cheek, or chin. Histologically, they have a paisley-tie appearance with dense red sclerotic stroma and must be differentiated from syringoma, morpheaform basal cell carcinoma, and desmoplastic trichoepithelioma.

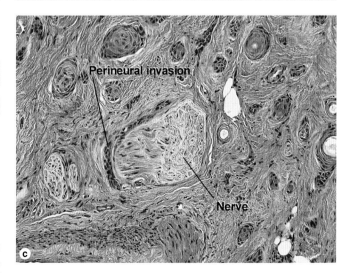

Fig. 5.10 Microcystic adnexal carcinoma

Table 5.2 Characteristics of microcystic adnexal carcinoma versus syringoma

Characteristic	Microcystic adnexal carcinoma	Syringoma
Paisley-tie pattern	Yes	Yes
Stroma	Red, sclerotic	Red, sclerotic
Horn cysts	Common	May occur
Size	Large	Small
Shape	Infiltrative	Round
Perineural extension	Yes	No
Basaloid islands	+/–	No
Clinical appearance	Plaque on upper lip, cheek, chin	Small papules on eyelids or eruptive papules

Table 5.3 Characteristics of microcystic adnexal carcinoma versus morpheaform basal cell carcinoma

Characteristic	Microcystic adnexal carcinoma	Morpheaform basal cell carcinoma
Paisley-tie pattern	Throughout tumor	Sometimes superficially
Stroma	Red, sclerotic	Red, sclerotic
Horn cysts	Common	Occasional
Deeply invasive	Yes	Yes
Perineural invasion	Yes	Yes
Clinical appearance	Plaque on upper lip, cheek, chin	Scarlike

Table 5.4 Characteristics of microcystic adnexal carcinoma versus desmoplastic trichoepithelioma

Characteristic	Microcystic adnexal carcinoma	Desmoplastic trichoepithelioma
Paisley-tie pattern	Yes	Yes
Stroma	Red, sclerotic	Red, sclerotic
Horn cysts	Common	Common
Calcification	Rare	Common
Lymphoid aggregates	Typical	Rare
Perineural extension	Yes	No
Central dell	No	Typical
Clinical appearance	Plaque on upper lip, cheek, chin	Firm doughnut

Sclerosing sweat duct carcinoma

Key Features

- Monophasic variant of MAC
- No pilar component
- Paisley-tie pattern of tadpole-shaped ducts with ample pink cytoplasm and horn cysts
- Dense pink to red sclerotic stroma
- Deeply invasive
- Lymphoid aggregates
- Perineural extension

Sclerosing sweat duct carcinoma has been described as the "syringoma from hell." Although small fields closely resemble syringoma,

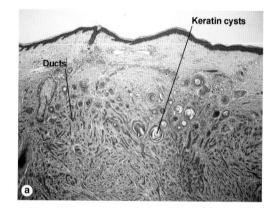

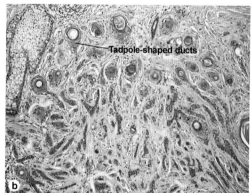

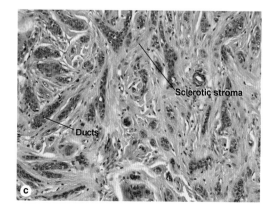

Fig. 5.11 Sclerosing sweat duct carcinoma

the tumor is deeply invasive and demonstrates perineural invasion. The clinical appearance is identical to that of a MAC. Perivascular nodular lymphoid aggregates are common in the tumor stroma.

Hidrocystoma

Key Features

- Simple cyst
- Lined by cuboidal or columnar cells
- Decapitation secretion may be noted

Hidrocystomas typically appear as bluish translucent papules on the cheeks or eyelids.

Endocrine mucin-producing sweat duct carcinoma of the eyelid

Key Features

- Arises within a hidrocystoma and progresses to mucinous carcinoma of the eyelid
- Solid to cystic nodule of round to oval cells with fine chromatin typical of neuroendocrine lesions
- Intracytoplasmic and extracellular mucin
- Positive for neuroendocrine markers such as synaptophysin and chromogranin
- Estrogen and progesterone receptor positive

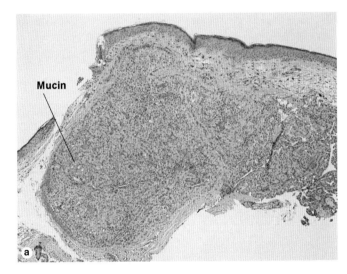

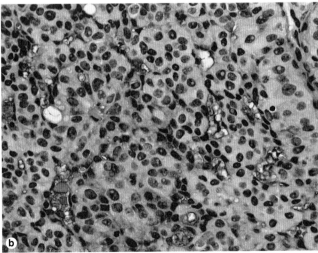

Fig. 5.13 Endocrine mucin-producing sweat duct carcinoma

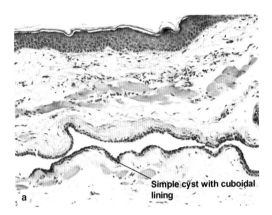

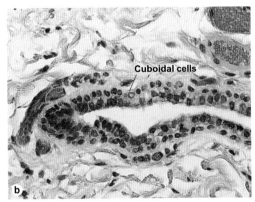

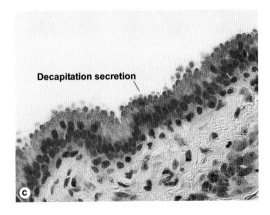

Fig. 5.12 Hidrocystoma

Mixed tumor (chondroid syringoma)

Key Features

- Sweat ducts with ample pink cytoplasm embedded in a mesenchymal stroma
- Secretory elements with blue nuclei and little cytoplasm may be present
- Cartilaginous differentiation common in stroma
- Bone formation may occur

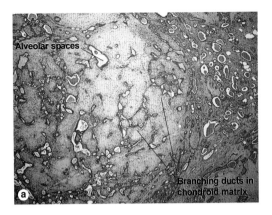

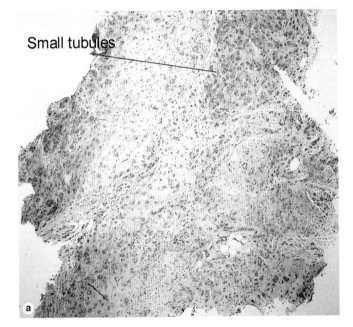

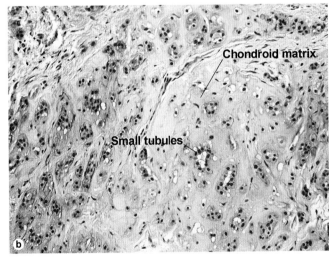

Fig. 5.14 Mixed tumor, small tubular type

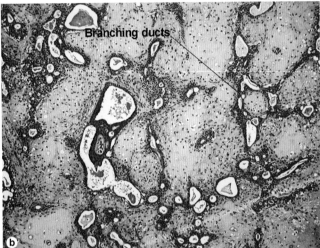

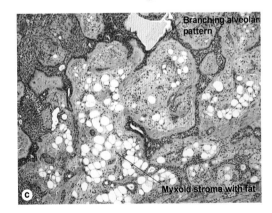

Fig. 5.15 Mixed tumor, branching alveolar type

Small tubular type

Key Features

- Sweat ducts with ample pink cytoplasm embedded in a mesenchymal stroma
- Cartilaginous differentiation common in stroma
- Small tubules resemble those of a syringoma

Branching alveolar type

Key Features

- Sweat ducts embedded in a mesenchymal stroma
- Cartilaginous differentiation common in stroma
- Tubules quite long, with a branching and alveolar pattern
- Decapitation secretion may be seen

Whereas the small tubular type of chondroid syringoma differentiates toward the sweat duct, the branching alveolar type shows differentiation toward both the secretory segment and duct. Mucin within the stroma is sulfated, giving it a deep gray-blue cartilaginous hue.

PEARL

Metachromatic stains for mucin include toluidine blue, methylene blue, and Giemsa (methylene blue plus eosin). Alcian blue and colloidal iron are not metachromatic stains. Chondroitin sulfate stains with Alcian blue and toluidine blue at both high and low pH.

Cutaneous myoepithelioma

Key Features

- Epithelioid, spindled, plasmacytoid, or clear cells in nests, cords, or sheets
- Hyalinized to chondromyxoid stroma
- No ducts

Myoepitheliomas are often considered in the spectrum with mixed tumor of the skin but lack ductal differentiation. Parachordomas belong to this spectrum but have more cytoplasmic vacuolization (physaliferous cells). Myoepithelioma has a propensity for the limbs of young adults. Expression of cytokeratin and/or EMA, as well as S100, is helpful in diagnosis. Calponin, SMA, and p63 may also be expressed. Malignant and benign tumors exist in this spectrum.

Malignant mixed tumor (malignant chondroid syringoma)

Key Features

- Similar to chondroid syringoma, but atypia, mitoses, and sometimes necrosis are noted

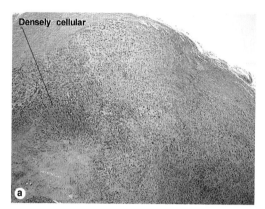
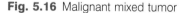
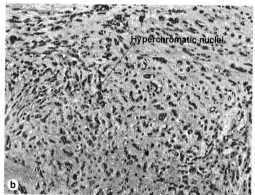

Fig. 5.16 Malignant mixed tumor

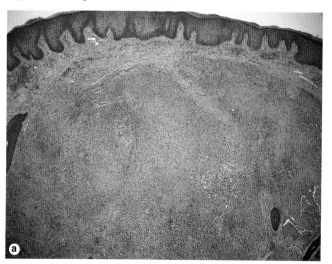
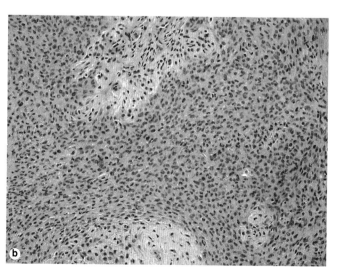

Fig. 5.17 Myoepithelioma

Acrospiromas

Key Features

- Differentiate toward the acrosyringium (the intraepidermal portion of the sweat duct)
- Cuboidal cells with ample pink cytoplasm
- Tendency toward clear cell degeneration

- Cuticle-lined ducts
- Pink sweat may be seen within ducts

Acrospiromas comprise a large family of sweat gland tumors that includes poromas, hidradenomas, dermal duct tumors, and hidroacanthoma simplex. They are all composed of cells that resemble those of the acrosyringium. They all demonstrate duct differentiation within tumor islands. Hybrid forms are common.

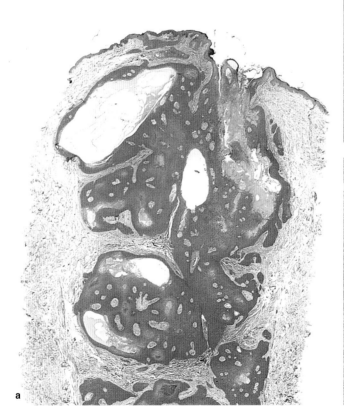

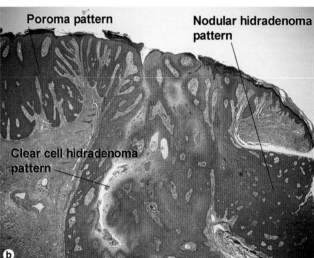

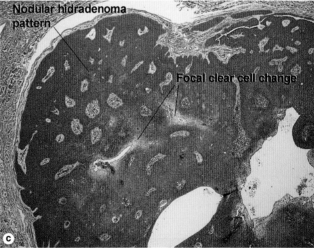

Fig. 5.18 Hybrid acrospiroma

Poroma

Key Features

- Cuboidal cells with ample pink cytoplasm
- Cuticle-lined ducts
- Connects with the epidermis
- Commonly found on the foot

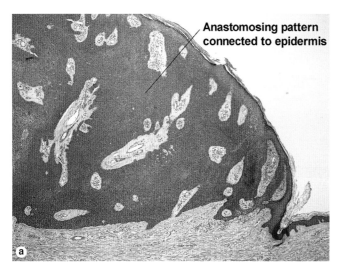

Anastomosing pattern connected to epidermis

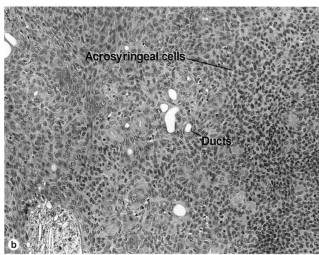

Acrosyringeal cells

Ducts

Fig. 5.19 Poroma

Hidroacanthoma simplex

Key Features

- Intraepidermal nests
- Cuboidal cells with ample pink cytoplasm
- Cuticle-lined ducts

Differential Diagnosis

Resembles clonal seborrheic keratosis, but contains ducts.

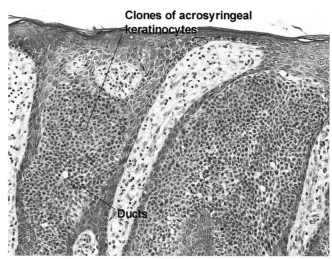

Clones of acrosyringeal keratinocytes

Ducts

Fig. 5.20 Hidroacanthoma simplex

Dermal duct tumor

Key Features

- Cuboidal cells with ample pink cytoplasm
- Cuticle-lined ducts
- Small dermal nodules

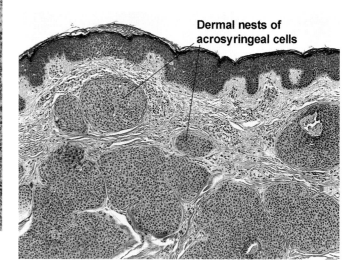

Dermal nests of acrosyringeal cells

Fig. 5.21 Dermal duct tumor

Nodular hidradenoma

Key Features

- Cuboidal cells with ample pink cytoplasm
- Cuticle-lined ducts
- Large dermal nodule
- Bright red zones of basement membrane zone reduplication commonly surround vessels

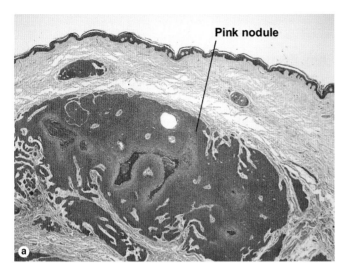

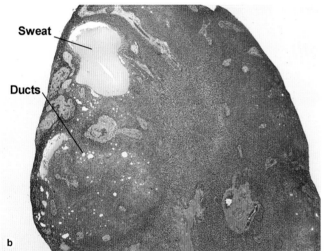

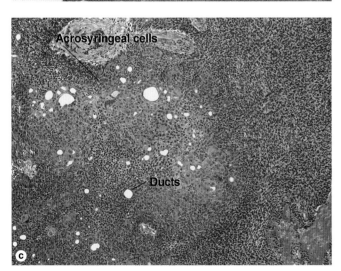

Fig. 5.22 Nodular hidradenoma

Clear cell hidradenoma

Key Features

- Cuboidal cells with ample pink cytoplasm
- Cuticle-lined ducts
- Large dermal nodule
- Clear cell degeneration
- Cystic degeneration common
- Bright red zones of basement membrane zone reduplication commonly surround vessels

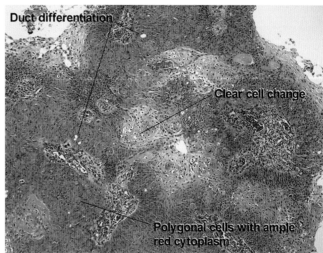

Fig. 5.23 Clear cell hidradenoma

Malignant acrospiroma (porocarcinoma, malignant poroma)

Key Features

- Invasive growth pattern
- Atypia, mitoses, and necrosis variable
- Some bland-appearing tumors metastasize

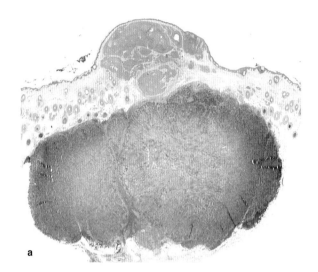

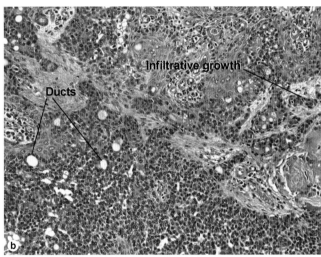

Fig. 5.24 Malignant acrospiroma (porocarcinoma)

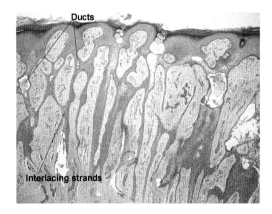

Fig. 5.25 Reactive syringofibroadenomatosis

Syringofibroadenoma of Mascaro

Key Features

- Most cases reactive; only a few are truly neoplastic
- Parallel or anastomosing ducts
- Fibromyxoid stroma

Most examples of syringofibroadenoma represent a reactive proliferation of eccrine ducts and would be better termed *reactive syringofibroadenomatosis*. Some cases have been associated with hidrotic ectodermal dysplasia and Schopf syndrome.

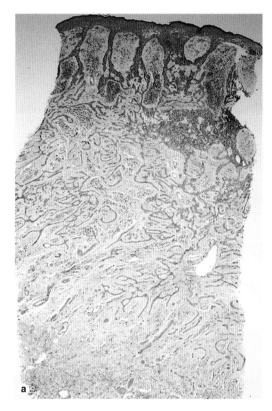

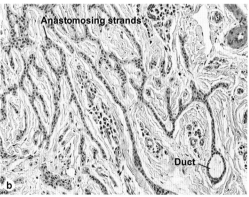

Fig. 5.26 Syringofibroadenoma of Mascaro, neoplastic type

Papillary "eccrine" adenoma (tubular apocrine adenoma)

Key Features

- No true distinction between papillary eccrine adenoma and tubular apocrine adenoma

- Differentiation toward both secretory segment and duct
- Dilated ductlike spaces
- Blue papillary projections into spaces variable

The variant called *papillary "eccrine" adenoma* is often found on the dorsal hand or foot of a black child. The tubular variant has a more varied presentation and may occur in the axilla, breast, cheek, or within a nevus sebaceus of Jadassohn.

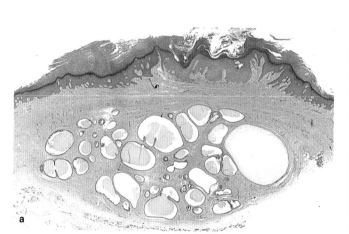

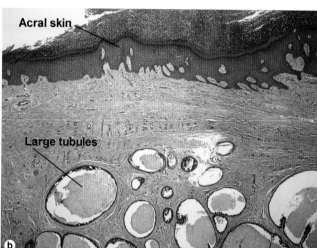

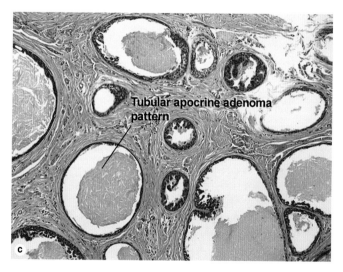

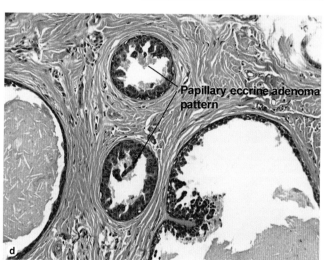

Fig. 5.27 Papillary "eccrine"/tubular apocrine adenoma

Adenoid cystic carcinoma

Key Features

- Sievelike (cribriform) appearance in some areas
- Tubular appearance in other areas
- Atypia and mitoses variable

Adenoid cystic carcinoma typically occurs in the vulva, breast, and salivary glands. Mucin is present in the cribriform areas, so the tumor has been likened to a pink sponge containing pale blue ink.

Differential Diagnosis

Trichoepithelioma is a blue tumor with a cribriform pattern. Adenoid cystic carcinoma is a red tumor with a cribriform pattern.

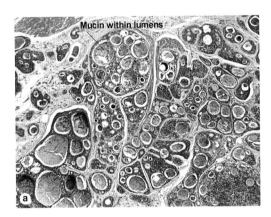

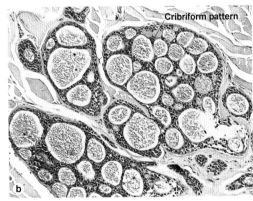

Fig. 5.28 Adenoid cystic carcinoma

Eccrine angiomatous hamartoma

Key Features

- Often present as tender, dusky nodules in children
- Mature sweat glands and vessels

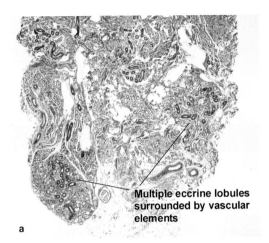

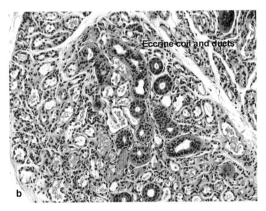

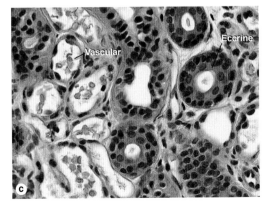

Fig. 5.29 Eccrine angiomatous hamartoma

Benign intraductal adenoma of the nipple

Key Features

- May present as erosive adenomatosis of the nipple
- Bland intraductal papillomatous neoplasm with preserved myoepithelial layer

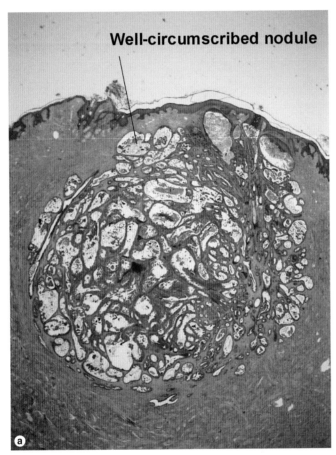

Well-circumscribed nodule

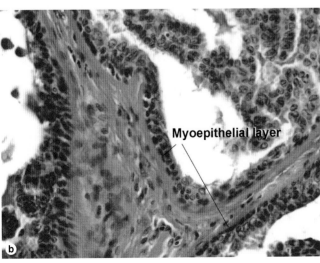

Myoepithelial layer

Fig. 5.30 Benign intraductal adenoma of the nipple

Supernumerary nipple (polythelia)

Key Features

- Subtle epidermal thickening with underlying pilosebaceous structures
- Surrounding scattered smooth muscle bundles typical of areola
- Central mammary duct may be visible

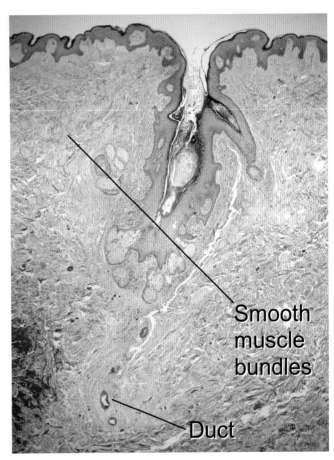

Smooth muscle bundles

Duct

Fig. 5.31 Supernumerary nipple

This developmental anomaly occurs anywhere along the embryonic milk line but has a predilection for the chest or upper abdomen. Histologically, polythelia resembles the normal nipple. Underlying breast tissue may be present.

Further reading

Ciarloni L, Frouin E, Bodin F, et al. Syringoma: a clinicopathological study of 244 cases. Ann Dermatol Venereol 2016;143(8–9):521–8.

Duke WH, Sherrod TT, Lupton GP. Aggressive digital papillary adenocarcinoma (aggressive digital papillary adenoma and adenocarcinoma revisited). Am J Surg Pathol 2000;24(6):775–84.

Fischer S, Breuninger H, Metzler G, et al. Microcystic adnexal carcinoma: an often misdiagnosed, locally aggressive growing skin tumor. J Craniofac Surg 2005;16(1):53–8.

Halachmi S, Lapidoth M. Approach to the rare eccrine tumors. Dermatol Surg 2011;37(8):1194–5.

Ishiko A, Shimizu H, Inamoto N, et al. Is tubular apocrine adenoma a distinct clinical entity? Am J Dermatopathol 1993;15(5):482–7.

Komine M, Hattori N, Tamaki K. Eccrine syringofibroadenoma (Mascaro): an immunohistochemical study. Am J Dermatopathol 2000;22(2):171–5.

Lago EH, Piñeiro-Maceira J, Ramos-e-Silva M, et al. Primary adenoid cystic carcinoma of the skin. Cutis 2011;87(5):237–9.

Mayo TT, Kole L, Elewski B. Eccrine poromatosis: case report, review of the literature, and treatment. Skin Appendage Disord 2015;1(2):95–8.

Melanocytic neoplasms

Dirk M. Elston

Solar lentigo

Key Features

- Thin rete with bulbous tips "dipped in chocolate"

Differential Diagnosis

Reticulated seborrheic keratosis looks similar to a lentigo but with anastomosis of rete and horn cysts.

Melanotic macule

Key Features

- Common on the lips and genitalia
- Rete are broad and squared-off with pigment at basal layer

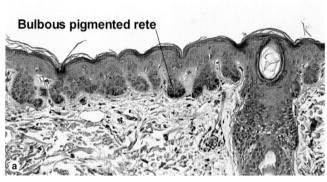

Bulbous pigmented rete

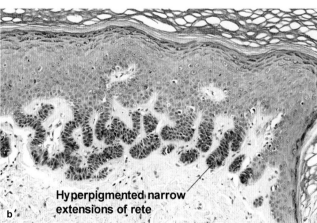

Hyperpigmented narrow extensions of rete

Fig. 6.1 Solar lentigo

Melanotic macules are typically light brown and evenly pigmented, but those in the genitalia may sometimes have strikingly irregular pigment. The histologic changes are the same, regardless of location and clinical appearance.

Benign melanocytic nevus

Key Features

- Sharply defined
- Well nested at the dermal–epidermal junction
- Round to oval nests at the tips and sides of rete ridges
- Matures[a]
- Disperses at the base of the lesion[a]
- No deep mitoses[a]
- No deep pigment in melanocytic nests[a]

[a]*These features are only present if there is a dermal component*

Benign nevi are bilaterally symmetrical from right to left, but they are asymmetrical from top to bottom. In contrast, melanoma metastases are radially symmetrical in all directions, like a cannonball.

A biopsy of a nevus demonstrates a discrete, well-nested melanocytic proliferation in the upper portion of the lesion. Melanocytes

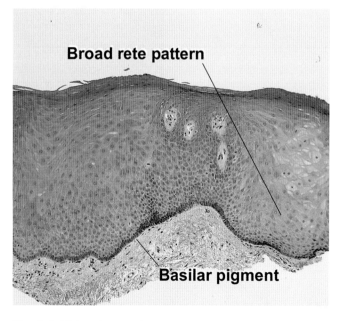

Broad rete pattern

Basilar pigment

Fig. 6.2 Melanotic macule

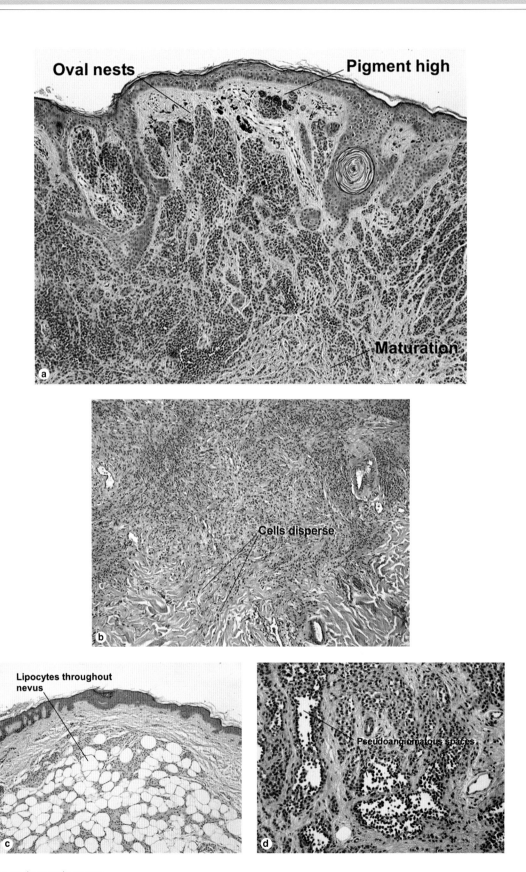

Fig. 6.3 Benign melanocytic nevus

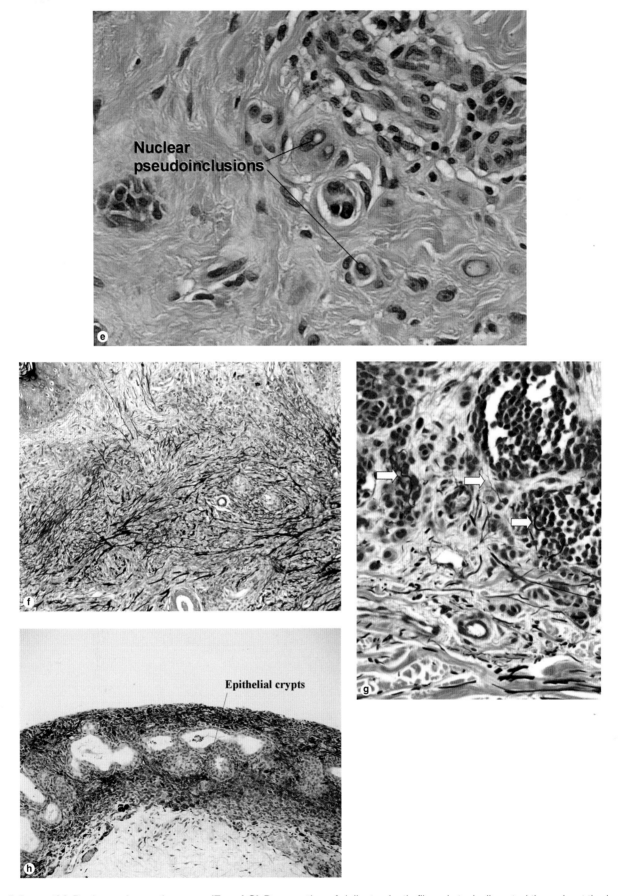

Fig. 6.3, cont'd Benign melanocytic nevus. **(F and G)** Preservation of delicate elastic fibers is typically noted throughout the lesion. See Fig. 6.29(J) for comparison with melanoma. **(H)** Conjunctival nevi characteristically demonstrate complex epithelial crypts. See Fig. 6.29(L) for comparison with conjunctival melanoma

disperse into individual units in the deeper portions of the lesion. Maturation refers to melanocytes becoming progressively smaller and spindled in the deeper portions of the lesion. Melanin should not be present in deep melanocytic nests, although melanophages may be present. In cases with questionable maturation, top-heavy HMB-45 immunostaining (loss of staining in the deep component) is a surrogate marker of maturation. Deep mitoses are absent. In unusual lesions, MIB-1 immunostaining is sometimes performed. MIB-1 is expressed in all active phases of the cell cycle—G1, M, G2, and S phase (but not resting G0)—and is not a mitotic marker. There should be no staining of deep melanocytic nuclei.

Table 6.1 gives general rules and is a good starting point for the evaluation of pigmented lesions. There are exceptions to the rules. For example, blue nevi show no evidence of maturation or dispersion. They are commonly deeply pigmented to the base of the lesion. They are readily recognized by their wedgelike or bulbous outline and characteristic cytologic features.

PEARLS

1. Broad junctional lesions on heavily sun-damaged skin are usually melanoma, regardless of how bland they appear.
2. Small, well-nested lesions are almost always benign.
3. Horn cysts can occur in the epidermis overlying melanocytic lesions. Horn cysts visible with dermoscopy are *not* diagnostic of seborrheic keratosis.
4. Epithelial crypts are common in conjunctival nevi.

Table 6.1 Characteristics of nevus versus melanoma

Characteristic	Nevus	Melanoma
Lateral circumscription	Sharp	Variable
Bilateral (right to left) symmetry	Yes	Commonly asymmetrical
Top to bottom symmetry	No	Variable
Size	Small	Usually quite broad
Dermal–epidermal junction	Well nested	Nonnested melanocytes usually outnumber nests in areas
Shape of junctional nests	Round to oval	Often elongated and bizarre
Location of junctional nests	Tips and sides of rete	Tops of dermal papillae often involved as well
Spacing of junctional nests	Regular	Usually irregular
Buckshot scatter in epidermis	Absent except in the center of Spitz nevi, pigmented spindle cell nevi, acral nevi, traumatized nevi, and sunburned nevi	Variable (present in superficial spreading malignant melanoma, usually not prominent in lentigo maligna and acral lentiginous malignant melanoma)
Maturation	Cells become smaller and more neuroid from top to bottom	Typically fails to mature
Dispersion	Disperses to single units at base of lesion	Generally remains nested at base
Junctional vs. dermal nests	Dermal nests smaller than junctional nests; from top to bottom, nests become smaller, melanocytes disperse	Dermal nests often larger than junctional nests
Deep mitoses	Rare	Variable
Deep pigment	No	Variable
HMB-45	Top heavy	Commonly stains strongly to base
MIB-1	No deep nuclei positive	Deep nuclei commonly positive
S100A6	Spitz nevi usually stain diffusely	Usually patchy

Balloon cell nevus

Key Features

- Balloon cells
- Sharply defined
- Well nested at the dermal–epidermal junction
- Matures
- Disperses at the base of the lesion
- No deep mitoses
- No deep pigment in melanocytic nests

Balloon change is a degenerative feature. Ultrastructurally, it is characterized by swelling of cellular organelles.

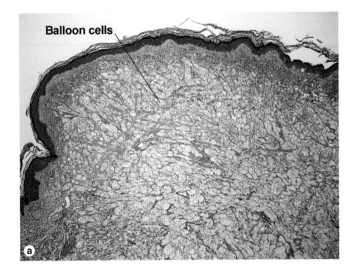

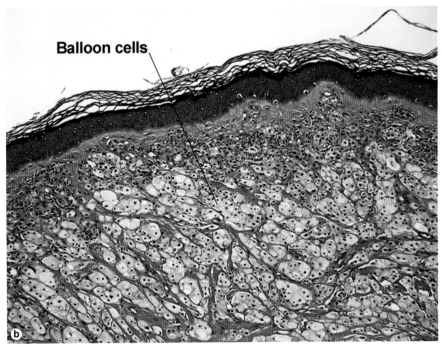

Fig. 6.4 Balloon cell nevus

"Neural" nevus

Key Features

- S-shaped spindle cells similar to those of a neurofibroma
- Nevic corpuscles resembling Meissner corpuscles
- Sharply defined
- Disperses at the base of the lesion
- No deep mitoses
- No deep pigment

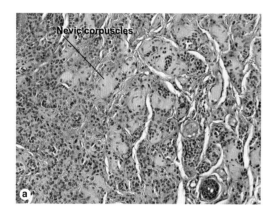

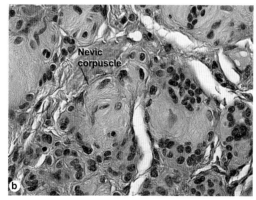

Fig. 6.5 Neural nevus

Congenital nevus

Key Features

- Broad
- Bland cytologically
- Matures
- Cells disperse at base
- Often within or aggregated about follicles, vessel walls, and nerves
- Patchy perivascular pattern
- Single-file interstitial pattern

A typical congenital nevus demonstrates a well-defined melanocytic proliferation with bland nuclei. The lesion is symmetrical from right to left, with a patchy perivascular, periadnexal, and interstitial pattern. Cells mature and disperse in the deeper portions of the lesion.

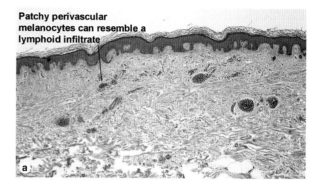

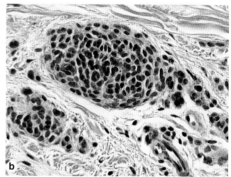

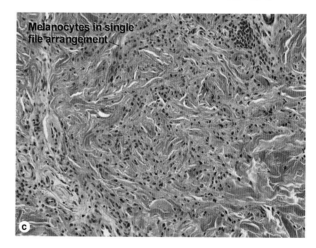

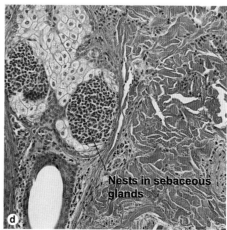

Fig. 6.6 Congenital nevus

Spitz nevus

Key Features

- Hyperkeratosis, hypergranulosis, pseudoepitheliomatous hyperplasia (PEH)[a]
- Well nested at the dermal–epidermal junction[a]
- Nests vertically oriented along rete ("raining-down pattern," "bananas on the tree")[a]
- Melanocytes within the nests share the vertical orientation[a]
- Clefts around nests[a]
- Kamino bodies[a]
- Large spindle and epithelioid cells
- Nuclei as large as or larger than keratinocyte nuclei
- Nuclei vesicular with prominent nucleoli
- Two-tone cytoplasm
- Sharply defined laterally
- Line symmetry from left to right
- Matures from top to bottom
- Disperses at the base of the lesion
- No deep mitoses
- No deep pigment in nests
- Buckshot scatter OK in center of lesion[a]
- These features are only present if there is a junctional component

[a]*These features are only seen if a dermal component is present.*

Benign spindle and epithelioid cell (Spitz) nevi occur in adults, but most commonly present as pink papules on the face or scalp of a child. Unfortunately, melanomas can demonstrate large spindle and epithelioid cells, hyperkeratosis, hypergranulosis, and pseudoepitheliomatous hyperplasia. These features are especially common among melanomas in the pediatric age group. Critical distinguishing features include sharp lateral circumscription, maturation, and dispersion, all of which should be present in benign Spitz nevi. Deep mitoses should be absent. Kamino bodies are dull pink areas of trapped basement membrane material within the epidermis. They stain blue to green with a trichrome stain and mark with immunostains for type IV collagen.

In lesions with any atypical feature, immunostaining is commonly performed. HMB-45 immunostaining should be top-heavy, and the lesion should stain diffusely for S100A6. MIB-1 staining should be absent in melanocyte nuclei at the base of the lesion.

Comparative genomic hybridization and chromosome deletion analysis by fluorescent in situ hybridization are promising techniques. The majority of Spitz nevi have a normal chromosome complement. Some large Spitz nevi have an 11p gain.

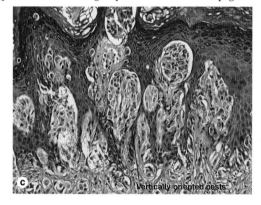

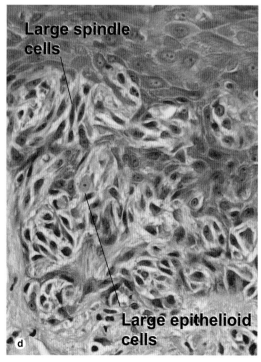

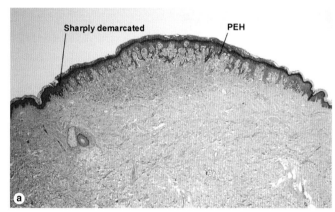

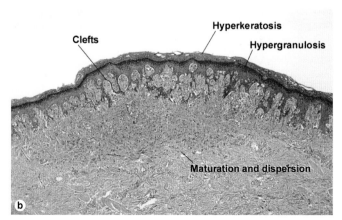

Fig. 6.7 Spitz nevus (*PEH,* pseudoepitheliomatous hyperplasia)

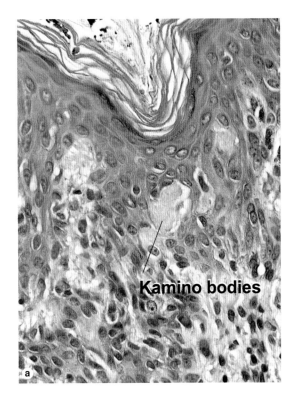

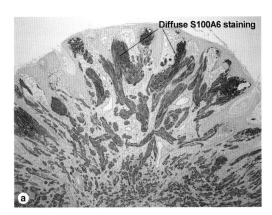

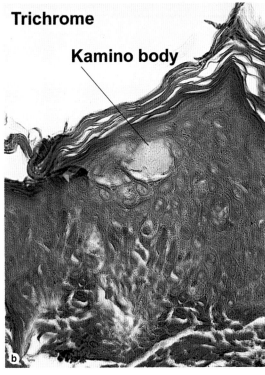

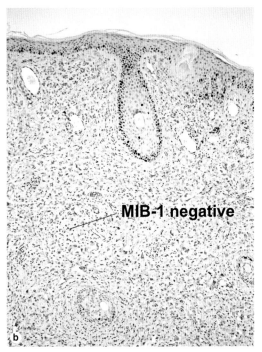

Fig. 6.8 Kamino body (trichrome stain)

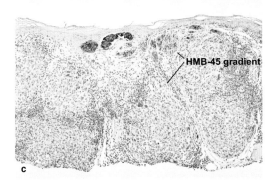

Fig. 6.9 Immunostaining pattern of Spitz nevus

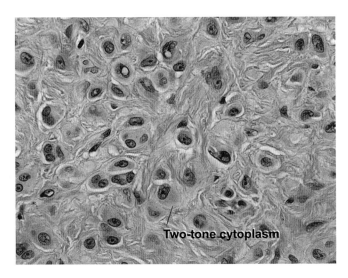

Fig. 6.10 Intradermal Spitz nevus

Pagetoid intraepidermal Spitz nevus

Key Features

- Buckshot intraepidermal scatter of large epithelioid melanocytes
- Hyperkeratosis variable
- Relatively small and very sharply circumscribed lesions of children and young adults
- Lack nuclear pleomorphism and hyperchromasia

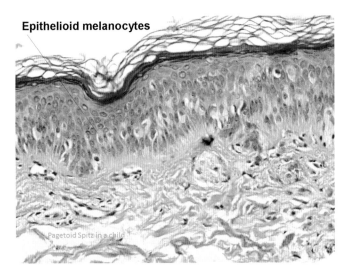

Fig. 6.11 Pagetoid intraepidermal Spitz nevus

Pigmented spindle cell nevus of Reed

Key Features

- Hyperkeratosis, hypergranulosis, pseudoepitheliomatous hyperplasia
- Well nested at the dermal–epidermal junction
- Clefts around nests variable
- Kamino bodies variable
- Small spindle cells
- Sharply defined
- Line symmetry from left to right
- Matures from top to bottom if compound
- Disperses at the base of the lesion if compound
- No deep mitoses
- No deep pigment in nests
- Buckshot scatter OK in center of lesion

Benign pigmented spindle cell nevus is considered by many to be a variant of Spitz nevus. They typically present as deeply pigmented macular lesions on the thighs or lower legs of young women. The spindled melanocytes are smaller than those in a Spitz nevus. Epithelioid cells are rare.

Table 6.2 Characteristics of Spitz nevus versus pigmented spindle cell nevus of Reed

Characteristic	Spitz nevus	Pigmented spindle cell nevus of Reed
Age	Children	Young women
Color	Usually pink	Usually dark brown
Location	Head	Legs
Hyperkeratosis, hypergranulosis, and pseudoepitheliomatous hyperplasia	Yes	Yes
Cytology	Large spindle and epithelioid cells	Small spindle cells
Kamino bodies	Common	Variable
Buckshot scatter in epidermis	Normal in center lesion	Normal in center lesion
S100A6	Strongly +	Weak and patchy

"Special site" nevus

Key Features

- Occur in the anogenital region, axillae, umbilicus, breast, scalp, ears
- One pattern resembles a dysplastic nevus
- Second pattern characterized by large junctional nests that appear poorly cohesive (white space surrounding each melanocyte)

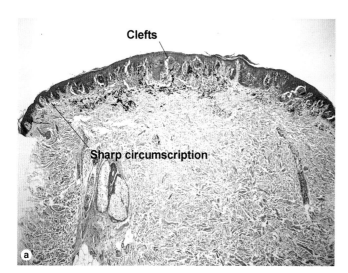

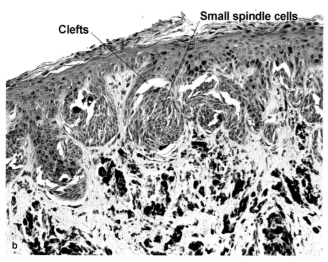

Fig. 6.12 Pigmented spindle cell nevus

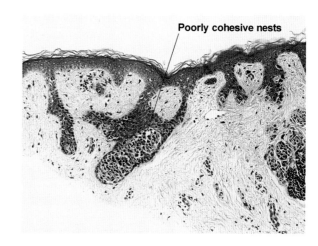

Fig. 6.13 Genital nevus

Acral nevus

Key Features

- On volar skin, nests are commonly elongated and follow dermatoglyphs
- Buckshot scatter OK in center of lesion
- Sharply defined
- Well nested at the dermal–epidermal junction
- Matures
- Disperses at the base of the lesion
- No deep mitoses
- No deep pigment in melanocytic nests

Within the central portion of an acral nevus, melanocytes are commonly noted above the dermal–epidermal junction. As long as it is confined to the center of the lesion, "buckshot scatter" by itself is not a worrisome feature in an acral nevus.

If volar nevi are bisected perpendicular to the dermatoglyphs, the nests will appear round. The rete pattern will be regular. If they are inappropriately sectioned parallel to the dermatoglyphs, the nests will appear long and confluent. The rete pattern may appear effaced in such sections. Oblique sections will give the appearance of irregular nesting and Swiss-cheese rete. It is important to communicate carefully with the laboratory when submitting a specimen from acral skin. Some clinicians prefer to bisect the specimen themselves, perpendicular to the dermatoglyphs.

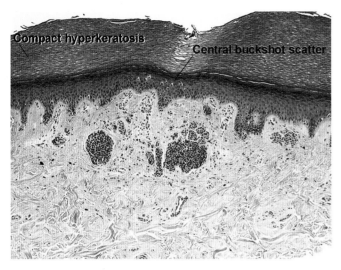

Fig. 6.14 Acral nevus

"Ancient" nevus

Key Features

- Large, hyperchromatic nuclei
- No confluent growth
- No expansile growth pattern
- No mitoses
- Sharply defined
- Well nested at the dermal–epidermal junction
- Matures
- Disperses at the base of the lesion
- No deep pigment in nests

The term *"ancient" atypia* has been applied to atypical nuclei in benign lesions. Mitoses, confluent growth, or an expansile growth pattern (nodule) should never be present.

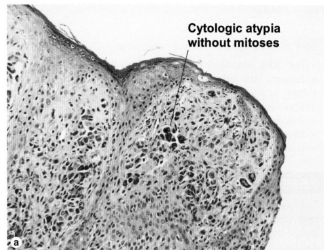

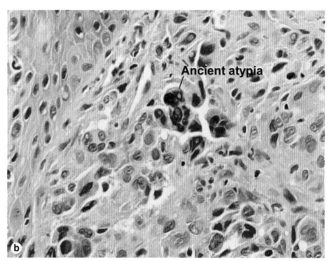

Fig. 6.15 Ancient nevus

Halo nevus

Key Features

- Bandlike lymphoid infiltrate through the lesion
- Sharply defined
- Well nested at the dermal–epidermal junction
- Matures
- Disperses at the base of the lesion
- No deep mitoses
- No deep pigment in nests (melanophages may be present)

PEARL

The pattern of the lymphoid infiltrate of a halo nevus resembles a cocktail party, with lymphocytes and melanocytes mingling together. In contrast, the pattern of the lymphoid infiltrate of a melanoma resembles a wall of riot police trying to hold back an angry mob (band of lymphocytes at the periphery of melanocytic nests).

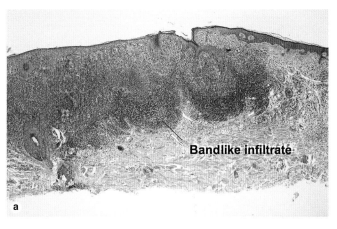

Bandlike infiltrate

a

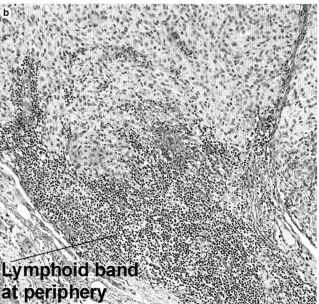

b

Lymphoid band at periphery

Fig. 6.17 Melanoma for comparison

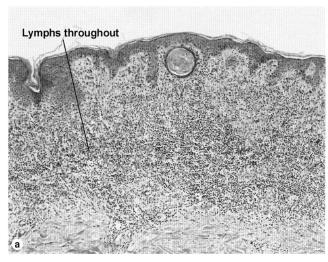

Lymphs throughout

a

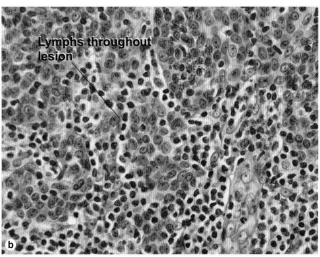

Lymphs throughout lesion

b

Fig. 6.16 Halo nevus

Blue nevus

Key Features

- Wedge or bulbous outline
- Pigment typically extends to base
- Melanocytes do not mature or disperse
- No deep mitoses
- No necrosis
- Typically has a distinctive sclerotic, red stroma
- Distinctive cytology

Variants of blue nevus are defined by the cytologic characteristics of the melanocytes. *Common blue nevi* are often seen on the dorsal hands and feet, face, and scalp. They are composed of dendritic melanocytes. *Cellular blue nevi* are commonly seen on the buttocks. They are composed of fusiform melanocytes with vesicular nuclei and prominent nucleoli. A closely related lesion referred to as an *epithelioid blue nevus* is associated with the Carney complex. It lacks the sclerotic stroma usually associated with blue nevi. *Deep penetrating nevi* are composed of melanocytes with small hyperchromatic nuclei, a smudged chromatin pattern, and inconspicuous nucleoli. Combined blue nevi are common. They include lesions with mixed features of different types of blue nevi, as well as lesions with components of blue and ordinary nevus. Dendritic "equine-type" melanomas are quite rare; they can be differentiated from blue nevi by the presence of nuclear atypia and the lack of sclerotic stroma.

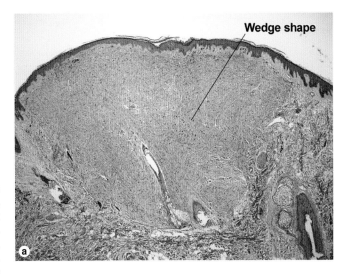

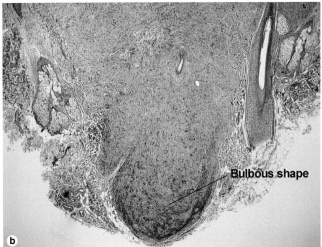

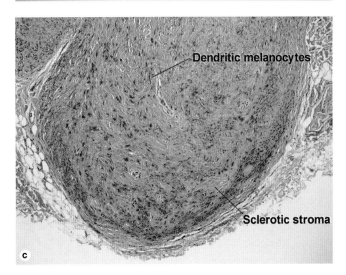

Fig. 6.18 Common blue nevus

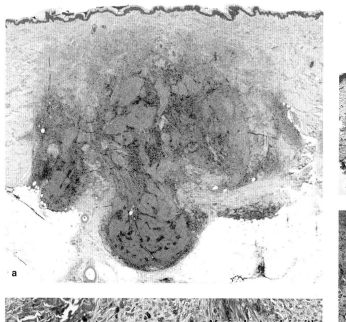

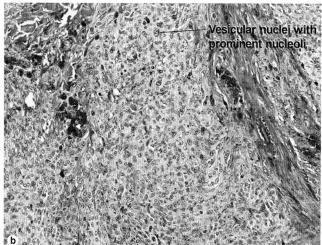

Fig. 6.19 Cellular blue nevus

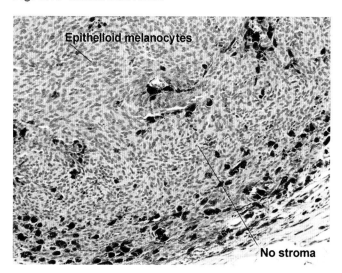

Fig. 6.20 Epithelioid blue nevus

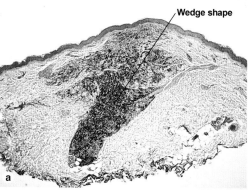

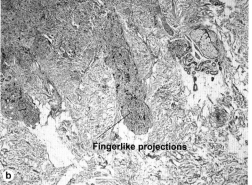

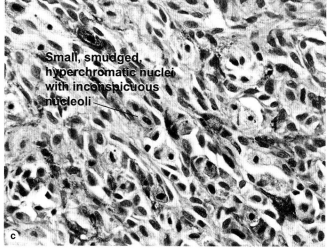

Fig. 6.21 Deep penetrating nevus

Combined nevus

Key Features

- Two or more populations of nevus cells

Combined nevi most commonly demonstrate a banal (ordinary) nevus component as well as a blue nevus component, but any variant of nevus can be represented within a combined nevus. Common combined nevus of Reed demonstrates "deep penetrating nevus" clones within a banal nevus.

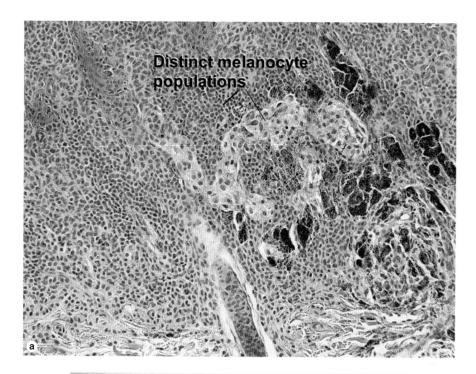

Distinct melanocyte populations

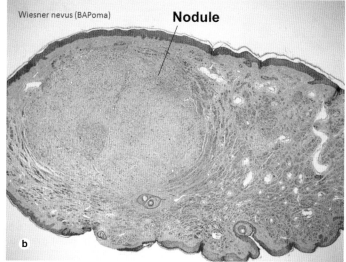

Wiesner nevus (BAPoma)

Nodule

Fig. 6.22 (A) Common combined nevus of Reed (deep penetrating nevus clones embedded within a banal nevus). **(B–E)** Wiesner nevus (BAP-1 mutated clone embedded within a banal nevus)

continued

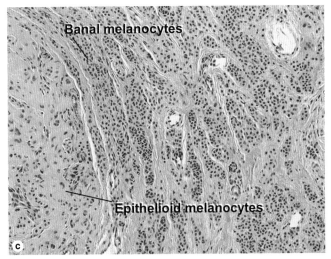

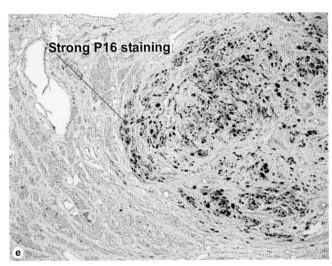

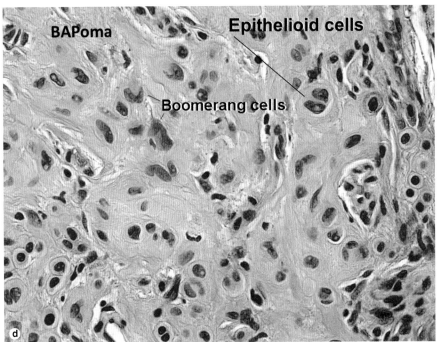

Fig. 6.22, cont'd

Wiesner nevus (benign BAPoma)

Key Features

- A unique type of combined nevus with a clone of epithelioid nevus cells embedded in a banal nevus
- Unlike Spitz nevi, the epithelioid population usually lacks vesicular nuclei, does not mature, and does not disperse at the base
- Some degree of hyperchromasia and pleomorphism is common and boomerang-shaped nuclei cells are frequently identified
- Occasional mitotic figures
- Low Ki-67 (MIB-1) proliferative fraction
- Retention of elastic fibers

- Strong expression of p16 and loss of BAP-1 within the clone
- Their behavior is benign, although they occur in families with uveal melanoma

Wiesner nevus (BAPoma) is associated with the familial uveal melanoma/renal carcinoma syndrome. The cutaneous nevi are unusual, but benign and malignant degeneration within a Wiesner nevus is rare. At scanning magnification, a dermal nodule of epithelioid melanocytes is present, typically surrounded by banal nevus. The epithelioid melanocytes differ from those of Spitz nevi by their lack of vesicular nuclei and less prominent nucleoli, as well as lack of maturation and dispersion. Unlike Spitz nevi, they do not demonstrate an HMB-45 staining gradient, but do demonstrate loss of BAP-1 staining, strong p16 staining, a low

MIB-1 fraction, and retention of elastic fibers within the clonal population. Loss of p16 staining may be evidence of progression to malignancy.

BAP-1 mutation on a background of BRAF mutation appears to produce a benign Wiesner nevus, whereas BAP-1 mutation on a background of GNAQ or GNA11 mutation produces uveal melanoma and blue nevus–like melanoma. Loss of both 9p21 and its protein product p16 is associated with malignant progression of a Wiesner nevus, whereas loss of 9p21 is not required for malignant behavior of a blue nevus-like melanoma.

Benign Clark nevus (dysplastic nevus)

Key Features

- Commonly large, oval, and multiple
- Irregular pigment common
- Fading border or fried-egg appearance clinically (central papule, surrounding macule)
- Fading macular border corresponds to the "shoulder" region
- Junctional component extends at least three retia beyond the intradermal component
- Club-shaped hyperplasia of the rete
- Horizontally oriented nests with bridging of adjacent rete
- Nests are at tips and sides of rete
- Concentric papillary dermal fibrosis
- Large oval melanocytes, especially in shoulder region
- Well nested at the dermal–epidermal junction
- Matures
- Disperses at the base of the lesion, except in some old fibrotic lesions
- No deep mitoses
- No deep pigment in nests

Dysplastic nevi occur in patients with the B-K mole/melanoma syndrome (dysplastic nevus syndrome) as well as sporadically. Any growing mole will have some features in common with a dysplastic nevus. "Special site" nevi can be indistinguishable from dysplastic nevi. Some refer to these as "atypical" nevi.

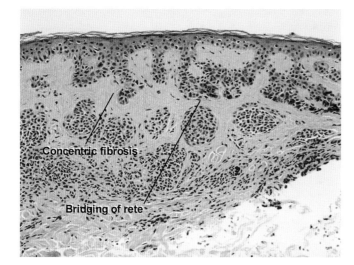

Fig. 6.23 Dysplastic nevus

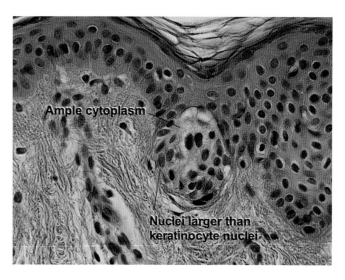

Fig. 6.24 Atypia in the shoulder region of a dysplastic nevus

Grading dysplastic nevi

- Low-grade: atypia restricted to shoulder region
- Moderate: atypia in both shoulder region and central portion, some irregularity and confluence of nests
- High-grade: high-grade cytologic atypia in areas, not entirely well nested at junction, irregular nests, may be marginal in distinction from malignant melanoma in situ

Some have questioned the significance of grading of dysplastic nevi. Others prefer to divide them into high-grade and low-grade lesions.

Management

The management of dysplastic nevi is controversial. Most of the atypical cells are found in the shoulder region at the lateral edges of the specimen. The shoulder extends beyond the clinically apparent edge of the specimen. A broad saucerization that includes a 0.5-mm margin of normal-appearing skin will provide the pathologist with the entire lesion, including the entire shoulder region, and reduce the likelihood of a positive margin.

In the author's opinion (DME), high-grade lesions are best managed like malignant melanoma in situ. The risk of melanoma arising in a lesion with low-grade or moderate atypia is low, but grading of moderate nevi is variable, and one pathologist's moderate dysplastic nevus could be another's melanoma. *My own practice when faced with a positive margin is to leave benign low-grade Clark nevi alone unless a lesion recurs clinically at the site. I perform a broader shave for lesions with moderate atypia and a positive margin and excise high-grade lesions.*

Junctional lentiginous nevus

Key Features

- Club-shaped epidermal hyperplasia
- Round to oval melanocytic nests at the dermal–epidermal junction
- Nests restricted to the tips and sides of rete

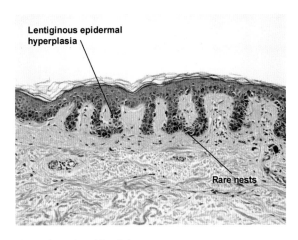

Fig. 6.25 Junctional lentiginous nevus

Recurrent nevus (persistent nevus, pseudomelanoma)

Key Features

- Confluent, poorly nested, or irregularly nested junctional melanocytic proliferation
- Underlying scar
- Melanocytic proliferation confined to the area overlying the scar
- May see residual bland nevus under scar

Recurrent nevi may simulate melanoma. History is critical, and review of the prior biopsy material may be necessary.

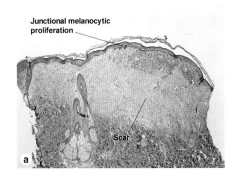

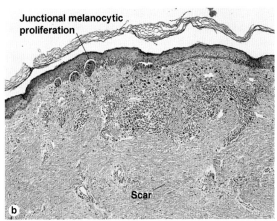

Fig. 6.26 Recurrent nevus

Nevus of Ota/nevus of Ito

Key Features

- Dendritic melanocytes scattered between collagen bundles in the upper third of the dermis
- Melanocytes oriented east to west
- No sclerotic stroma

A biopsy will demonstrate a subtle band of dendritic melanocytes in the upper dermis. There is no associated sclerotic stroma. Clinically, they present as deep blue patches on the face (Ota) or shoulder (Ito).

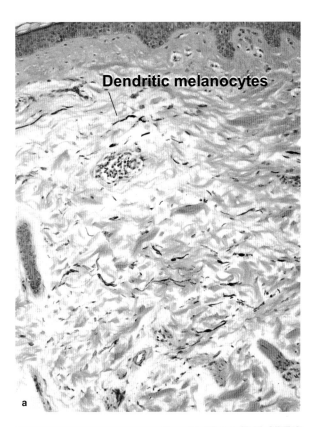

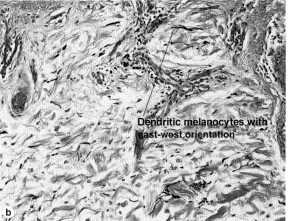

Fig. 6.27 Nevus of Ota

Mongolian spot

Key Features

- Dendritic melanocytes scattered between collagen bundles in the lower half of the dermis
- Melanocytes oriented east to west
- No sclerotic stroma

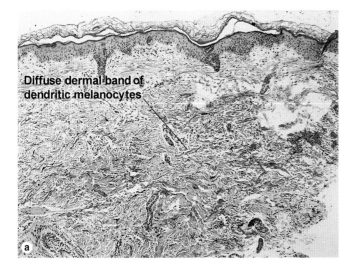

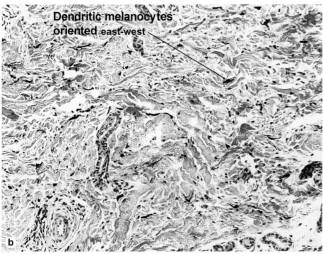

Fig. 6.28 Mongolian spot

Malignant melanoma

Key Features

- Usually are broad and asymmetrical
- Poorly nested epidermal melanocytes
- Irregularly spaced, irregularly shaped nests not just at tips and sides of rete
- Areas of confluence
- May show adnexal extension
- Lack of maturation and dispersion
- May have deep mitoses and deep pigment in nests
- Atypia is variable

PEARLS

1. Compared with nevi, melanomas are more likely to demonstrate multiple nucleoli, peripheral nucleoli, a clumped "peppered moth" chromatin pattern, solid hyperchromasia, nuclear molding or a round nucleus adjacent to a flattened nucleus, epidermal consumption, a parallel theque pattern at the base of the lesion, and atypical mitoses.
2. Pigment within the stratum corneum overlying a benign volar nevus typically forms columns over the dermatoglyph furrows. In contrast, the pigment within the stratum corneum present overlying a volar melanoma is more diffuse and is overpresent overlying the dermatoglyph ridges, which correspond to the arches between rete ridges. The rhyme "ridges are risky; furrows are fine" has been used in dermoscopy, but also applies to histopathology.
3. On volar skin, the presence of hyperchromatic, angulated melanocytes with irregular dendrites, no matter how few in number, suggests a diagnosis of acral melanoma.
4. Nevi tend to involve the tips and sides of rete ridges, whereas melanoma often involves the arches. Melanoma is your "arch" enemy.
5. Conjunctival melanomas are typically broad, with a flattened epithelium and junctional confluence of atypical melanocytes. Pagetoid scatter may occur. Benign conjunctival nevi differ by sharp circumscription, lack of atypia, and lack of elastosis. They often exhibit hyperplasia of the epithelium with prominent crypts.
6. In lentiginous types of melanoma, the atypical melanocytes within the epidermis proliferate predominantly at the dermal–epidermal junction, with little to no buckshot scatter.
7. The vertical growth phase is an expansile dermal nodule. It typically invades the reticular dermis (into the zone of bundled collagen or solar elastosis) or appears as a dermal nest larger than the largest junctional nest. Mitoses or necrosis may be noted in the nodule. The vertical growth phase may have different cytologic features from the radial growth phase. Metastases typically resemble the vertical growth phase cytologically.
8. Measure the depth of invasion from the granular layer, the base of an ulcer, or the inner root sheath (if invading outward from a follicle).
9. Clark levels are no longer included in standard staging, but are included here for historical context:
   I. Confined to the epidermis (in situ melanoma)
   II. Into the papillary dermis
   III. To the papillary dermis–reticular dermis interface
   IV. Into the reticular dermis
   V. Into the subcutaneous fat

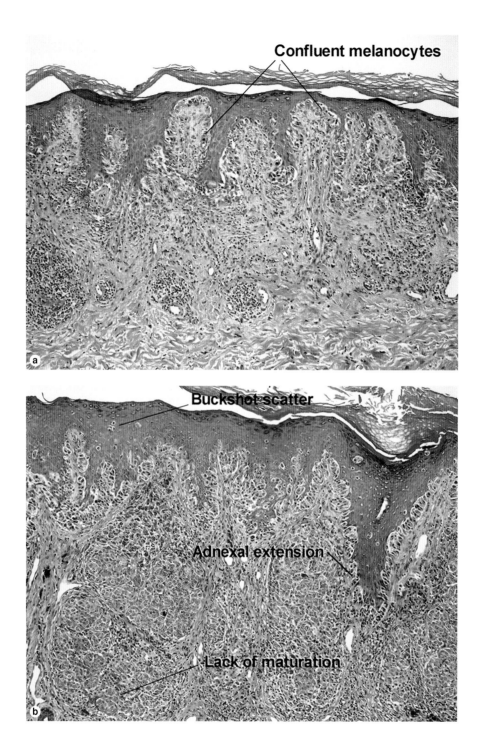

Fig. 6.29 Malignant melanoma

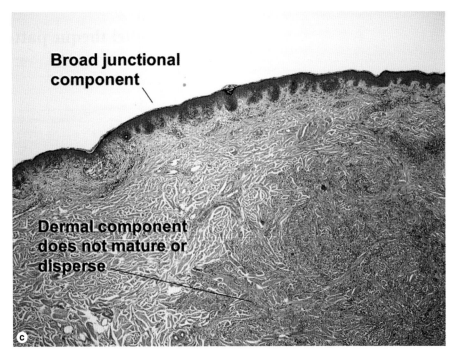

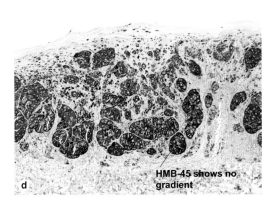

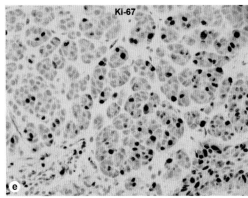

Fig. 6.29, cont'd

continued

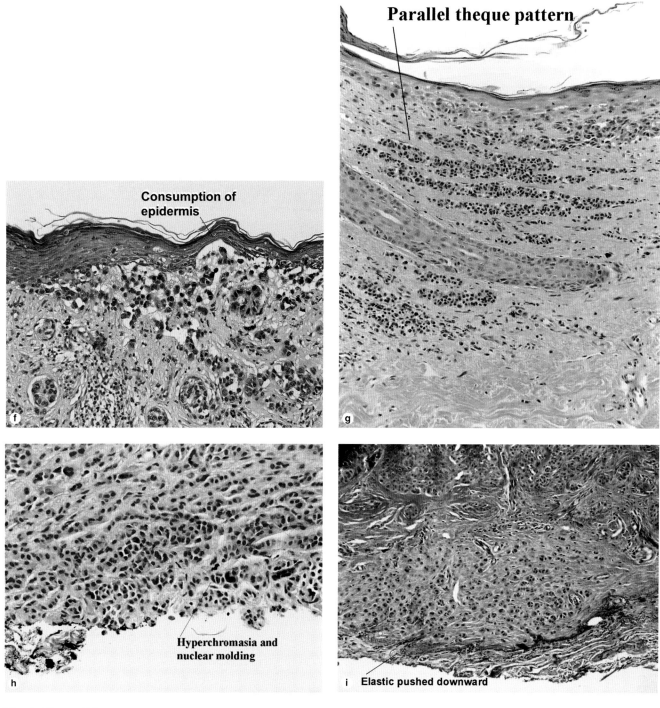

Parallel theque pattern

Consumption of epidermis

Hyperchromasia and nuclear molding

Elastic pushed downward

Fig. 6.29, cont'd

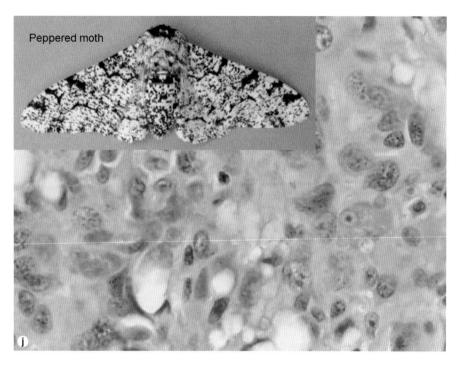

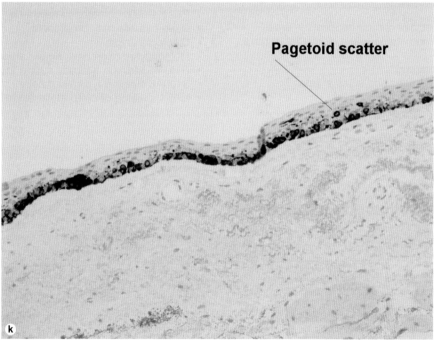

Fig. 6.29, cont'd Malignant melanoma. Confluent melanocytes involving the arches between rete. **(J)** Elastic tissue is displaced downward (snowplow effect). **(K)** Peppered moth chromatin pattern characteristic of advanced melanoma. (Image of peppered moth courtesy of David Tomlinson, Professor Emeritus, Faculty of Life Sciences, University of Manchester)

Table 6.3 Distinguishing features of melanomas

Type of melanoma	Distinguishing features	Type of melanoma	Distinguishing features
Superficial spreading melanoma	Radial growth phase characterized by buckshot scatter in epidermis	Acral lentiginous melanoma	Poorly nested and confluent melanocytes at the dermal–epidermal junction
Nodular melanoma	Lacks radial growth phase	Desmoplastic melanoma	Commonly arises in subtle in situ lesions of a lentiginous type
Lentigo maligna	Malignant melanoma in situ		Desmoplastic stroma
	Poorly nested and confluent melanocytes at the dermal–epidermal junction		Spindle cells with variable atypia
			Nodular lymphoid aggregates
	Adnexal extension	Mucosal melanoma	Oral, genital, or conjunctival mucosa
	Heavily sun-damaged skin		
Lentigo maligna melanoma	Lentigo maligna with vertical growth phase		Often has a lentiginous growth pattern

Superficial spreading malignant melanoma

Key Features

- Broad lesion
- Buckshot scatter of atypical melanocytes within the epidermis
- Nonnested melanocytes outnumber nests in areas
- Nests vary in size and shape (often elongated, bizarre, or confluent)
- Nests not evenly spaced
- Nests not confined to tips and sides of rete
- Typically not symmetrical (right to left)

- Typically fails to mature from top to bottom
- Typically fails to disperse at base
- Dermal nests often larger than junctional nests
- Deep pigment may be present within melanocytic nests
- Lymphoid infiltrate frequent at base, walling off lesion ("riot police")
- Plasma cells common in infiltrate
- Deep mitoses may be present
- Cytologic atypia
- Melanocytes often have ample amphophilic cytoplasm
- HMB-45 staining typically strong to base
- S100A6 staining typically patchy
- MIB-1 staining of deep melanocyte nuclei common

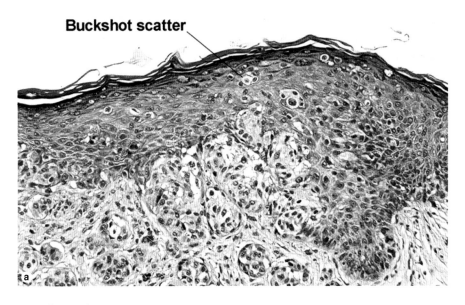

Buckshot scatter

Fig. 6.30 Superficial spreading melanoma

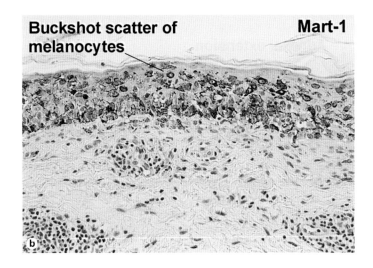

Fig. 6.30, cont'd

Lentigo maligna

Key Features

- Broad lesion on sun-damaged skin
- Rete ridge pattern commonly effaced
- Predominantly junctional growth of atypical melanocytes
- Multinucleated giant cells (starburst giant cells) may be seen at dermal–epidermal junction (DEJ)
- Nonnested melanocytes usually outnumber nests in areas
- Nests vary in size and shape (often elongated, bizarre, or confluent)
- Nests not evenly spaced
- Extends down adnexal structures
- Nests not confined to tips and sides of rete
- Often lacks sharp lateral circumscription
- Often not symmetrical (right to left)
- Cytologic atypia

Lentigo maligna typically exhibits asymmetrical growth. Because the atypical melanocytes are only one cell thick at the DEJ, the lateral borders are poorly defined clinically. The lesion often extends far beyond the clinically apparent margin.

PEARLS

1. Small biopsies are likely to result in misdiagnosis. Skip areas are common. Lichenoid regression can mimic a lichenoid actinic keratosis or benign lichenoid keratosis. Benign pigmented lesions (pigmented actinic keratosis and solar lentigo) occur in collision with lentigo maligna in about half of all cases. Small biopsies may sample only the benign lesion. The false-negative rate of a small biopsy is up to 80%. The best biopsy technique for a large macular facial lesion may be a broad thin shave, or multiple small shave biopsies, to sample every color within the lesion.
2. Although effacement of the rete is typical, lentiginous epidermal hyperplasia may occur, and lentigo maligna may closely resemble a junctional lentiginous nevus or junctional dysplastic nevus. A broad junctional lesion on sun-damaged skin is probably melanoma in situ.

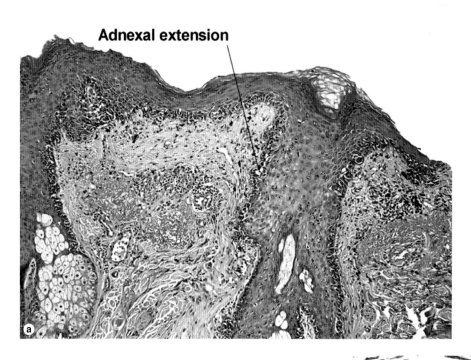

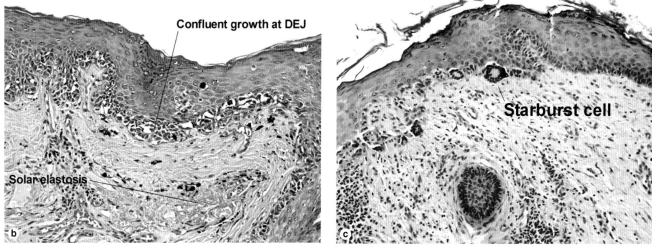

Fig. 6.31 Lentigo maligna (*DEJ,* dermal–epidermal junction)

Lentigo maligna melanoma

Key Features

- Lentigo maligna with a vertical growth phase
- Vertical growth phase may be epithelioid, spindled, or desmoplastic

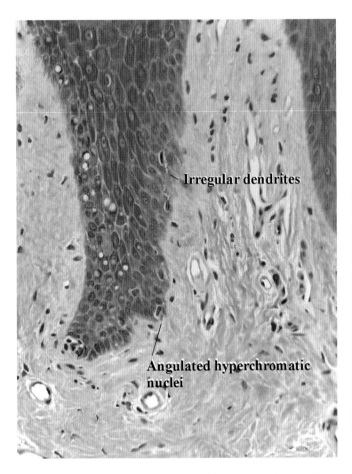

Fig. 6.32 Acral lentiginous melanoma: Hyperchromatic, angulated dendritic melanocytes on acral sites are highly suspicious for acral lentiginous melanoma. They often fail to exhibit a confluent growth pattern, so the diagnosis can be easily missed

Spindle cell melanoma

Key Features

- Spindled cytology
- Most reliable immunostains are S100 and SOX10

Differential Diagnosis

Spindled melanomas can closely resemble other spindle cell neoplasms. The microscopic differential diagnosis for an atypical spindle cell tumor *SLAM*med up against the epidermis includes:

- *S*quamous cell carcinoma (keratin positive)
- *L*eiomyosarcoma (smooth muscle actin positive, desmin positive)
- *A*typical fibroxanthoma (diagnosis of exclusion)
- *M*elanoma (S100 positive)

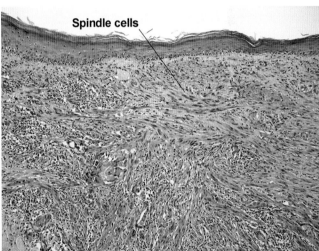

Fig. 6.33 Spindle cell melanoma

Desmoplastic melanoma

Key Features

- Dense desmoplastic stroma
- Nodular lymphoid aggregates

- May see a subtle overlying lentigo maligna
- S100 and SOX10 are generally reliable, but other immunostains like HMB-45 are unreliable in desmoplastic melanoma
- Atypia of spindle cells is variable
- Perineural extension common

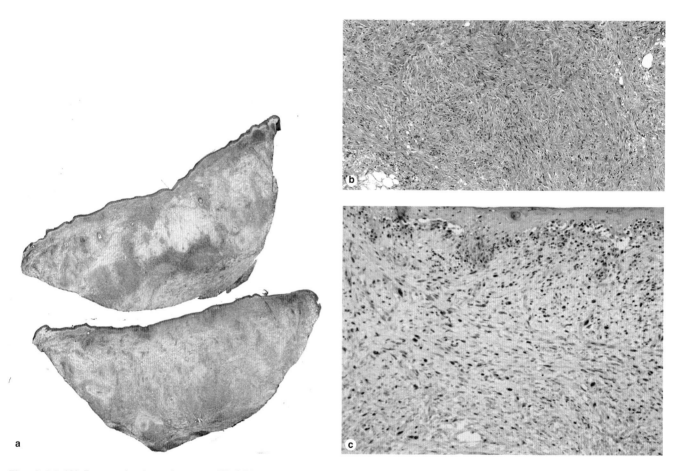

Fig. 6.34 (A) Desmoplastic melanoma. **(C)** SOX-10 staining of desmoplastic melanoma

Nodular melanoma

Key Features

- No apparent radial growth phase
- May be symmetrical in all directions
- Typically fails to mature from top to bottom
- Typically fails to disperse at base
- Deep pigment may be present in melanocytic nests

- Lymphoid infiltrate frequent at base, walling off lesion ("riot police")
- Plasma cells commonly present in infiltrate
- Deep mitoses may be present
- Cytologic atypia
- Necrosis
- HMB-45 staining typically strong to base
- S100A6 staining typically patchy
- MIB-1 staining of deep melanocyte nuclei common

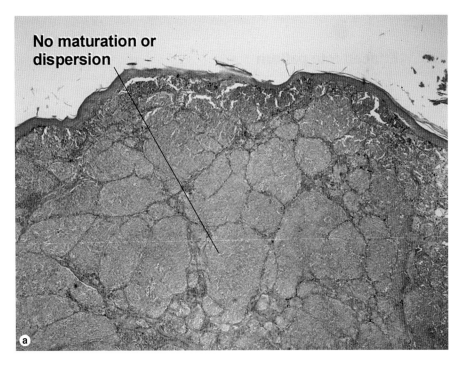

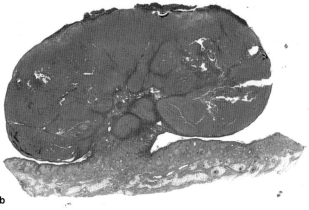

Fig. 6.35 Nodular melanoma

Regressing melanoma

- Lichenoid regression may occur in lentigo maligna
- Regression in other melanomas is probably secondary to genomic instability rather than inflammatory response
- May appear as zones of fibrosis and melanophages
- Adverse prognostic indicator
- "Tumoral melanosis" may be regressed melanoma

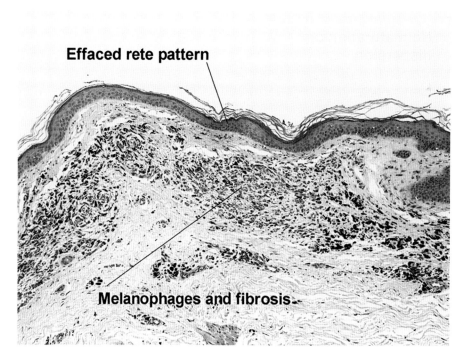

Effaced rete pattern

Melanophages and fibrosis

Fig. 6.36 Regressing melanoma

Metastatic melanoma

Key Features

- May be a radially symmetrical "cannonball"
- May be epidermotropic and nevoid
- Atypical cells may be noted in lymphatic vessels
- Cytologic atypia may be marked
- Mitoses common
- Necrosis common

- MIB-1 positivity common
- HMB-45 positive to base, or may be patchy or negative

Epidermotropic nevoid metastases typically fail to mature or disperse well at the base. This helps to distinguish them from nevi. In lymph nodes, metastatic melanoma is typically subcapsular in location. Nodal nevi occur, but are typically located within the capsule and are composed of bland nuclei.

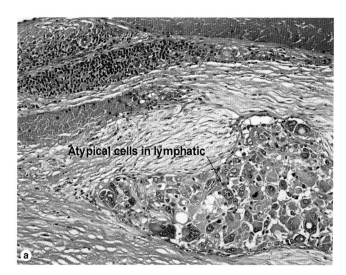

Atypical cells in lymphatic

a

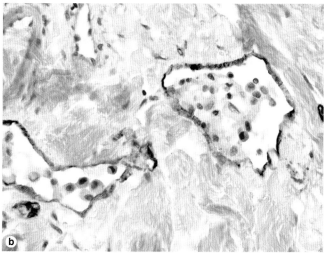

b

Fig. 6.37 Metastatic melanoma (part B demonstrates D2-40 staining confirming the presence of intralymphatic melanoma)

Clear cell sarcoma

Key Features

- Soft tissue tumor
- Clear cytoplasm
- Nuclear atypia
- S100 positive

Clear cell sarcoma is regarded by some as a form of primary soft tissue clear cell melanoma. The tumor is also defined by a characteristic chromosome translocation t(12;22)(q13;q12).

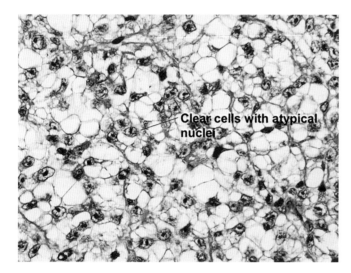

Fig. 6.38 Clear cell sarcoma

Further reading

Bauer J, Bastian BC. Distinguishing melanocytic nevi from melanoma by DNA copy number changes: comparative genomic hybridization as a research and diagnostic tool. Dermatol Ther 2006;19(1):40–9.

Boyd AS, Rapini RP. Acral melanocytic neoplasms: a histologic analysis of 158 lesions. J Am Acad Dermatol 1994;31(5 Pt 1):740–5.

Cerroni L. A new perspective for spitz tumors? Am J Dermatopathol 2005;27(4):366–7.

Cesinaro AM. Clinico-pathological impact of fibroplasia in melanocytic nevi: a critical revision of 209 cases. APMIS 2012;120(8):658–65.

Dalton SR, Gardner TL, Libow LF, et al. Contiguous lesions in lentigo maligna. J Am Acad Dermatol 2005;52(5):859–62.

Farrahi F, Egbert BM, Swetter SM. Histologic similarities between lentigo maligna and dysplastic nevus: importance of clinicopathologic distinction. J Cutan Pathol 2005;32(6):405–12.

Ferrara G, De Vanna AC. Fluorescence in situ hybridization for melanoma diagnosis: a review and a reappraisal. Am J Dermatopathol 2016;38(4):253–69.

Griewank KG, Ugurel S, Schadendorf D, et al. New developments in biomarkers for melanoma. Curr Opin Oncol 2013;25(2):145–51.

Kapur P, Selim MA, Roy LC, et al. Spitz nevi and atypical Spitz nevi/tumors: a histologic and immunohistochemical analysis. Mod Pathol 2005;18(2):197–204.

Lee CY, Gerami P. Molecular techniques for predicting behaviour in melanocytic neoplasms. Pathology 2016;48(2):142–6.

Massi D, De Giorgi V, Mandalà M. The complex management of atypical Spitz tumours. Pathology 2016;48(2):132–41.

Moore DA, Pringle JH, Saldanha GS. Prognostic tissue markers in melanoma. Histopathology 2012;60(5):679–89.

Stefanaki C, Stefanaki K, Chardalias L, et al. Differential diagnosis of Spitzoid melanocytic neoplasms. J Eur Acad Dermatol Venereol 2016;30(8):1269–77.

Strungs I. Common and uncommon variants of melanocytic naevi. Pathology 2004;36(5):396–403.

Tannous ZS, Mihm MC Jr, Sober AJ, et al. Congenital melanocytic nevi: clinical and histopathologic features, risk of melanoma, and clinical management. J Am Acad Dermatol 2005;52(2):197–203.

Urso C. A new perspective for spitz tumors? Am J Dermatopathol 2005;27(4):364–6.

Xu X, Elder DE. A practical approach to selected problematic melanocytic lesions. Am J Clin Pathol 2004;121:S3–32.

Interface dermatitis

Dirk M. Elston

Lichenoid interface dermatitis

Key Features

- Basal layer is destroyed
- Civatte bodies
- Sawtooth rete pattern

Causes of lichenoid interface dermatitis

- Lichen planus
- Benign lichenoid keratosis (BLK, lichen planus–like keratosis)
- Lichenoid drug eruption
- Lichenoid graft-versus-host disease (GvHD)
- Hypertrophic lupus erythematosus
- Lichenoid regression of a melanocytic lesion (usually lentigo maligna)

The biopsy in each of these conditions demonstrates a sawtooth rete ridge pattern with destruction of the basal layer, a bandlike lymphoid infiltrate, and presence of Civatte bodies. Compact hyperkeratosis and beaded hypergranulosis are typically present.

The cells of the stratum spinosum are enlarged and more eosinophilic than the normal epidermis. Vacuoles may be present in the lowest cells of stratum spinosum, but the basal layer is gone. An underlying bandlike lymphoid infiltrate is common.

If neither parakeratosis nor eosinophils is noted, the changes are consistent with lichen planus. Lichenoid interface dermatitis with neither eosinophils nor parakeratosis may also be seen in BLK (lichen planus–like keratosis), lichenoid drug eruption, lichenoid GvHD, hypertrophic lupus erythematosus, and lichenoid regression of lentigo maligna. Clinical correlation is essential. Direct immunofluorescence (DIF) will distinguish hypertrophic lupus erythematosus (continuous granular band of immunoglobulins and complement plus cytoid bodies) from lichen planus (shaggy fibrin, cytoid bodies).

When parakeratosis is present, lichen planus is very unlikely. The differential diagnosis still includes BLK, lichenoid drug eruption, lichenoid GvHD, and lichenoid regression of a melanocytic lesion. Hypertrophic lupus erythematosus rarely demonstrates parakeratosis.

The presence of eosinophils strongly favors a diagnosis of lichenoid drug eruption. The presence of eosinophils weighs strongly against a diagnosis of lichen planus. They are rarely seen in hypertrophic lupus erythematosus, BLK, lichenoid GvHD, or lichenoid regression of a melanocytic lesion.

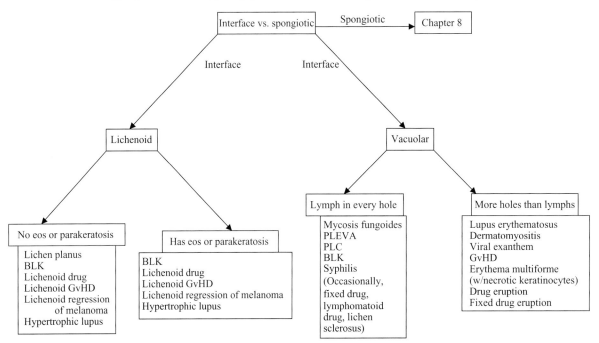

Fig. 7.1 Interface versus spongiotic dermatitis (*EOS*, eosinophils; *PLC*, pityriasis lichenoides chronica; *PLEVA*, pityriasis lichenoides et varioliformis acuta)

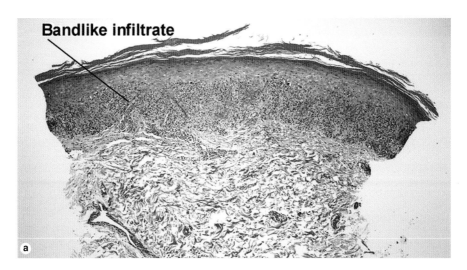

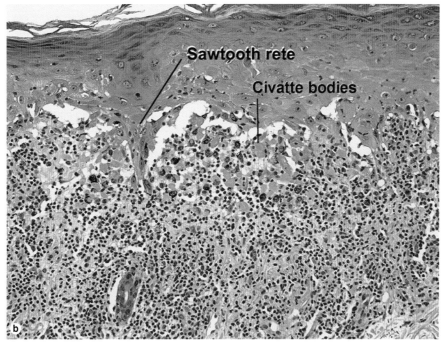

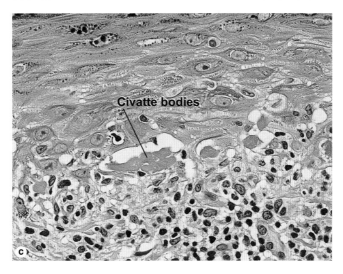

Fig. 7.2 Lichenoid interface dermatitis (lichen planus)

Late-phase (burnt-out) lichenoid dermatitis

Key Features

- Effacement of the rete pattern
- Melanin pigment incontinence (melanoderma)
- Civatte bodies

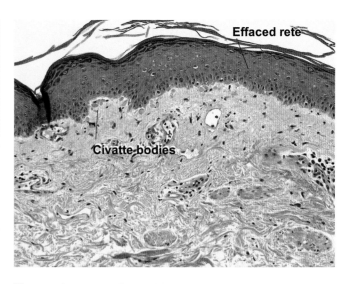

Fig. 7.4 Late-stage lichenoid dermatitis

Lichen planus

Key Features

- Lichenoid interface dermatitis
- No parakeratosis or eosinophils
- Sawtooth rete ridges

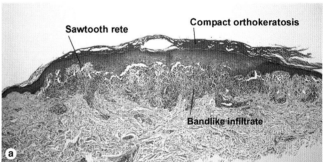

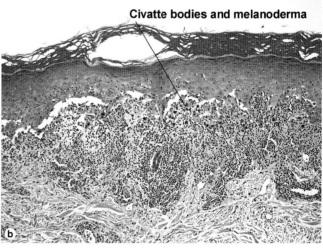

Fig. 7.5 Lichen planus

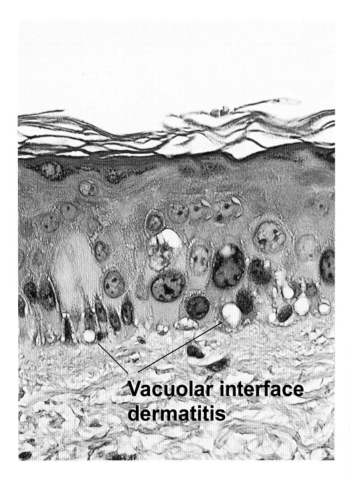

Fig. 7.3 Vacuolar interface dermatitis for comparision (graft-versus-host disease)

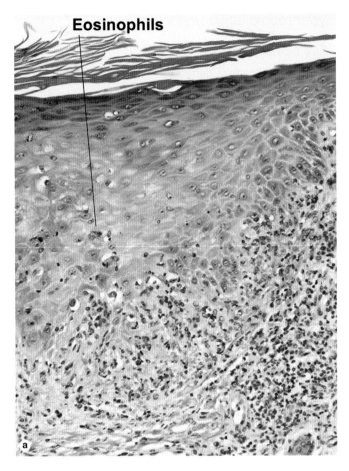

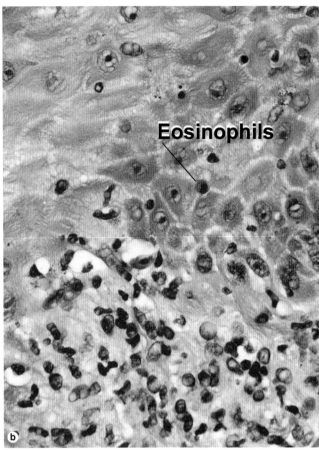

Fig. 7.6 Lichenoid drug eruption

Lichenoid drug eruption

Key Features

- Lichenoid interface dermatitis
- Typically has eosinophils
- Often has parakeratosis

Benign lichenoid keratosis

Key Features

- Lichenoid interface dermatitis
- May have parakeratosis
- Stratum corneum not homogeneous
- Rarely has eosinophils
- Solar lentigo commonly present at the margin

BLK usually presents as a solitary pearly pink macule on the trunk or an extremity. The biopsy is usually performed to rule out basal cell carcinoma. Most lesions represent lichenoid regression of benign solar lentigines. The earliest stage of evolution may show vacuolar interface dermatitis with a lymphocyte in every vacuole.

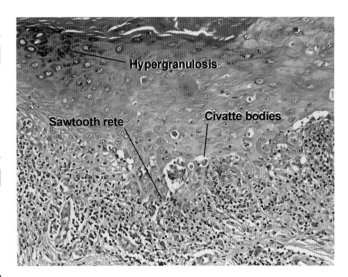

Fig. 7.7 Benign lichenoid keratosis

Lichenoid graft-versus-host disease

Key Features

- Lichenoid interface dermatitis
- May have parakeratosis
- Rarely has eosinophils

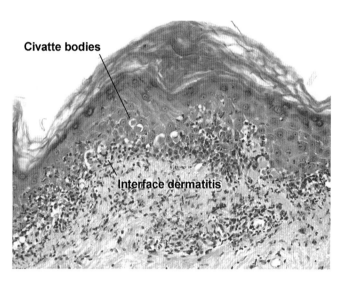

Fig. 7.8 Lichenoid GvHD

Hypertrophic lupus erythematosus

Key Features

- Lichenoid interface dermatitis
- Rarely has parakeratosis
- Rarely has eosinophils
- DIF: continuous granular band of immunoglobulin (Ig) G/A/M and C3 (full house) at the basement membrane zone (BMZ)
- Superficial and deep infiltrate
- Follicular plugging
- Many CD123+ plasmacytoid dendritic cells adjacent to epithelium (helps differentiate from squamous cell carcinoma in situ)

Hypertrophic lupus erythematosus is lichenoid histologically. It is distinguished from lichen planus by the DIF pattern, by the occasional presence of BMZ thickening or dermal mucin, and by clinical history and serologic findings. This is the form of chronic cutaneous lupus erythematosus that is most likely to give rise to invasive squamous cell carcinoma.

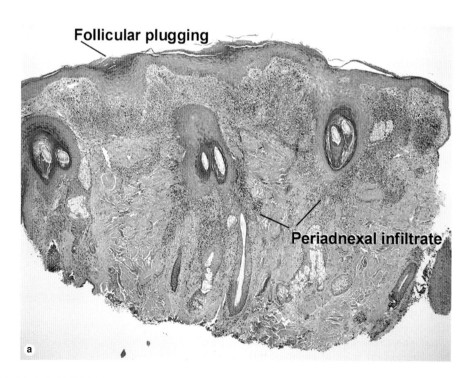

Fig. 7.9 Hypertrophic lupus erythematosus

Lichenoid regression of lentigo maligna

Key Features

- Lichenoid interface dermatitis
- Heavily sun-damaged skin
- Adjacent rete pattern may be effaced
- May have parakeratosis
- Rarely has eosinophils

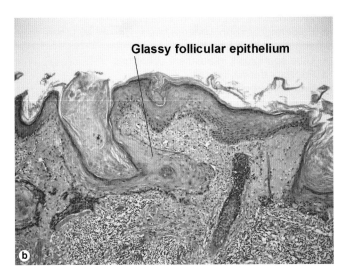

Fig. 7.9, cont'd

Porokeratosis

Key Features

- Cornoid lamella (column of parakeratosis at 45-degree angle, dyskeratotic cells below)
- Zone between cornoid lamellae may appear lichenoid or psoriasiform

Vacuolar interface dermatitis

Key Features

- Basal layer intact
- Vacuoles within basal layer
- Rounded rete pattern

Vacuolar interface dermatitis with a lymphocyte in nearly every vacuole

Vacuolar interface dermatitis with a lymphocyte in nearly every vacuole is characteristic of mycosis fungoides (MF), pityriasis lichenoides, and the early evolving stage of a BLK. Rarely, a similar pattern may be seen in fixed drug eruption, lymphomatoid drug eruption, or lichen sclerosus.

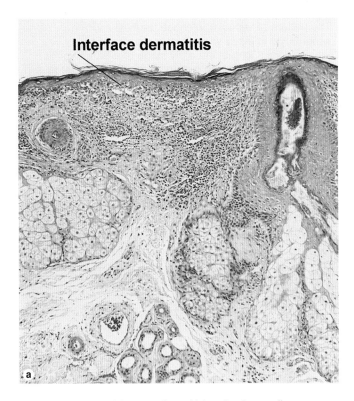

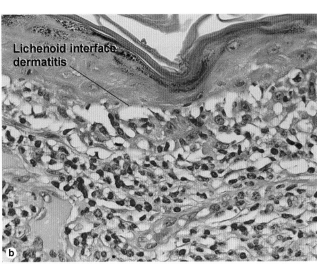

Fig. 7.10 Lichenoid regression within a lentigo maligna

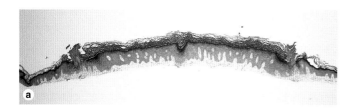

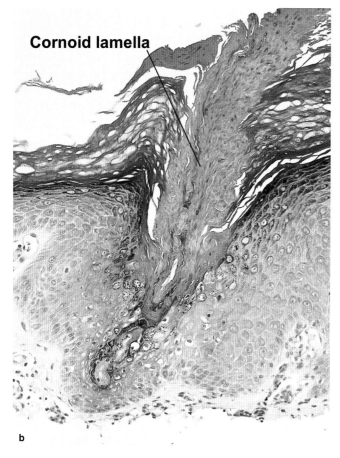

Cornoid lamella

b

Fig. 7.11 Porokeratosis

Mycosis fungoides

Key Features

- Vacuolar interface dermatitis
- A lymphocyte in nearly every vacuole ("a lymph in every hole")
- Lymphocytes hyperchromatic and surrounded by white space (lump of coal on a pillow)
- Lymphocytes tend to line up along the dermal–epidermal junction (DEJ)
- Lymphocytes tend to form small aggregates
- Epidermal lymphocytes are larger, darker, and more angulated than lymphocytes in dermis
- Little spongiosis in adjacent epidermis
- Papillary dermal fibrosis
- Bare underbelly sign
- Pautrier microabscess

The biopsy demonstrates epidermotropism of large atypical lymphocytes with little accompanying spongiosis. These lymphocytes show some tendency to form small aggregates and to line up along the DEJ. Papillary dermal fibrosis is prominent. The bare underbelly sign refers to the tendency for the superficial perivascular lymphoid infiltrate to predominate above the vessel, with few lymphocytes below the vessel. It has been likened to a vacuum cleaner sucking the lymphocytes toward the surface. Immunostaining and gene rearrangement studies can be helpful. Selective loss of CD7 expression in the atypical intraepidermal lymphocytes is a common finding. As the disease progresses from patch, to plaque, to tumor stage, atypical cells appear in the dermal infiltrate and epidermotropism is lost.

Differential Diagnosis

The pattern of vacuolar interface dermatitis with a lymphocyte in every vacuole may also be seen in pityriasis lichenoides, the early stage of a BLK, syphilis, and sometimes fixed drug eruption and lichen sclerosus. The pattern of large dark nuclei with surrounding vacuoles at the DEJ may also be seen in lentigo maligna and lymphomatoid drug eruption.

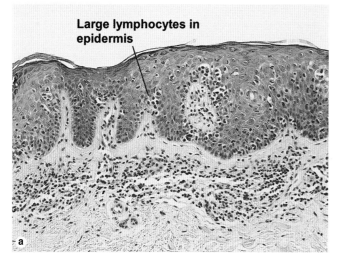

Large lymphocytes in epidermis

a

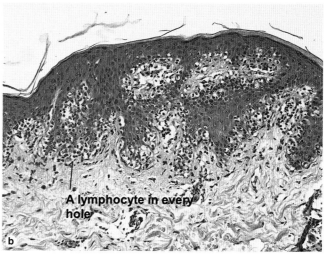

A lymphocyte in every hole

b

Fig. 7.12 Mycosis fungoides

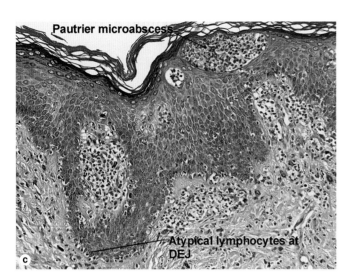

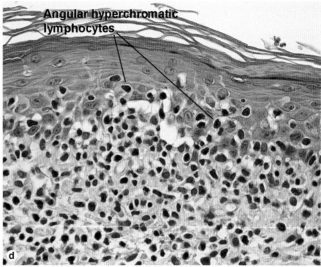

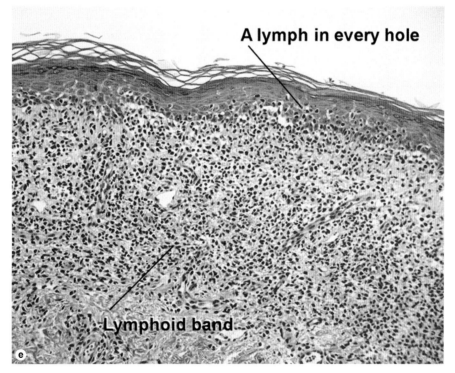

Fig. 7.12, cont'd

Pityriasis lichenoides et varioliformis acuta (PLEVA)

Key Features

- Vacuolar interface dermatitis
- A lymphocyte in nearly every vacuole
- Compact stratum corneum ± ulceration or crust
- No papillary dermal fibrosis
- Erythrocyte extravasation
- Transepidermal elimination of erythrocytes
- Neutrophil margination within dermal vessels

The biopsy demonstrates vacuolar interface dermatitis with a lymphocyte in every vacuole. Keratinocyte necrosis, central ulceration, and crusting may be noted. Erythrocyte extravasation with transepidermal elimination of erythrocytes is common. The infiltrate is purely lymphoid, with both a superficial and deep perivascular pattern. Prominent intravascular margination of neutrophils is typical. The infiltrate in PLEVA is characterized by CD8-positive cytotoxic T cells. A clone can often be detected by gene rearrangement studies.

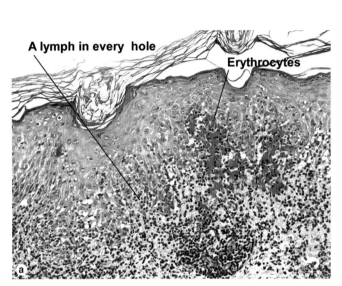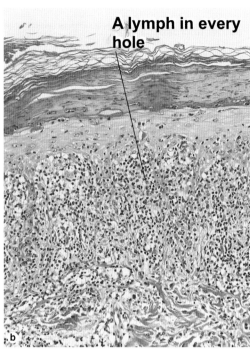

Fig. 7.13 Pityriasis lichenoides et varioliformis acuta (PLEVA) (Note neutrophils within "dirty" scale crust.)

Pityriasis lichenoides chronica

Key Features

- Vacuolar interface dermatitis
- A lymphocyte in nearly every vacuole
- Transepidermal elimination of erythrocytes variable

Early stage of benign lichenoid keratosis

Key Features

- Vacuolar interface dermatitis
- A lymphocyte in nearly every vacuole

Vacuolar interface dermatitis with vacuoles or cell death out of proportion to lymphocytes

Lupus erythematosus

Key Features

- Interface change usually vacuolar, but may be lichenoid (as in hypertrophic lupus erythematosus)
- Compact hyperkeratosis
- Follicular hyperkeratosis
- BMZ thickening
- Melanin pigment incontinence (melanoderma) underlying the DEJ
- Vertical columns of lymphocytes within fibrous tract remnants

- Perivascular lymphoid aggregates
- Lymphoid aggregates within the eccrine coil
- Dermal mucin between collagen bundles
- Underlying lupus panniculitis may be present
- DIF: continuous granular band of IgG/A/M and C3 (full house) at the BMZ

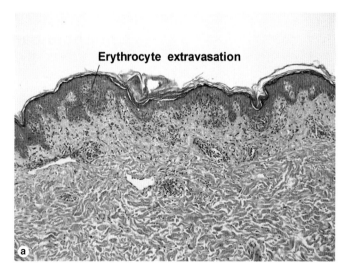

Fig. 7.14 Pityriasis lichenoides chronica

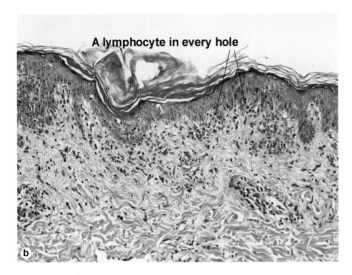

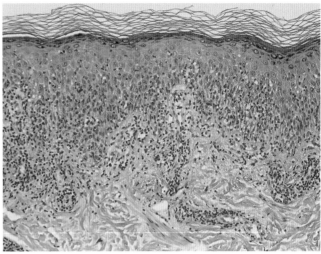

Fig. 7.15 Early benign lichenoid keratosis (*BLK,* lichen planus–like keratosis)

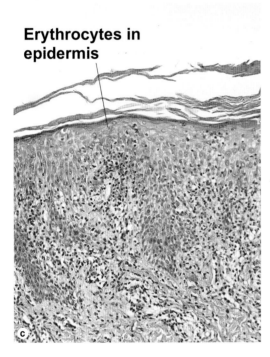

Fig. 7.14, cont'd

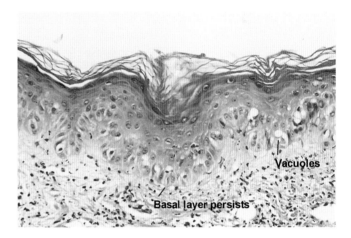

Fig. 7.16 Acute lupus erythematosus

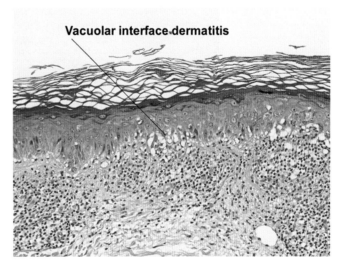

The features of discoid lupus erythematosus appear in a time-dependent fashion. Biopsies of acute lupus erythematosus show only vacuolar interface dermatitis. DIF will usually be negative at this stage. Subacute lesions of lupus erythematosus show vacuolar interface dermatitis, hyperkeratosis, and follicular plugging, as well as a variable dermal infiltrate. DIF is positive in about one third of cases. Well-established discoid lesions (of at least 3 months' duration) typically demonstrate strong DIF. Histologically, established discoid lupus erythematosus lesions are characterized by hyperkeratosis, follicular plugging, vacuolar interface dermatitis, BMZ thickening, both a patchy superficial and deep perivascular and periadnexal lymphoid infiltrate, and interstitial mucin. Underlying lupus panniculitis may be present.

Fig. 7.17 Subacute lupus erythematosus

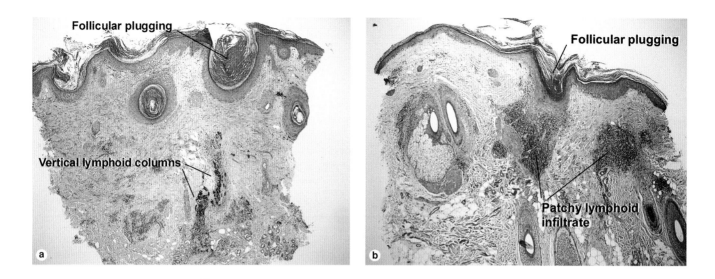

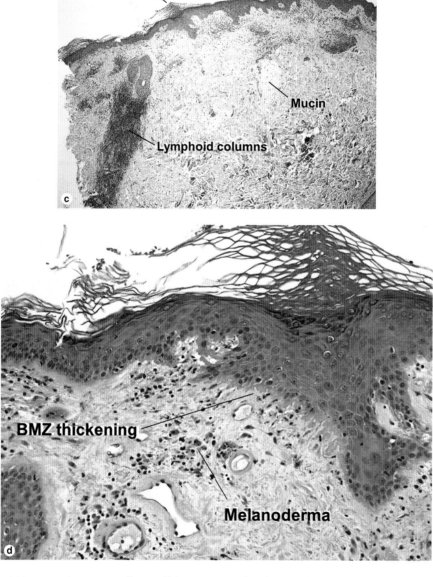

Fig. 7.18 Chronic discoid lupus erythematosus (Image F demonstrates the characteristic shaggy fibrin and coarse, granular, bandlike staining of complement and immunoglobulins. The presence of immunofluorescence with every component is referred to as a *full house*)

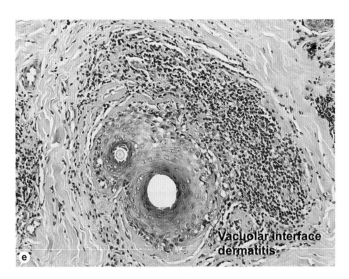

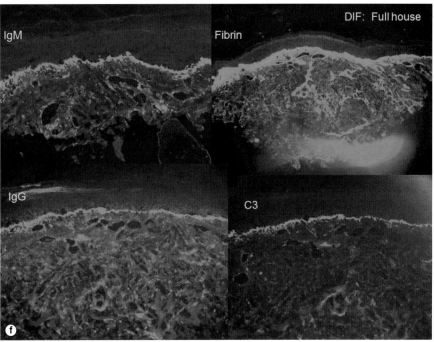

Fig. 7.18, cont'd

Differential Diagnosis

1. Dermatomyositis may look identical to lupus erythematosus, although the former usually demonstrates epidermal atrophy.
2. Tumid lupus lacks interface changes.
3. Lichen striatus lacks dermal mucin.
4. Differential diagnosis of nodular lymphoid infiltrate—the seven *L*s:

*L*upus
*L*ight (polymorphous light eruption): papillary dermal edema usually prominent
*L*ymphoma
*L*ymphocytoma cutis
*L*ichen striatus (eccrine coil involved like lupus)
*L*ymphocytic eruption of Jessner–Kanof
*L*ues (vacuolar interface dermatitis typically paired with elongation of rete, interstitial busy dermis, endothelial swelling, lymphocytes with ample cytoplasm or plasma cells)

5. Viral exanthem (may have erythrocyte extravasation; lacks hyperkeratosis, papillary dermal fibrosis)
6. Drug eruption (may be mix of inflammatory patterns, lacks hyperkeratosis, papillary dermal fibrosis)
7. Phototoxic eruption (lacks hyperkeratosis, papillary dermal fibrosis)

Polymorphous light eruption

Key Features

- Plaque variant has papillary dermal edema and dense perivascular lymphoid infiltrate
- Epidermal to dermal separation can occur due to edema rather than lichenoid or vacuolar damage
- Papulovesicular variant is spongiotic

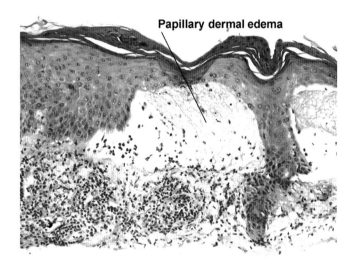

Fig. 7.19 Polymorphous light eruption

Lichen striatus

Key Features

- Lichenoid interface dermatitis
- Blaschkoid interface dermatitis
- Lymphoid aggregates perivascular and in eccrine coil

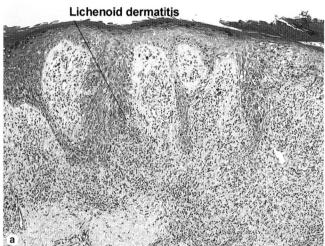

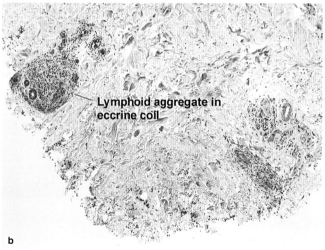

Fig. 7.20 Lichen striatus

Dermatomyositis

Key Features

- Vacuolar interface dermatitis
- Similar to lupus erythematosus
- Typically demonstrates epidermal atrophy

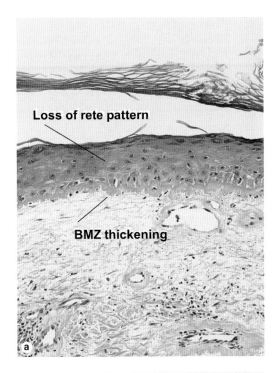

Loss of rete pattern

BMZ thickening

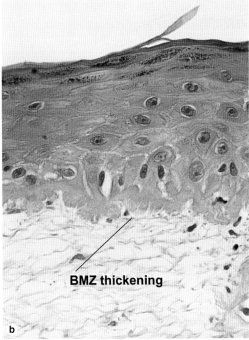

BMZ thickening

Fig. 7.21 Dermatomyositis

Syphilis

Key Features

- Vacuolar or lichenoid interface dermatitis together often with slender acanthosis
- Vacuolar interface dermatitis together with an interstitial pattern (busy dermis)
- Interface-predominant pattern may have an atrophic epidermis
- Neutrophils in the stratum corneum
- Plasma cells present in about two thirds of cases
- Endothelial swelling obliterates the lumen of small vessels
- Perivascular lymphocytes and histiocytes with visible cytoplasm

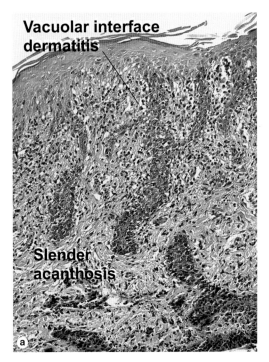

Vacuolar interface dermatitis

Slender acanthosis

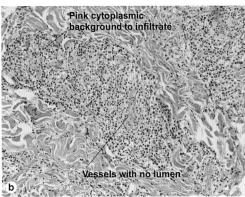

Pink cytoplasmic background to infiltrate

Vessels with no lumen

Fig. 7.22 Lues (syphilis). Part D demonstrates interstitial "busy dermis." Part E demonstrates *Treponema pallidum* immunostain

continued

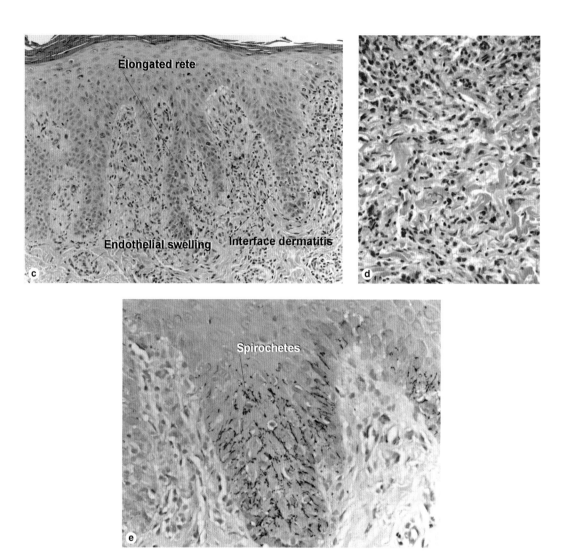

Fig. 7.22, cont'd

Erythema multiforme

Key Features

- Acute (normal) basket-weave stratum corneum
- Vacuolar interface dermatitis with individual necrotic keratinocytes above the basal layer
- May progress to confluent epidermal necrosis
- Cell death out of proportion to lymphocytes
- In late stage, bulla and reepithelialization occur

The typical picture of erythema multiforme includes a normal stratum corneum with "death and squalor" in the underlying epidermis. In the acute stage, the infiltrate is purely lymphoid.

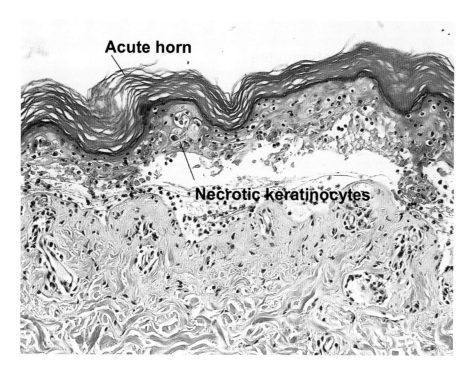

Fig. 7.23 Erythema multiforme

Toxic epidermal necrolysis

Key Features

- Looks like erythema multiforme

Paraneoplastic pemphigus

Key Features

- Acantholysis may or may not be present
- May be lichenoid
- May look like erythema multiforme (see Chapter 9)

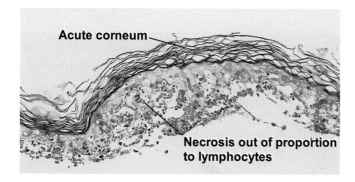

Fig. 7.24 Toxic epidermal necrolysis

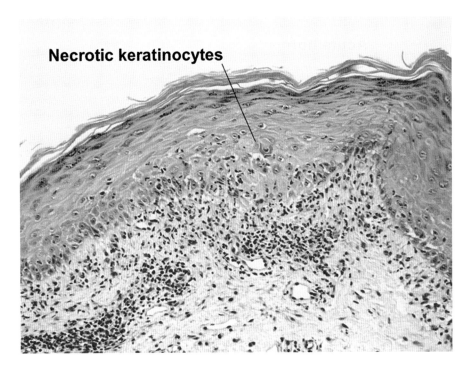

Necrotic keratinocytes

Fig. 7.25 Paraneoplastic pemphigus

Fixed drug eruption

Key Features

- Vacuolar interface dermatitis
- Proportion of lymphocytes and vacuoles variable
- Polymorphous infiltrate (typically with eosinophils)
- Acute (normal) stratum corneum
- Chronic dermal changes:
  - Papillary dermal fibrosis
  - Melanin pigment incontinence in perivascular location

The most important diagnostic feature is the mismatch between the normal stratum corneum and chronic changes in the superficial dermis. Fixed drug eruption is episodic. The biopsy is likely to occur during an acute inflammatory phase, but dermal changes from past episodes are present. The result is a normal stratum corneum consistent with an acute process. In contrast, there is papillary dermal fibrosis consistent with a chronic process. Pigment has had time to be carried to a perivascular location. The polymorphous infiltrate typically includes eosinophils and may include neutrophils.

> **PEARL**
>
> The normal stratum corneum whispers, "Look at me, I'm an acute process." The papillary dermal fibrosis and pigment around vessels respond, "Liar! There are chronic changes in the dermis."

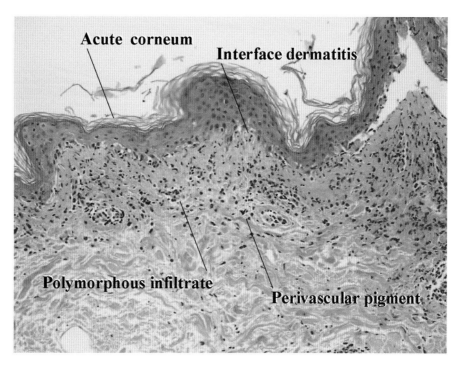

Fig. 7.26 Fixed drug eruption

Graft-versus-host disease (GVHD)

Key Features

Subacute (fairly compact) stratum corneum
Vacuolar interface dermatitis

Necrotic keratinocytes
Epithelial atypia and disorder
The features listed above are those for acute GvHD, chronic GvHD may be lichenoid or sclerodermoid.

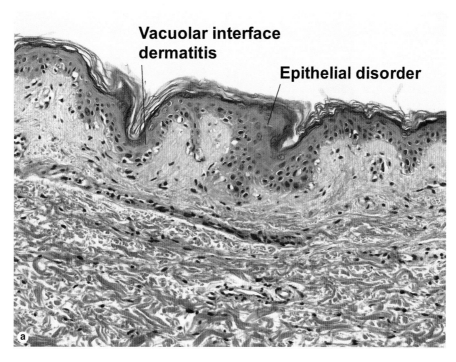

Fig. 7.27 Graft-versus-host disease (GvHD)

continued

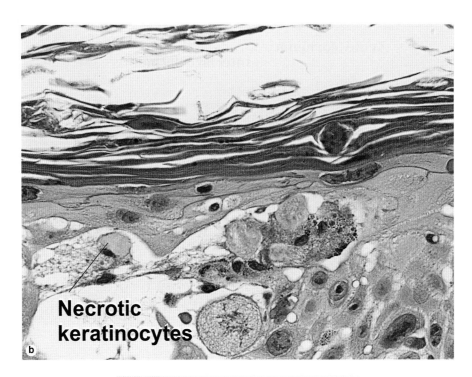

Necrotic keratinocytes

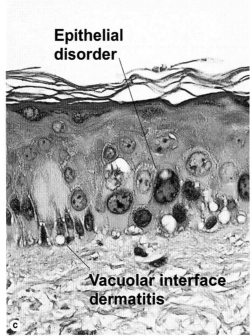

Epithelial disorder

Vacuolar interface dermatitis

Fig. 7.27, cont'd

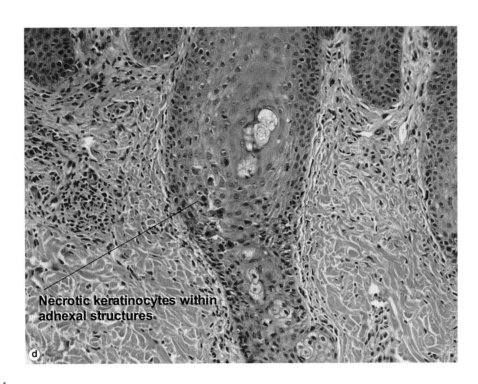

Fig. 7.27, cont'd

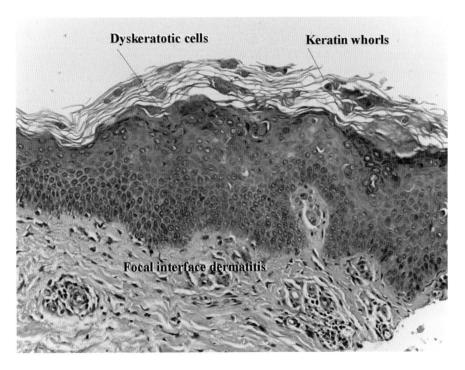

Fig. 7.28 Still's disease

Still's disease

Key features

Acute lesions: Perivascular neutrophilic infiltrate with little karyorrhexis

Chronic lesions: Keratin whorls in corneum and dyskeratotic "dead reds" scattered through the epidermis. Focal interface dermatitis may be present.

Acute lesions of Still's disease may resemble urticaria or erythema marginatum. Chronic lesions may appear and erythematous and slightly hyperpigmented macules and papules. Like urticaria, the acute lesions demonstrate neutrophils with little karyorrhexis. Chronic lesions have many dyskeratotic cells similar to the second stage of incontinentia pigmenti, but with characteristic whorls of keratin in the stratum corneum.

Further reading

Agozzino M, Gonzalez S, Ardigó M. Reflectance confocal microscopy for inflammatory skin diseases. Actas Dermosifiliogr 2016;107(8):631–9.

Brönnimann M, Yawalkar N. Histopathology of drug-induced exanthems: is there a role in diagnosis of drug allergy? Curr Opin Allergy Clin Immunol 2005;5(4):317–21.

Dalton SR, Chandler WM, Abuzeid M, et al. Eosinophils in mycosis fungoides: an uncommon finding in the patch and plaque stages. Am J Dermatopathol 2012;34(6):586–91.

Dalton SR, Fillman EP, Altman CE, et al. Atypical junctional melanocytic proliferations in benign lichenoid keratosis. Hum Pathol 2003;34(7):706–9.

Flamm A, Parikh K, Xie Q, et al. Histologic features of secondary syphilis: A multicenter retrospective review. J Am Acad Dermatol 2015;73(6):1025–30.

Kaley J, Pellowski DM, Cheung WL, et al. The spectrum of histopathologic findings in cutaneous eruptions associated with influenza A (H1N1) infection. J Cutan Pathol 2013;40(2):226–9.

Massone C, Kodama K, Kerl H, et al. Histopathologic features of early (patch) lesions of mycosis fungoides: a morphologic study on 745 biopsy specimens from 427 patients. Am J Surg Pathol 2005;29(4):550–60.

Morgan MB, Stevens GL, Switlyk S. Benign lichenoid keratosis: a clinical and pathologic reappraisal of 1040 cases. Am J Dermatopathol 2005;27(5):387–92.

Smith SB, Libow LF, Elston DM, et al. Gloves and socks syndrome: early and late histopathologic features. J Am Acad Dermatol 2002;47(5):749–54.

Yawalkar N, Pichler WJ. Immunohistology of drug-induced exanthema: clues to pathogenesis. Curr Opin Allergy Clin Immunol 2001;1(4):299–303.

Zhang Y, Wang Y, Yu R, et al. Molecular markers of early-stage mycosis fungoides. J Invest Dermatol 2012;132(6): 1698–706.

Psoriasiform and spongiotic dermatitis

Dirk M. Elston

Psoriasis

Key Features

- Neutrophils above parakeratosis in stratum corneum
- Little to no serum in stratum corneum
- Alternating neutrophils and parakeratosis in the stratum corneum (sandwich sign)
- Neutrophilic spongiform pustules
- Little spongiosis in adjacent epidermis
- Tortuous blood vessels in dermal papillae

The appearance of psoriasis depends on the stage of the lesion and type of lesion. Early guttate lesions demonstrate no acanthosis. Established plaques demonstrate a characteristic pattern of regular acanthosis. Pustular psoriasis may never demonstrate acanthosis. Acral and intertriginous lesions of psoriasis commonly demonstrate a background of spongiosis, but spongiosis is distinctly absent from the surrounding epidermis in most other locations. *Reiter disease* and *geographic tongue* histologically look like psoriasis.

PEARL

Collections of neutrophils within the stratum corneum:
- Psoriasis, tinea, impetigo, *Candida*, seborrheic dermatitis, syphilis (PTICSS)

Plaque psoriasis

Key Features

- Regular, bulbous, club-shaped acanthosis
- Thin superpapillary plates
- Alternating neutrophils and parakeratosis in the stratum corneum (sandwich sign)
- Little to no serum in stratum corneum
- Neutrophilic spongiform pustules
- Little spongiosis in adjacent epidermis

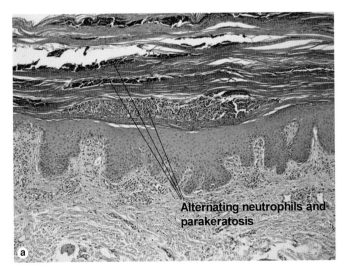

Alternating neutrophils and parakeratosis

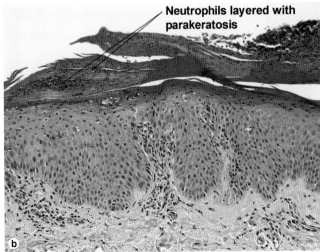

Neutrophils layered with parakeratosis

Fig. 8.1 Plaque psoriasis

continued

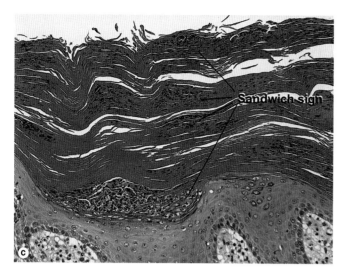

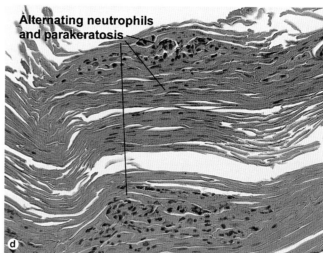

Fig. 8.1, cont'd

Pustular psoriasis

Key Features

- Collections of neutrophils within stratum corneum
- Subcorneal pustules
- Spongiform pustules

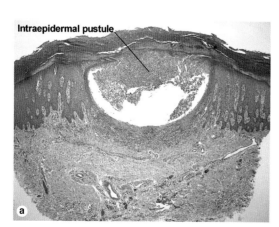

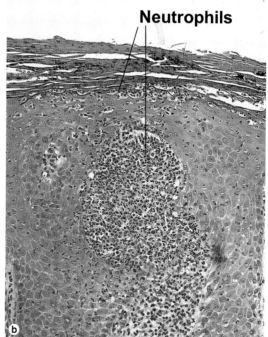

Fig. 8.2 Pustular psoriasis

Guttate psoriasis

Key Features

- Neutrophils above parakeratosis

The key histologic feature of guttate psoriasis is a focus of neutrophils on top of parakeratosis (half of the sandwich sign, jelly up). The neutrophilic focus may be small and only visible in step sections. The focus often has a humplike configuration or resembles a child's drawing of a seagull.

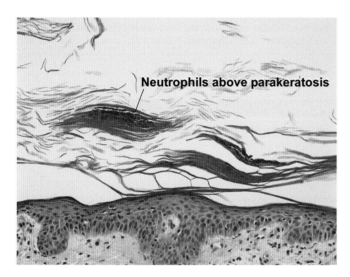

Fig. 8.3 Guttate psoriasis

Inflammatory linear verrucous epidermal nevus (ILVEN)

Key Features

- Alternating orthokeratosis and parakeratosis from left to right
- Areas of orthokeratosis have a prominent granular layer
- Areas of parakeratosis lack an underlying granular layer (see Chapter 2)

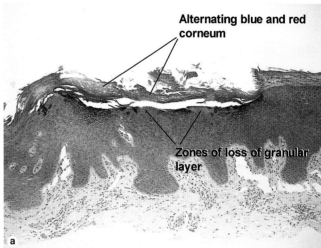

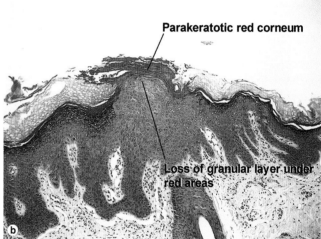

Fig. 8.4 Inflammatory linear verrucous epidermal nevus (ILVEN)

Mycosis fungoides

Key Features

- Epidermal collections of lymphocytes
- Lymphocytes hyperchromatic and surrounded by white space (lump of coal on a pillow)
- Epidermal lymphocytes larger, darker, and more angulated than lymphocytes in dermis
- Little spongiosis in adjacent epidermis
- Papillary dermal fibrosis
- In areas, lymphocytes may also line up along the dermal epidermal junction
- Bare underbelly sign (see Chapters 7 and 24)

Syphilis

Key Features

- Vacuolar interface dermatitis together with elongated psoriasiform acanthosis
- Vacuolar interface dermatitis together with interstitial dermal infiltrate (busy dermis)
- Neutrophils in the stratum corneum
- Plasma cells present in about two thirds of cases
- Endothelial swelling obliterates the lumen of small vessels
- Perivascular lymphocytes and histiocytes with visible cytoplasm (see Chapters 7 and 17)

PEARL

Plasma cells are commonly associated with:

Diagnoses:
- Kaposi sarcoma
- Syphilis
- Leishmaniasis
- Rhinoscleroma
- Melanoma
- Squamous cell carcinoma

Body locations that recruit plasma cells:
- Face
- Mucosa
- Back of neck
- Axillae
- Breasts
- Anogenital area
- Shins

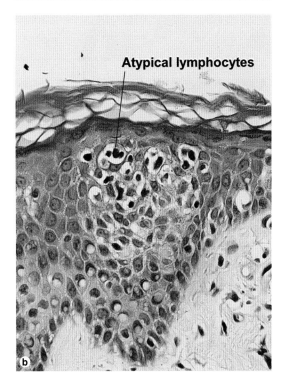

Fig. 8.5 Psoriasiform mycosis fungoides

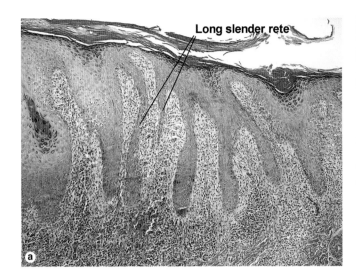

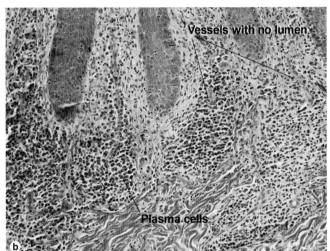

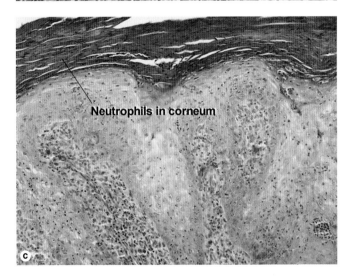

Fig. 8.6 Syphilis

Necrolytic erythemas/nutritional deficiency dermatitis

Key Features

- Pallor and ballooning of upper epidermis

Causes include glucagonoma (necrolytic migratory erythema), necrolytic acral erythema associated with hepatitis C, pellagra, and acrodermatitis enteropathica. Although pallor and ballooning of the upper epidermis are characteristic, many biopsies demonstrate only nonspecific dermatitis with diffuse parakeratosis.

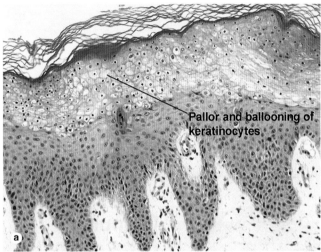

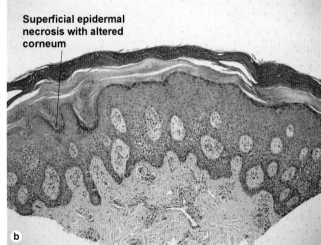

Fig. 8.7 (A) Necrolytic migratory erythema. **(B)** Necrolytic acral erythema

Granular parakeratosis

Key Features

- Compact hyperkeratosis with parakeratosis
- Granules in stratum corneum
- Granular layer preserved

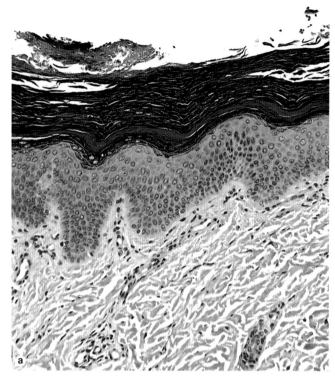

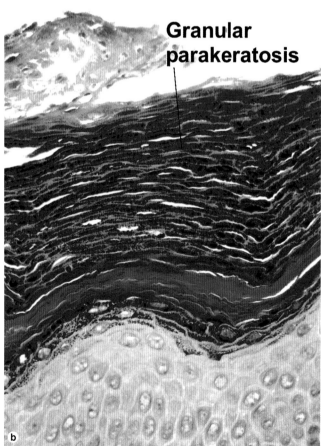

Granular parakeratosis

Fig. 8.8 Granular parakeratosis

Porokeratosis

Key Features

- Cornoid lamella (column of parakeratosis at 45-degree angle, dyskeratotic cells below)
- Zone between cornoid lamellae may appear lichenoid or psoriasiform (see Chapter 7)

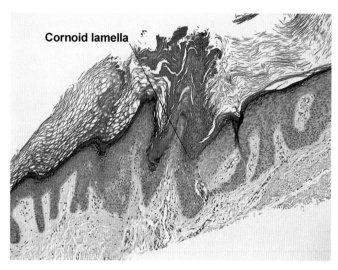

Cornoid lamella

Fig. 8.9 Porokeratosis

Acute spongiotic dermatitis

Key Features

- Spongiosis (intercellular edema)
- Exocytosis of lymphocytes

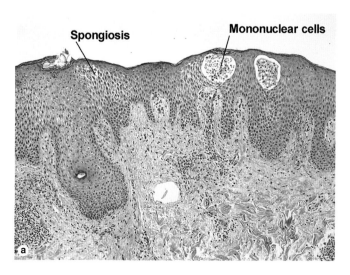

Spongiosis   Mononuclear cells

Fig. 8.10 Acute spongiotic dermatitis

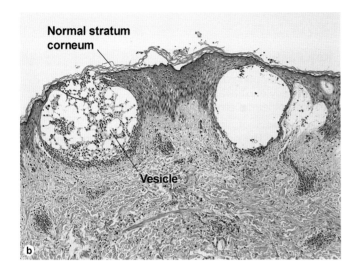

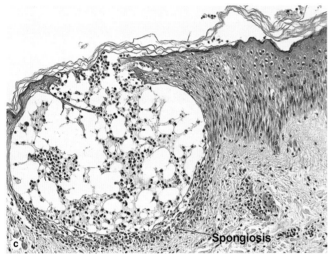

Fig. 8.10, cont'd

Seborrheic dermatitis

Key Features

- Psoriasiform spongiotic dermatitis
- Neutrophilic scale/crust at edges of follicular ostium

Subacute spongiotic dermatitis

Key Features

- Parakeratosis
- Acanthosis
- Spongiosis (intercellular edema)
- Exocytosis of lymphocytes

Common causes of spongiotic dermatitis:
- Allergic contact dermatitis
- Dyshidrotic dermatitis
- Nummular dermatitis
- Stasis dermatitis
- Id reaction

- Pityriasis rosea
- Spongiotic pigmenting purpura
- Tinea

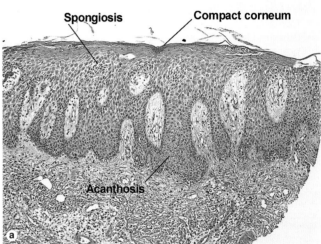

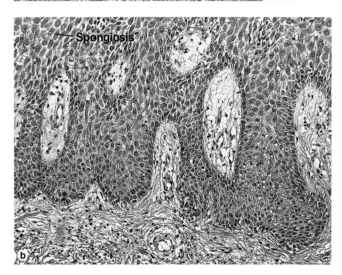

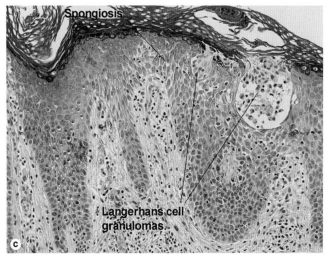

Fig. 8.11 Subacute spongiotic dermatitis

Chronic dermatitis (lichen simplex chronicus)

Key Features

- Compact stratum corneum
- Stratum lucidum as in volar skin, but follicles are present (hairy palm appearance)
- Irregular acanthosis
- Papillary dermal fibrosis

The histologic findings of chronic dermatitis are those of lichen simplex chronicus. Excoriation commonly produces focal superficial epidermal necrosis. Papillary dermal fibrosis is commonly accompanied by capillary proliferation (angiofibroplasia). Vertical streaking of papillary dermal collagen is common.

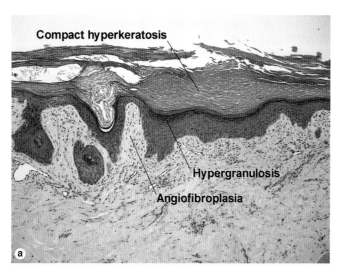

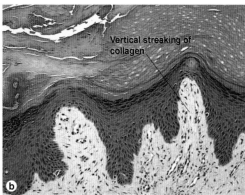

Fig. 8.12 Lichen simplex chronicus

Pityriasis rosea

Key Features

- Subacute spongiotic dermatitis
- Erythrocyte extravasation
- Transepidermal elimination of erythrocytes

The herald patch of pityriasis rosea is broad and fairly uniform in appearance. The subsequent lesions demonstrate a migrating spongiotic focus, followed by a trailing scale. The focus and scale form a roughly 45-degree angle.

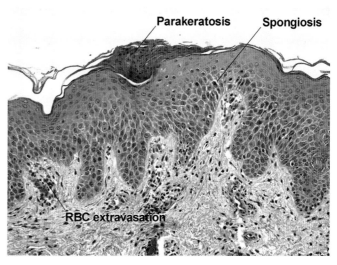

Fig. 8.13 Pityriasis rosea (*RBC*, red blood cell)

Spongiotic pigmented purpuric eruption (PPE)

Key Features

- Spongiosis
- Inflammation purely lymphoid
- Surrounds capillaries (centered above the level of the postcapillary venule)
- Erythrocyte extravasation
- Hemosiderin deposits over time

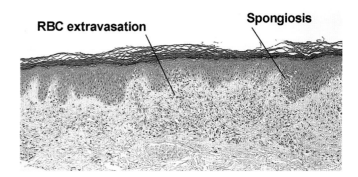

Fig. 8.14 Pigmented purpuric eruption (*RBC*, red blood cell)

Stasis dermatitis

Key Features

- Subacute spongiotic dermatitis
- Cannonball-like angioplasia in the superficial dermis
- Hemosiderin

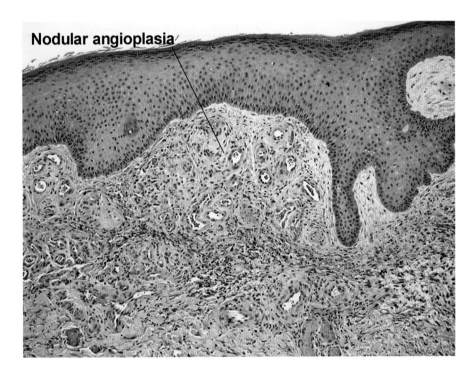

Nodular angioplasia

Fig. 8.15 Stasis dermatitis

Spongiotic dermatitis with intraepidermal eosinophils

Key Features

- Spongiosis
- Eosinophils within the epidermis ("eosinophilic spongiosis")

PEARL

Causes include herpes gestationis, arthropod bite, allergic contact dermatitis, pemphigus, pemphigoid, incontinentia pigmenti, erythema toxicum (spongiosis adjacent to a follicle) (HAAPPIE).

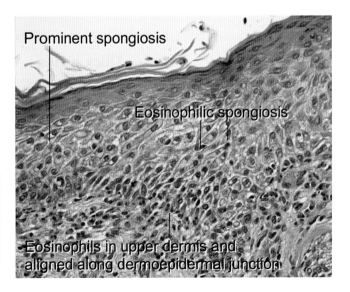

Prominent spongiosis

Eosinophilic spongiosis

Eosinophils in upper dermis and aligned along dermoepidermal junction

Fig. 8.16 Pemphigoid

Zoon balanitis

Key Features

- Spongiosis
- Flattened, diamond-shaped keratinocytes
- Dermal plasma cells

Zoon balanitis (balanitis circumscripta plasmacellularis) demonstrates subacute spongiotic mucositis with an underlying dense, plasmacytic infiltrate and flattened keratinocytes with intercellular edema.

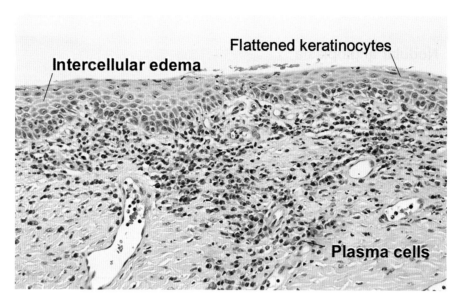

Fig. 8.17 Zoon balanitis

Pityriasis rubra pilaris

Key Features

- Acanthosis with thick superpapillary plates
- Parakeratosis adjacent to follicles
- Vertical and horizontal alternating (checkerboard) orthokeratosis and parakeratosis
- Occasional spongiosis
- Occasional acantholysis in follicles or eccrine ducts

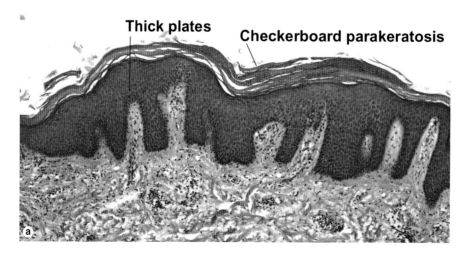

Fig. 8.18 Pityriasis rubra pilaris

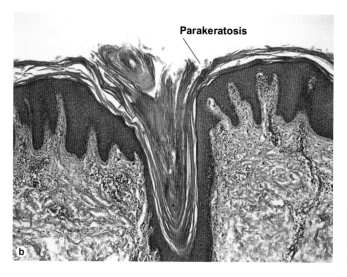

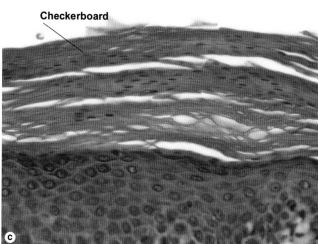

Fig. 8.18, cont'd

Toxic shock syndrome

Key Features

- Mild spongiosis with neutrophils
- Sparse karyorrhectic debris in epidermis and surrounding vessels

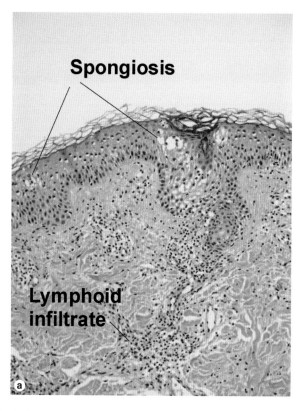

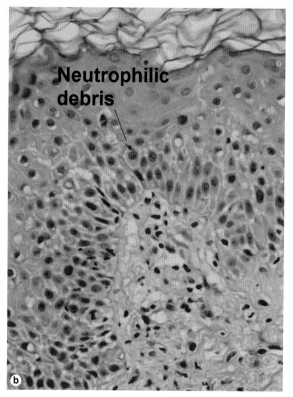

Fig. 8.19 Toxic shock syndrome

Further reading

Behrhof W, Springer E, Bräuninger W, et al. PCR testing for Treponema pallidum in paraffin-embedded skin biopsy specimens: test design and impact on the diagnosis of syphilis. J Clin Pathol 2008;61(3):390–5.

Chen CY, Chi KH, George RW, et al. Diagnosis of gastric syphilis by direct immunofluorescence staining and real-time PCR testing. J Clin Microbiol 2006;44(9):3452–6.

Hugel H. Histological diagnosis of inflammatory skin diseases. Use of a simple algorithm and modern diagnostic methods. Pathologe 2002;23(1):20–37.

Meymandi S, Silver SG, Crawford RI. Intraepidermal neutrophils – a clue to dermatophytosis? J Cutan Pathol 2003;30(4):253–5.

Pujol RM, Wang CY, el-Azhary RA, et al. Necrolytic migratory erythema: clinicopathologic study of 13 cases. Int J Dermatol 2004;43(1):12–18.

Blistering diseases

Whitney A. High

Subcorneal vesiculobullous disorders

Pemphigus foliaceus

Key Features

- Subcorneal split
- Acantholysis (loss of attachments between keratinocytes)
- Dyskeratosis may occur within the granular layer
- Direct immunofluorescence demonstrates "netlike" deposition of immunoglobulin (Ig) G and C3 between keratinocytes in upper epidermis

Pemphigus foliaceus is a subcorneal vesiculobullous disorder caused by autoantibodies directed at an intercellular keratinocyte adhesion protein: desmoglein 1 (160 kD). The disease usually presents with superficial crusted erosions upon the face and upper trunk. The superficial nature of the blisters makes them fragile, and upon presentation most patients lack intact bullae.

The presence of a subcorneal blister, with acantholytic cells and scattered eosinophils, is highly suggestive of pemphigus foliaceus. Direct immunofluorescence (DIF) is diagnostic and demonstrates intercellular IgG and C3 deposition, primarily confined to the upper half of the epidermis. The split occurs in the granular layer, as in staphylococcal scalded-skin syndrome. Pemphigus foliaceus may demonstrate neutrophils within the vesicle, making distinction from bullous impetigo difficult. A tissue Gram stain may be helpful, but the presence of an impetiginized crust does not wholly exclude pemphigus foliaceus.

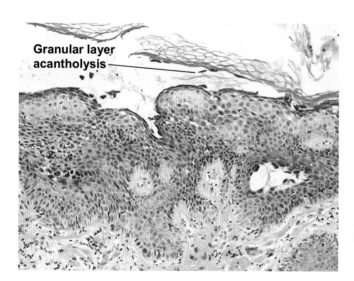

Granular layer acantholysis

Fig. 9.1 Pemphigus foliaceus

Pemphigus erythematosus blends the immunohistologic findings of pemphigus foliaceus with those of lupus erythematosus. Patients often have a positive serum antinuclear antibody (ANA). Immunofluorescence studies demonstrate intercellular deposition of immunoreactants and a "lupus band" of granular immunoreactants at the dermoepidermal junction.

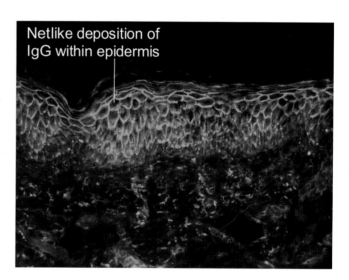

Netlike deposition of IgG within epidermis

Fig. 9.2 Direct immunofluorescence of "netlike" staining in the upper epidermis of pemphigus foliaceus

Subcorneal pustular dermatosis (Sneddon–Wilkinson disease)

Key Features

- Subcorneal pustule
- Pustule "sits" or "floats" upon the epidermis without depressing it
- Superficial mixed perivascular infiltrate with occasional neutrophils
- Dyskeratosis is uncommon
- Immunofluorescence is negative (distinguishing it from IgA pemphigus)

Cases of subcorneal pustular dermatosis with intercellular deposition of IgA have been reclassified as IgA pemphigus. Subcorneal pustular dermatosis may represent a subclass of pustular psoriasis, although mitotic figures within the underlying epidermis, common to psoriasis, are not identified in subcorneal pustular dermatosis. The classic patient is an older woman with annular or polycyclic lesions of the trunk or groin with pustules at the periphery.

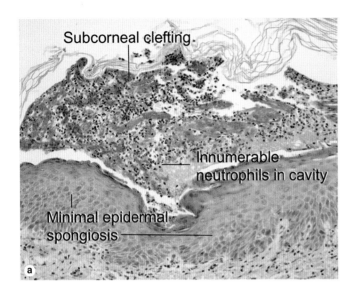

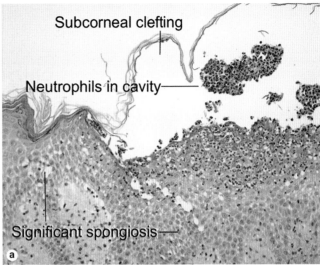

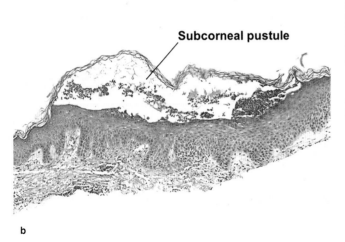

Fig. 9.3 (A) Subcorneal pustular dermatosis. **(B)** "Subcorneal pustular dermatosis" type of IgA pemphigus

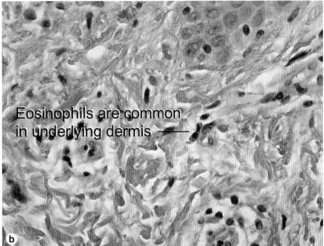

Fig. 9.4 Acute generalized exanthematous pustulosis

Acute generalized exanthematous pustulosis

Key Features

- Subcorneal or superficial epidermal pustules
- Mild spongiosis in the surrounding epidermis
- Superficial mixed infiltrate in an edematous papillary dermis
- Occasional eosinophils within the dermal infiltrate
- Immunofluorescence is negative

Acute generalized exanthematous pustulosis (AGEP) is an uncommon reaction to exogenous medications. Beta-lactam antibiotics and macrolides are most often implicated, but a myriad of other drug associations have been reported. The presence of eosinophils in the inflammatory infiltrate helps distinguish the condition from pustular psoriasis. Early pustules may be associated with hair follicles or sweat ducts.

Intraepidermal vesiculobullous disorders

Pemphigus vulgaris

Key Features

- Split immediately above basal layer leaves a "tombstone row" of basal keratinocytes
- Tracking of separation down hair follicles ("follicular extension")
- Eosinophils may occur in spongiotic foci or within the blister cavity
- Superficial lymphocytic inflammatory infiltrate in dermis
- Eosinophils may be seen within the dermal infiltrate
- Direct immunofluorescence demonstrates "netlike" deposition of IgG and C3 between keratinocytes in lower epidermis

Pemphigus vulgaris is an intraepidermal vesiculobullous disorder caused by autoantibodies directed at an intercellular keratinocyte adhesion protein: desmoglein 3 (130 kD). The disease presents with erosions of the skin and mucosa. Often the disease begins in the posterior oropharynx weeks before cutaneous lesions are noted. Most patients lack intact bullae upon presentation. Erythematous skin shears easily when lateral pressure is applied (Nikolsky sign).

Clefting above the basal layer, with acantholysis of the remaining basilar keratinocytes, leads to a visual impression likened to "rows of tombstones" sitting upon the dermal papillae. Tracking of the blistering down adnexal structures is often demonstrated. Direct immunofluorescence is diagnostic and demonstrates intercellular IgG and C3 deposition in a "netlike" pattern, primarily confined to the lower half of the epidermis. Pemphigus antibodies can also be measured via enzyme-linked immunosorbent assay (ELISA)–based technology and generally titer to disease activity. DIF studies on plucked hairs have also been recently suggested to monitor for remission/recurrences.

Pemphigus vegetans is a related disorder that demonstrates vegetative cutaneous lesions with epidermal hyperplasia and lesser vesiculation. Suprabasilar crypts of eosinophils may be identified within the acanthotic epidermis.

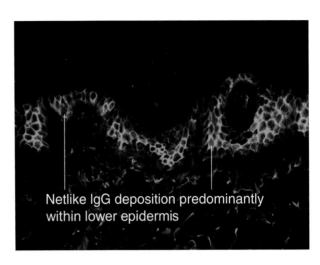

Fig. 9.6 Direct immunofluorescence of pemphigus vulgaris

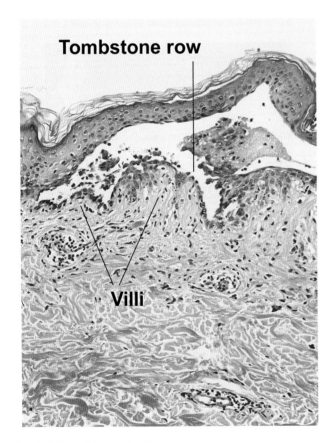

Fig. 9.5 Pemphigus vulgaris

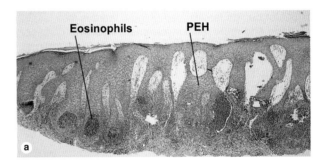

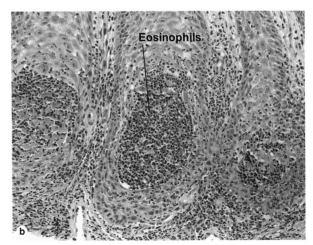

Fig. 9.7 Pemphigus vegetans–pseudoepitheliomatous hyperplasia (PEH) and eosinophils

Familial benign chronic pemphigus (Hailey–Hailey disease)

Key Features

- An inherited disorder with defective cell–cell adhesion
- Not antibody mediated
- Acantholysis at all levels of the epidermis resembles a "dilapidated brick wall"
- Acanthosis
- Red, dyskeratotic rim surrounds nucleus
- Immunofluorescence is negative

Hailey–Hailey disease is an autosomal-dominant, inherited disease caused by mutations in the *ATP2C1* gene. This gene encodes for a portion of a calcium pump essential for proper keratinocyte differentiation and adhesion. Skin of the intertriginous areas is most often affected, and the appearance has been likened to "wet tissue paper." Acantholysis at all levels of the epidermis yields the histologic appearance of a "dilapidated brick wall." Although the disease itself is not immunologically mediated, superinfection of macerated skin by bacteria or yeast may engender an inflammatory infiltrate in the superficial dermis.

Differential Diagnosis

The Hailey–Hailey variant of Grover disease has similar histologic findings; however, in contrast to the broad lesions of benign familial pemphigus, there is less extensive and more focal involvement in Grover disease.

The negative DIF and observed dyskeratosis and follicular sparing in Hailey–Hailey disease allow distinction from pemphigus vulgaris. The acanthosis of benign familial pemphigus is a feature not typically identified in other blistering disorders.

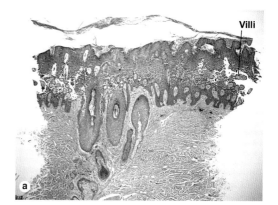

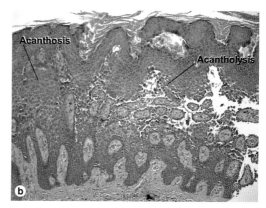

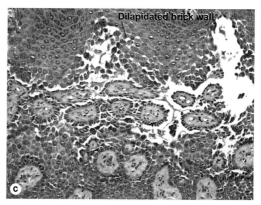

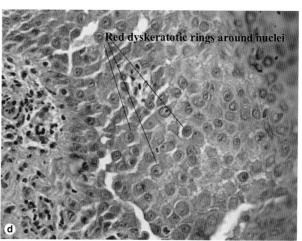

Fig. 9.8 Hailey–Hailey disease

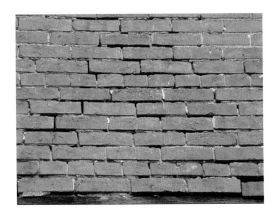

Fig. 9.9 Dilapidated brick wall for comparison to classic Hailey-Hailey disease

Keratosis follicularis (Darier disease)

Key Features

- Acantholytic dyskeratosis
- Acantholysis accentuated in the lower epidermis, yielding suprabasilar clefting
- More dyskeratosis than Hailey–Hailey disease
- Less acantholysis than Hailey–Hailey disease
- Grains (basophilic keratinocytes with elongated nuclei in or near the granular layer)
- Corps ronds (dyskeratotic keratinocytes with a round nucleus surrounded by a blue rim or clear halo)
- Hyperkeratosis and parakeratosis in the overlying stratum corneum
- Immunofluorescence studies are negative

PEARL

- Dyskeratotic keratinocytes in Hailey–Hailey disease have a red rim around the nucleus, whereas those in Darier disease usually have a blue or clear rim

---

The acantholysis results in suprabasal clefts (lacunae) that contain projections of papillary dermis covered by a single layer of basal cells (villi). There are two types of dyskeratotic cells. The granular layer and horny layer contain corps ronds, round dyskeratotic cells with pyknotic nuclei, a clear perinuclear halo, and pale to bright eosinophilic cytoplasm. Grains are seen in the granular layer as flattened, basophilic, dyskeratotic cells.

Darier disease is an autosomal-dominant disorder with greasy, yellow-brown, crusted, and hyperkeratotic lesions in the seborrheic areas. Other cutaneous findings include cobblestone papules of the mucosa, palmoplantar pits, verrucous lesions on the dorsal hands and feet (acrokeratosis verruciformis of Hopf), and red and white longitudinal nail streaks with distal "V" nicking. Similar to Hailey–Hailey disease, the gene responsible, *ATP2A2*, encodes a calcium pump.

Differential Diagnosis

The differential diagnosis of acantholytic dyskeratosis includes the Darier type of Grover disease where the degree of dyskeratosis is less extensive and more localized. The acantholysis and dyskeratosis of warty dyskeratoma are isolated to a solitary, cup-shaped, follicular configuration. Acantholytic dyskeratosis unrelated to Darier disease may occur in the genital region (vulvocrural dyskeratosis).

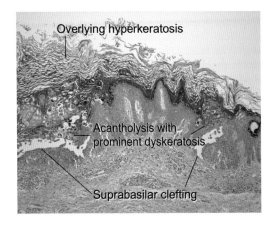

Fig. 9.10 Darier disease

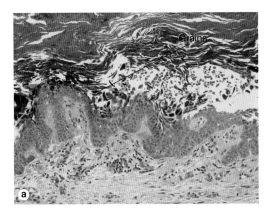

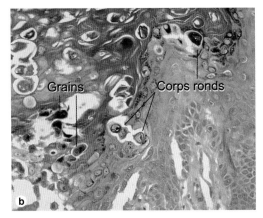

Fig. 9.11 Darier disease, corps ronds and grains

Transient acantholytic dermatosis (Grover disease)

Key Features

- Darier pattern with acantholysis and dyskeratosis
- Hailey–Hailey-like, full-thickness acantholysis
- Pemphigus pattern with partial-thickness acantholysis
- Spongiotic pattern with rare acantholytic cells

More than one of these patterns may be found in the same specimen. The clinical presentation, the mixture of histologic patterns, and the focal nature of the lesions help to distinguish the disease from histologic mimics. Eosinophils, if present, aid in differentiation from Darier disease. DIF is typically negative, in contrast to pemphigus.

Grover disease is an acquired, pruritic disorder most commonly affecting older men on the trunk. Typically there is a sudden onset of discrete, crusted papules. Despite the name, the eruption may or may not be transient. Heat, fever, and sweating precipitate this disorder. Despite histologic similarities to some genodermatoses, Grover disease is not an inherited disorder.

Paraneoplastic pemphigus

Key Features

- Variable intraepidermal acantholysis
- Dermal infiltrate of lymphocytes, which is often heavy and bandlike ("lichenoid")

- Interface reaction with necrotic keratinocytes and vacuolar change
- Subepidermal clefting is possible, though less common
- Focal epidermal spongiosis is possible
- DIF demonstrates "netlike" epidermal deposition of IgG and C3 (similar to pemphigus) and linear deposition at the dermoepidermal junction
- Indirect immunofluorescence on rat bladder epithelium is used for screening purposes

Paraneoplastic pemphigus demonstrates a wide variety of histologic patterns. The most common form represents a hybrid of classic pemphigus (intraepidermal acantholysis) and erythema multiforme (lichenoid lymphocytic infiltrate with interface reaction and necrotic keratinocytes). In one single study, 27% of cases had only suprabasilar acantholysis alone.

Multiple autoantibodies have been detected in paraneoplastic pemphigus, including those directed at desmoglein 1 (160 kD), desmoglein 3 (130 kD), desmoplakin I (250 kD), bullous pemphigoid antigen 1 (230 kD), envoplakin (210 kD), periplakin (190 kD), and an unnamed 170-kD antigen. In fact, as a screening measure, one can measure both pemphigus antibodies (DG1 and DG3) and bullous pemphigoid antibodies (BP230), and positivity for all three antibodies, at the same time and in the appropriate clinical setting, suggests the diagnosis.

Paraneoplastic pemphigus is more severe and recalcitrant to treatment than is pemphigus vulgaris. The disease often remits with cancer remission and recurs with cancer recurrence.

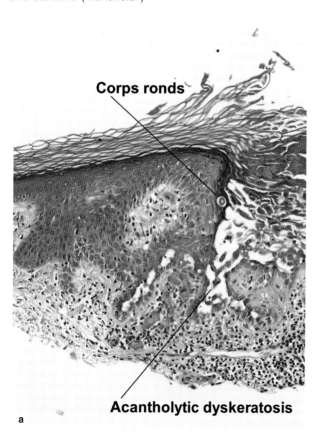

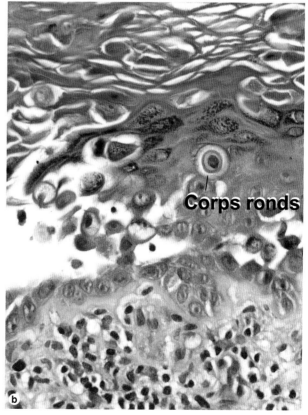

Fig. 9.12 Darier-type Grover disease

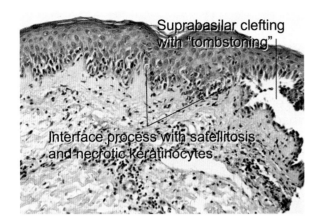

Fig. 9.13 Paraneoplastic pemphigus with intraepidermal acantholysis and interface dermatitis

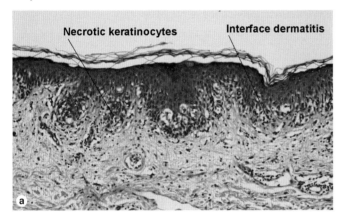

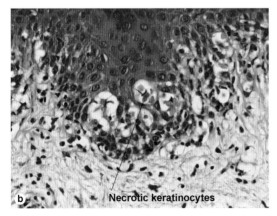

Fig. 9.14 Paraneoplastic pemphigus

Subepidermal vesiculobullous disorders: pauciinflammatory subepidermal conditions

Porphyria cutanea tarda

Key Features

- Subepidermal vesiculation
- Acral skin with compact orthokeratosis

- Solar elastosis (due to patient age and characteristic acral location)
- Minimal inflammatory infiltrate
- Protuberance of rigid dermal papillae into blister cavity ("festooning")
- Entrapped amphophilic basement membrane within the overlying epidermis ("caterpillar bodies")
- Perivascular hyaline material deposited in superficial dermis
- Periodic acid–Schiff staining may accentuate the perivascular deposition of hyaline material
- DIF demonstrates IgM and C3 in vessels (adsorbed by the hyaline material like a sponge)

Porphyria cutanea tarda is the most common form of porphyria in the United States. It is commonly associated with hepatitis C, alcohol ingestion, and iron overload. Inherited types result from reduced activity of uroporphyrinogen decarboxylase, an enzyme involved in heme synthesis. Blisters, erosions, and milia occur on the hands and other photoexposed locations.

Pseudoporphyria results in *essentially identical* clinical and histopathologic changes, but it is instead due to an exogenous medication. Naproxen sodium causes the majority of cases. No disturbance of porphyrin synthesis has been detected in pseudoporphyria. Pseudoporphyria may occur in young patients, and solar elastosis may not be demonstrated. Limited evidence suggests that occasional eosinophils may be more common in pseudoporphyria and festooning of the papillary dermis may not be as prominent.

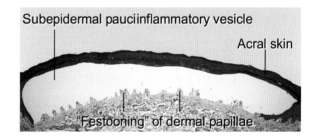

Fig. 9.15 Porphyria cutanea tarda (PCT)

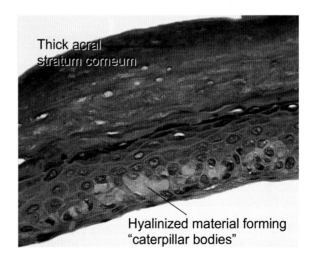

Fig. 9.16 PCT: caterpillar bodies

Epidermolysis bullosa acquisita

Key Features

- Subepidermal vesiculation
- Fibrin deposition in the floor of the blister cavity
- Some cases may show neutrophils within the papillary dermis, whereas other cases are histologically indistinguishable from bullous pemphigoid
- Dermal fibrosis (scar) may be present in the dermis
- Milia formation may be seen in late lesions
- DIF of adjacent skin demonstrates linear deposition of IgG and C3 at the dermoepidermal junction in a U-serrated pattern; IgA has been demonstrated in a significant number of cases

Epidermolysis bullosa acquisita (EBA) is caused by an antibody to type VII collagen, a major component of the anchoring fibrils. It is thought that deposition of immune complexes leads to the neutrophilic inflammation that is observed in some specimens.

The histology may overlap with bullous pemphigoid. Indirect immunofluorescence performed upon salt-split skin may be used to distinguish these overlapping conditions when the typical "U-shaped" and serrated pattern of EBA is not apparent by DIF.

In bullous pemphigoid, immunoreactants are deposited within the basement membrane zone and highlight the "roof" of salt-split skin, whereas in epidermolysis bullosa (and most forms of cicatricial pemphigoid), the immunoreactants mark the "floor" of salt-split skin.

Toxic epidermal necrolysis/Stevens–Johnson syndrome

Key Features

- Subepidermal vesiculation/sloughing with confluent necrosis of the epidermis
- Minimal inflammatory infiltrate
- Some cases may show a sparse superficial perivascular inflammatory infiltrate
- Overlap between toxic epidermal necrolysis and Stevens–Johnson syndrome exists
- Immunofluorescence is negative

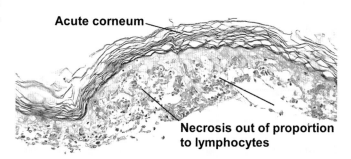

Fig. 9.18 Toxic epidermal necrolysis

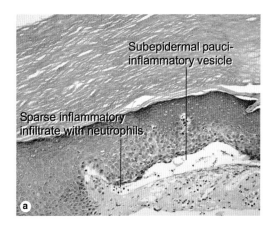

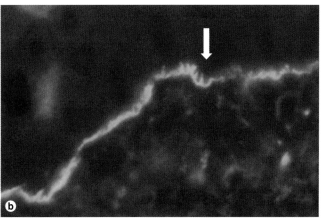

Fig. 9.17 (A) Epidermolysis bullosa acquisita. (B) Epidermolysis bullosa acquisita, DIF showing characteristic U-serrated pattern (*arrow*)

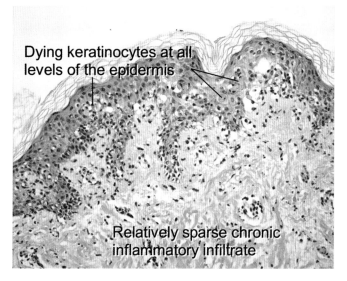

Fig. 9.19 Stevens–Johnson syndrome

Inflammatory subepidermal conditions

Bullous pemphigoid

Key Features

- Subepidermal bulla
- Eosinophils typically present within blister cavity
- In some patients, neutrophils predominate in the blister cavity
- Early lesions may demonstrate exocytosis of eosinophils within a mildly spongiotic epidermis ("eosinophilic spongiosis")
- Urticarial lesions may demonstrate eosinophils "lined up" along the dermoepidermal junction
- DIF of adjacent skin demonstrates linear deposition of C3 and IgG along the dermoepidermal junction in an N-serrated pattern
- Indirect immunofluorescence on salt-split skin demonstrates immunoreactants in the roof of the blister (compared with the same test in epidermolysis bullosa acquisita, which marks the floor)

Bullous pemphigoid usually occurs in older patients, although children are occasionally affected. The disease is associated with autoantibodies to bullous pemphigoid antigen I (230 kD) and/or bullous pemphigoid antigen II (180 kD). The latter antigen is most clearly linked to pathogenesis. Antibodies for BPI and BPII can be measured via ELISA-based technology, and in general, the levels titer to disease activity.

The subepidermal vesiculation of bullous pemphigoid results in firm and tense blisters. Intensely pruritic urticarial plaques, without clinically apparent vesiculation, may predate frankly bullous lesions ("urticarial pemphigoid"). Mucosal involvement is sometimes present, but, unlike pemphigus, it is rarely the first site of involvement.

Pemphigoid gestationis (also known as *herpes gestationis*) is a related vesiculobullous condition occurring in gravid women; it has essentially identical histopathologic and immunohistologic findings.

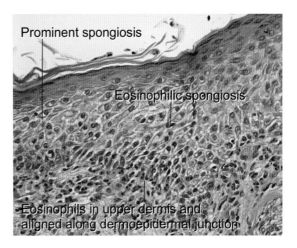

Fig. 9.21 Urticarial pemphigoid

Cicatricial pemphigoid

Key Features

- Subepidermal vesiculation
- Variable degree of inflammation in the dermis
- Neutrophilic microabscesses in the dermis may be identified in new lesions
- Cicatricial pemphigoid usually demonstrates fewer eosinophils than bullous pemphigoid
- Direct immunofluorescence of adjacent skin demonstrates linear deposition of IgG and C3 along the dermoepidermal junction in 80% of cases (also seen along appendageal structures)

Cicatricial pemphigoid refers to a heterogeneous group of scarring, subepidermal blistering disorders caused by a variety of autoantibodies. Tense bullae that heal with scarring are a common theme. Most subtypes involve oral or ocular mucosa. Lesions often recur at the same site, and this may lead to extensive dermal scarring. Paraneoplastic variants have been described in the literature.

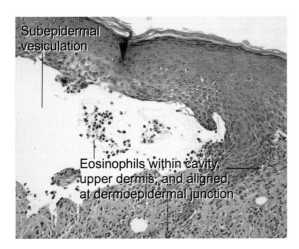

Fig. 9.20 Bullous pemphigoid

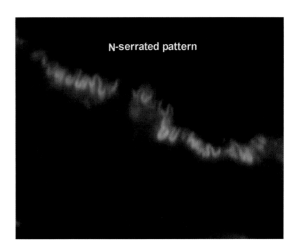

Fig. 9.22 Direct immunofluorescence of bullous pemphigoid showing linear deposition of IgG at the dermoepidermal junction

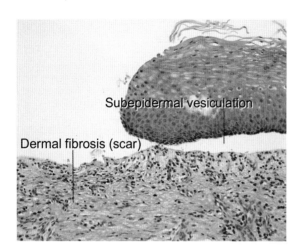

Fig. 9.23 Cicatricial pemphigoid

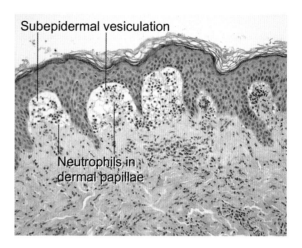

Fig. 9.24 Dermatitis herpetiformis

Dermatitis herpetiformis

Key Features

- Subepidermal vesiculation
- Neutrophilic abscesses in tips of dermal papillae
- Slight fibrin deposition in the tips of dermal papillae at points of vesiculation
- DIF demonstrates granular deposition of IgA within dermal papillae ± along dermoepidermal junction. Granules have a vertical "picket-fence" appearance

Dermatitis herpetiformis is an intensely pruritic, vesiculobullous disorder. Lesions are common upon the elbows, knees, buttocks, and scalp. Recent research indicates that epidermal transglutaminase-3 is the autoantigen in dermatitis herpetiformis. The disease is highly correlated with celiac disease (gluten-sensitive enteropathy). Essentially, all patients have some level of gastrointestinal pathology, even if it is subclinical. Strict gluten-free diets prevent clinical manifestations of the disease.

Granular deposition of IgA distinguishes dermatitis herpetiformis from linear IgA bullous dermatosis. Deposition is most marked in perilesional skin, with the densest deposits in dermal papillae. A vertical "picket fence" granule pattern may be apparent. Other immunoglobulins may be present in dermatitis herpetiformis; IgM is identified concurrently in up to 30% of cases.

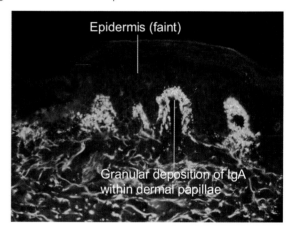

Fig. 9.25 Direct immunofluorescence of dermatitis herpetiformis showing granular deposition of IgA in the dermal papillae

Linear IgA bullous dermatosis

Key Features

- Subepidermal vesiculation
- Neutrophils are the predominant inflammatory cell
- Some cases may demonstrate scattered eosinophils and a mild perivascular lymphocytic inflammatory infiltrate
- DIF of adjacent skin demonstrates linear deposition of IgA along the dermoepidermal junction (the only immunoreactant present in 80% of cases)

Linear IgA is a heterogeneous, subepidermal, vesiculobullous disorder. In children, the disease is referred to as *chronic bullous dermatosis of childhood*. Both disorders are caused by autoantibodies targeting proteins (97–120 kD) that form as degradation products of bullous pemphigoid antigen II. Classically, the disease results in grouped annular lesions of tense bullae, which have been likened to a "string of pearls" or "clutch of jewels." Vancomycin may cause a drug-induced form of the disease.

By light microscopy, linear IgA bullous dermatosis overlaps significantly with dermatitis herpetiformis. It may be difficult to separate the two conditions without DIF examination.

PEARL

The differential diagnosis for neutrophils within dermal papillae or subepidermal collections of neutrophils:

Plaid
- Bullous **p**emphigoid
- **L**upus (bullous)
- EB**A**
- Linear **i**mmunoglobulin A bullous dermatosis (LABD)
- **D**ermatitis herpetiformis

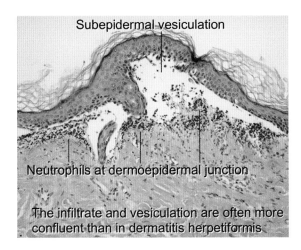

Fig. 9.26 Linear IgA bullous dermatosis

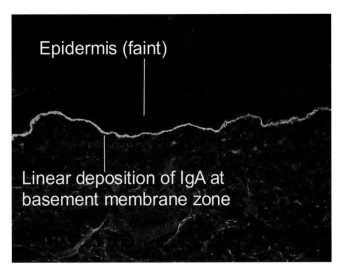

Fig. 9.27 Direct immunofluorescence showing linear deposition of IgA along dermoepidermal junction

Bullous lupus erythematosus

Key Features

- Subepidermal bulla with neutrophils
- Immunoreactants on floor of salt-split skin
- Other features of lupus may be present

Key Features

- Midepidermal necrosis
- Serum may be present

Further reading

Chhabra S, Minz RW, Saikia B. Immunofluorescence in dermatology. Indian J Dermatol Venereol Leprol 2012;78(6):677–91.

Connor BL, Marks R, Jones EW. Dermatitis herpetiformis: histologic discriminants. Trans St Johns Hosp Dermatol Soc 1972;58:191–8.

Fung MA, Murphy MJ, Hoss DM, et al. The sensitivity and specificity of "caterpillar bodies" in the differential diagnosis of subepidermal blistering disorders. Am J Dermatopathol 2003;25:287–90.

Horn TD, Anhalt GJ. Histologic features of paraneoplastic pemphigus. Arch Dermatol 1992;128:1091–5.

Jeong SJ, Lee CW. Bullous pemphigoid: persistent lesions of eczematous/urticarial erythemas. Cutis 1995;56:225–6.

Letko E, Papaliodis DN, Papaliodis GN, et al. Stevens–Johnson syndrome and toxic epidermal necrolysis: a review of the literature. Ann Allergy Asthma Immunol 2005;94:419–36.

Liu AY, Valenzuela R, Helm TN, et al. Indirect immunofluorescence on rat bladder transitional epithelium: a test with high specificity for paraneoplastic pemphigus. J Am Acad Dermatol 1993;28:696–9.

Nishioka K, Hashimoto K, Katayama I, et al. Eosinophilic spongiosis in bullous pemphigoid. Arch Dermatol 1984;120:1166–8.

Quirk CJ, Heenan PJ. Grover's disease: 34 years on. Australas J Dermatol 2004;45:83–6.

Sardy M, Karpati S, Merkl B, et al. Epidermal transglutaminase (TGase 3) is the autoantigen of dermatitis herpetiformis. J Exp Med 2002;195:747–57.

Schmidt E, Zillikens D. Pemphigoid diseases. Lancet 2013;381(9863):320–32.

Tsuruta D, Dainichi T, Hamada T, et al. Molecular diagnosis of autoimmune blistering diseases. Methods Mol Biol 2013;961:17–32.

Yeh SW, Ahmed B, Sami N, et al. Blistering disorders: diagnosis and treatment. Dermatol Ther 2003;16:214–23.

Granulomatous and histiocytic diseases

Tammie Ferringer

Granulomas are discrete collections of histiocytes with or without multinucleate giant cells. Histiocytes are bone marrow derived or mesenchymal. In granulomas, their cytoplasmic membranes touch with no intervening connective tissue. Infectious etiologies, especially fungal and mycobacterial, should be excluded with special stains in any granulomatous process without obvious etiology. Examination under polarized light is required to exclude birefringent foreign material.

Granulomas can be categorized into sarcoidal, tuberculoid, palisading, and suppurative. Sarcoidal granulomas, composed of epithelioid histiocytes, are "naked" granulomas with a paucity of surrounding infiltrate. Tuberculoid granulomas are associated with a peripheral mononuclear infiltrate and may show central caseous necrosis. Palisading granulomas surround devitalized collagen (necrobiosis), mucin, or foreign material. Suppurative granulomas have a central collection of neutrophils (stellate abscess).

Granuloma annulare

Key Features

Interstitial pattern
• Patchy interstitial histiocytes, lymphocytes, and mucin give the appearance of a "busy dermis" at low power

Palisading pattern
• Histiocytes surround altered dermal collagen and mucin

Granuloma annulare typically involves the upper- to mid-reticular dermis. The mucin in palisading lesions is usually apparent with routine staining as faint feathery blue material; however, colloidal iron or other mucin stains can be used for confirmation. Sparse multinucleate histiocytes are typically identified, and eosinophils occur in approximately half of cases. Rarely, perforation of the process through the epidermis (transepidermal elimination) occurs.

The subcutaneous tissue can be involved. Subcutaneous or deep granuloma annulare typically consists of histiocytes palisading around fibrin rather than mucin. It may be indistinguishable from rheumatoid nodule, resulting in its designation as pseudorheumatoid nodule. This subtype of granuloma annulare typically occurs on the lower legs, hands, head, and buttock in young individuals without rheumatoid disease.

The microscopic differential diagnosis of granuloma annulare and other palisading granulomas includes epithelioid sarcoma. Clues to this malignant neoplasm include necrosis and mild cytologic atypia. Epithelioid sarcoma demonstrates a biphasic pattern with transition between epithelioid and spindle cells. Cells stain for both keratin and vimentin.

Table 10.1 shows distinctions between granuloma annulare and necrobiosis lipoidica.

Table 10.1 Features of granuloma annulare and necrobiosis lipoidica

Feature	Granuloma annulare	Necrobiosis lipoidica
Distribution	Focal and patchy	Diffuse and full thickness
Granuloma	Palisaded or interstitial	Horizontal tiers (layers)
Mucin	Yes	No
Shape of punch biopsy	Tapered	Rectangular
Plasma cells	Rare	Common
Cholesterol clefts	No	Occasional

Differential Diagnosis

The microscopic differential for a "busy dermis" includes (see Appendix 1):
• Blue nevus
• Dermatofibroma
• Dermal Spitz nevus
• Metastatic breast carcinoma
• Kaposi sarcoma (patch stage)
• Granuloma annulare
• Scleromyxedema
• Neurofibroma

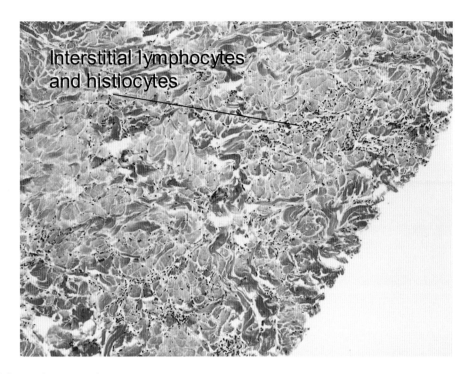

Fig. 10.1 Interstitial granuloma annulare

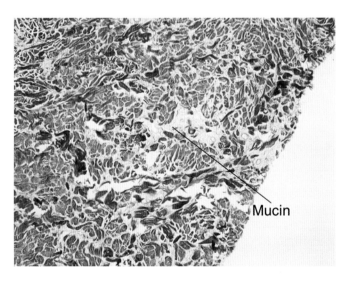

Fig. 10.2 Interstitial granuloma annulare (colloidal iron)

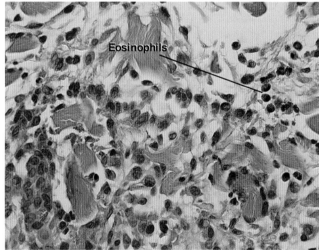

Fig. 10.3 Granuloma annulare

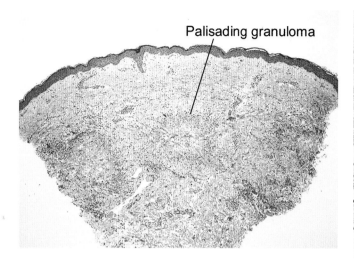

Fig. 10.4 Palisading granuloma annulare

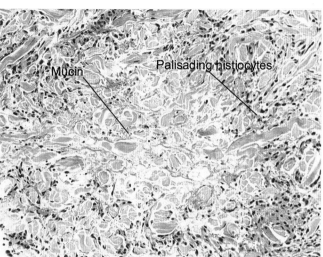

Fig. 10.5 Palisading granuloma annulare

Actinic granuloma

Key Features

- Solar elastosis
- Similar palisade to granuloma annulare but no mucin
- Elastic fibers are engulfed by palisading giant cells and histiocytes (elastolysis)
- Central loss of elastic tissue

These lesions occur on areas of chronic sun damage such as the face, neck, hands, and arms. They have a raised border and an atrophic, finely wrinkled center. The granulomas consume actinically damaged elastic tissue. Other names have included Miescher facial granuloma, atypical necrobiosis lipoidica of the face and scalp, and annular elastolytic giant cell granuloma. Some consider it to be a variant of granuloma annulare on sun-damaged skin. The central loss of elastic tissue, absence of mucin, and conspicuous multinucleated histiocytes are the primary basis for distinguishing these lesions.

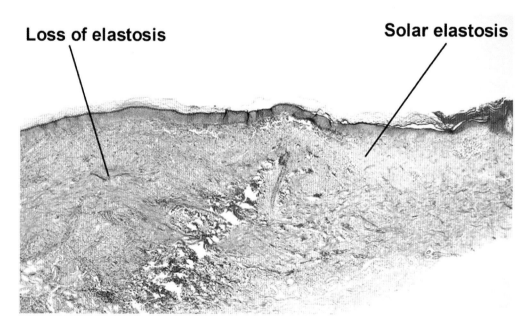

Fig. 10.6 Actinic granuloma

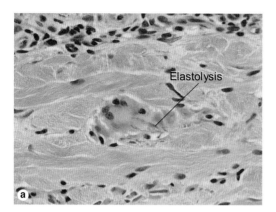

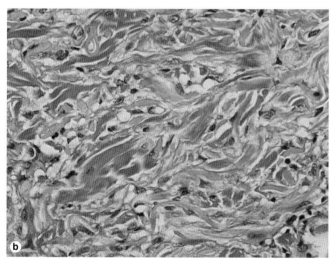

Fig. 10.7 Actinic granuloma

Necrobiosis lipoidica

Key Features

- Horizontal, acellular, pale, degenerated collagen between layers of granuloma
- Top-to-bottom and side-to-side involvement
- Plasma cells common in the deep dermis
- No mucin
- Rectangular punch due to sclerosis
- May see cholesterol clefts or lymphoid nodules
- Very early lesions can resemble interstitial granuloma annulare

A large proportion of patients with necrobiosis lipoidica have diabetes, thus the original name necrobiosis lipoidica diabeticorum. However, fewer than 1% of patients with diabetes have necrobiosis lipoidica. The pretibial area is the most common site, but other areas of the lower extremities, arms, hands, and trunk can rarely be involved.

Necrobiosis lipoidica is considered a palisading granulomatous dermatitis. The palisade is horizontally arranged in tiers like the layers of lasagna. The full thickness of the dermis and often the subcutis is involved.

The term *necrobiosis* refers to alteration of dermal connective tissue with loss of definition, pale staining, and absence of nuclei.

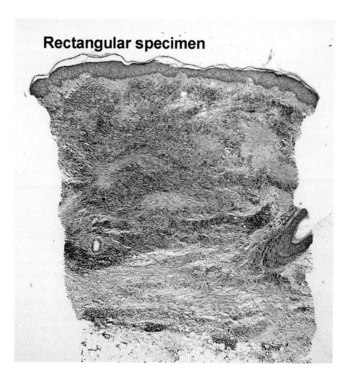

Fig. 10.8 Necrobiosis lipoidica

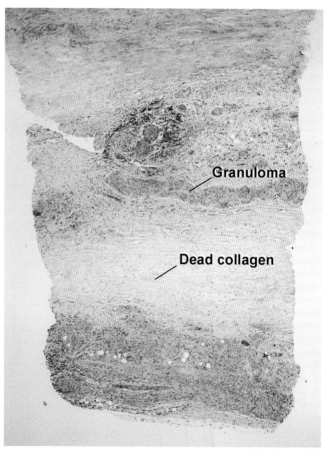

Fig. 10.9 Necrobiosis lipoidica

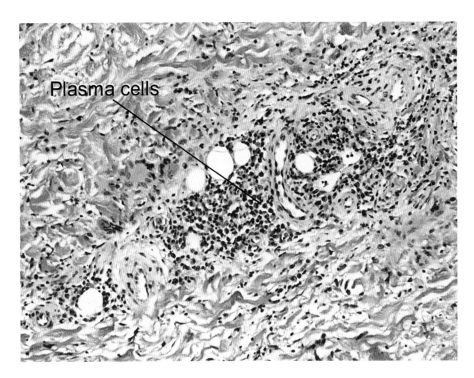

Fig. 10.10 Necrobiosis lipoidica

Rheumatoid nodule

Key Features

- Large palisading granuloma surrounding deeply staining eosinophilic fibrin

- Deep dermis and subcutis
- No mucin

The histology mimics subcutaneous granuloma annulare and rheumatic fever nodules. Rarely similar nodules occur in systemic lupus erythematosus.

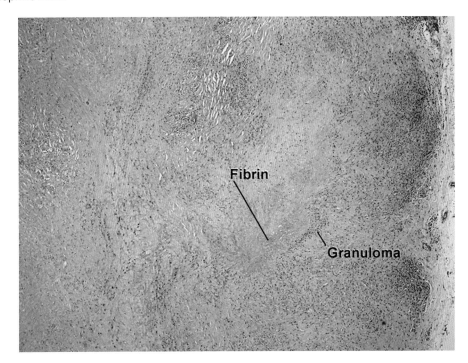

Fig. 10.11 Rheumatoid nodule

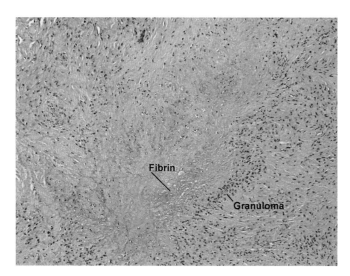

Fig. 10.12 Rheumatoid nodule

Lupus miliaris disseminatus faciei (LMDF: acne agminata)

Key Features

- Small, pealike palisaded granuloma with central caseous necrosis

Despite its histologic resemblance to miliary tuberculosis, LMDF is a variant of rosacea. LMDF can be distinguished from miliary tuberculosis by the absence of acid-fast bacilli.

Caseation has a dull, pale pink amorphous appearance, unlike the deeply staining fibrin of a rheumatoid nodule.

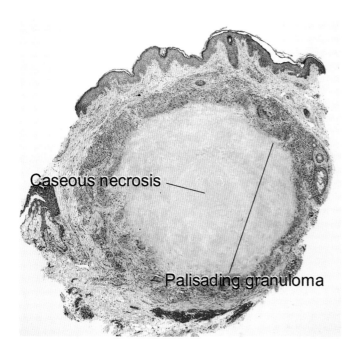

Fig. 10.13 Lupus miliaris disseminatus faciei (LMDF)

Sarcoidosis

Key Features

- Epithelioid histiocytes forming discrete "naked" granulomas with minimal lymphocytic infiltrate
- No necrosis

Cutaneous lesions are present in up to one quarter of patients with systemic sarcoidosis, but cutaneous lesions can occur in the absence of systemic disease in one quarter of patients.

Asteroid bodies and Schaumann bodies can be found in sarcoidosis but are not specific and have been observed in other granulomas such as tuberculosis, leprosy, and berylliosis. An eosinophilic star-burst inclusion within a giant cell is an asteroid body. Schaumann bodies are cytoplasmic, laminated calcifications.

Sarcoidosis is a diagnosis of exclusion requiring clinicopathologic correlation. Infectious etiologies, including acid-fast bacilli and fungi, should be sought with special stains. The granulomas should be polarized to rule out foreign body. However, the presence of small crystalline refractile silica material does not exclude the possibility of sarcoidosis. In fact, silica granulomas may be the earliest manifestation of sarcoidosis ("scar sarcoid").

Differential Diagnosis

The microscopic differential for "naked" granulomas includes:
- Sarcoidosis
- Cutaneous Crohn disease: perioral or perianal lesions with bowel symptoms
- Cheilitis granulomatosa (Melkersson–Rosenthal syndrome): on the lip
- Tuberculoid leprosy: granulomas follow nerves and acid-fast bacilli may be present
- Silica granuloma/scar sarcoid: polarizable material
- Granulomatous rosacea: adjacent to follicles
- Zirconium and beryllium granulomas: require high index of suspicion and spectrographic analysis

Necrobiotic xanthogranuloma (NXG)

Key Features

- X-shaped red zones of necrosis within granulomatous nodule (X-shaped necrosis in N**X**G)
- Lipidized histiocytes and multinucleate wreath giant cells, including Touton giant cells
- Dermis and subcutis involved
- Neutrophilic debris within necrotic areas
- Cholesterol clefts
- Plasma cells and lymphoid follicles

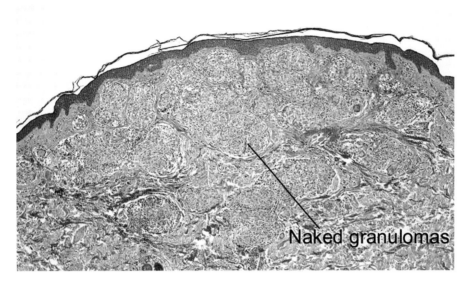

Fig. 10.14 Sarcoidosis

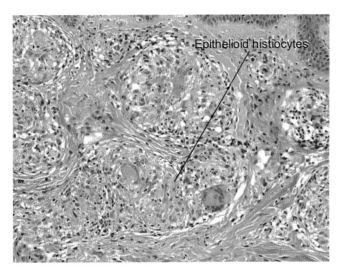

Fig. 10.15 Sarcoidosis

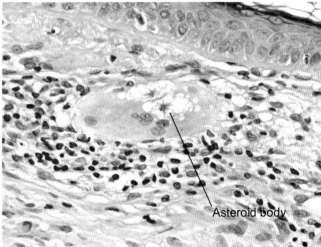

Fig. 10.16 Asteroid body

If the layered appearance of necrobiosis lipoidica is likened to strips of bacon, then the appearance of NXG resembles "pepper bacon" or "dirty cholesterol-laden bacon," with karyorrhectic debris making up the "pepper" or "dirt." The differentiation from necrobiosis lipoidica can be made clinically by the periorbital predominance and associated immunoglobulin (Ig) G (usually kappa) paraproteinemia in NXG. NXG is more cellular, has a greater proportion of foamy histiocytes, and contains more giant cells than necrobiosis lipoidica.

Touton giant cells have a ring of nuclei and a peripheral rim of foamy cytoplasm. Touton giant cells are also common in juvenile xanthogranuloma, dermatofibroma, and NXG.

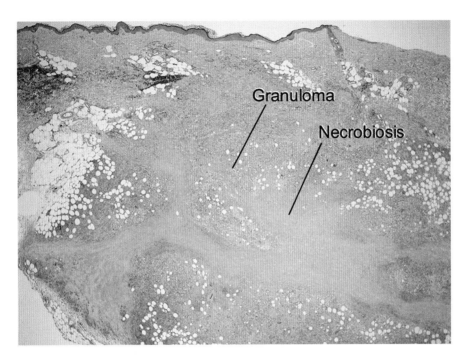

Fig. 10.17 Necrobiotic xanthogranuloma: The zones of necrosis typically intersect, producing an X shape in NXG

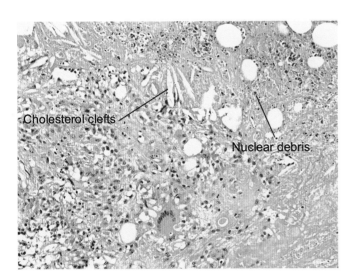

Fig. 10.18 Necrobiotic xanthogranuloma

Xanthogranuloma

Key Features

- Early: sea of purple histiocytes in the papillary and reticular dermis
- Later: wreath giant cells appear
- Late: lipidized histiocytes and Touton giant cells
- Secondarily inflamed with lymphocytes and eosinophils

Xanthogranulomas can be seen at any age, but are most common in children, giving rise to the name *juvenile xanthogranulomas*.

Early xanthogranulomas are clinically red and consist of numerous histiocytes with abundant cytoplasm, giving the impression of a sea of lavender histologically. Over time, the histiocytes become lipidized and the lesion clinically becomes yellow-orange. At this point, Touton giant cells, with a wreath of nuclei surrounded by foamy cytoplasm, are identified. Regressing lesions show a proliferation of fibroblasts and fibrosis. In contrast to those in dermatofibromas, the Touton giant cells in xanthogranulomas don't contain hemosiderin.

In children with multiple xanthogranulomas, an eye exam should be considered, as ocular involvement can result in glaucoma or anterior-chamber hemorrhage. Visceral xanthogranulomas with pericarditis have been reported. An association between xanthogranuloma, neurofibromatosis I, and juvenile chronic myelogenous leukemia has been reported.

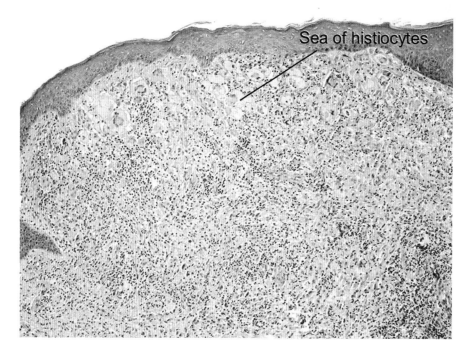

Fig. 10.19 Xanthogranuloma

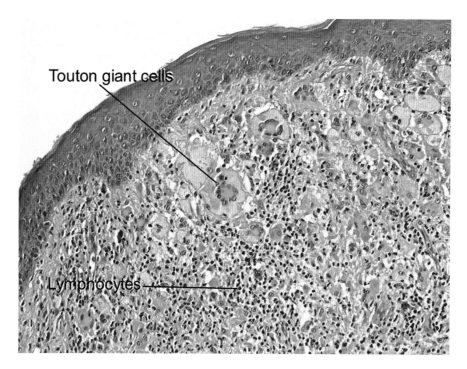

Fig. 10.20 Xanthogranuloma

Reticulohistiocytic granuloma (solitary reticulohistiocytoma)

Key Features

- Sea of purple histiocytes in dermis
- Each histiocyte often sits in a punched-out lacuna
- Cytoplasm of histiocyte is two-toned with darker and lighter areas
- Cytoplasm is dusty rose or ground glass
- Binucleate and multinucleate cells occur

Multinucleate cells typically have irregularly arranged vesicular nuclei containing prominent nucleoli. There are admixed lymphocytes and lesser numbers of eosinophils and neutrophils. Older lesions are less inflammatory and reveal cells with artifactual halos around them due to retraction.

Lesions can be solitary or multiple. When multiple they may be associated with systemic findings. Multicentric reticulohistiocytosis consists of multiple lesions with deforming arthritis, coral beading around the nail folds, and an associated internal malignancy in 10% of cases.

Differential Diagnosis

Xanthogranulomas have more foamy cells, including Touton giant cells, and are much less likely to have cells with ground-glass cytoplasm.

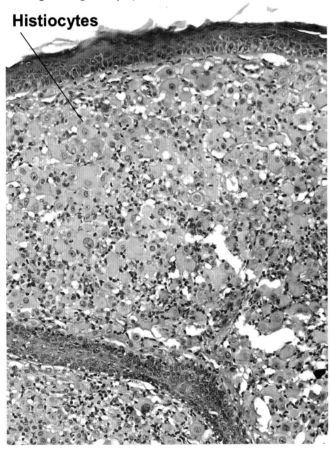

Fig. 10.21 Reticulohistiocytic granuloma

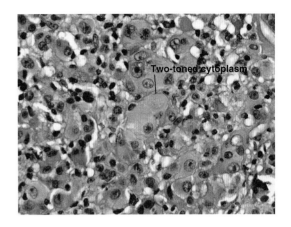

Fig. 10.22 Reticulohistiocytic granuloma

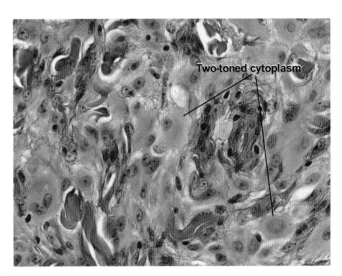

Fig. 10.23 Reticulohistiocytic granuloma

Rosai–Dorfman disease (sinus histiocytosis with massive lymphadenopathy)

Key Features

- Fibrotic nodules showing light and dark areas
- Sheets of histiocytes (light areas) with nodules of lymphoytes (dark areas)
- Emperipolesis (intact cells, especially lymphocytes and plasma cells, passing through histiocytes)
- S100 positive, CD1a negative, CD68 positive

Rosai–Dorfman disease typically occurs in the first two decades of life as painless cervical adenopathy and fever. There is extranodal involvement in one third of cases. Skin lesions are found in approximately 10% with a predilection for the eyelids and the malar area. Occasionally, the skin is the only site of involvement. Emperipolesis is a phenomenon where lymphocytes and plasma cells pass through histiocytes, but are not found within phagolysosomes.

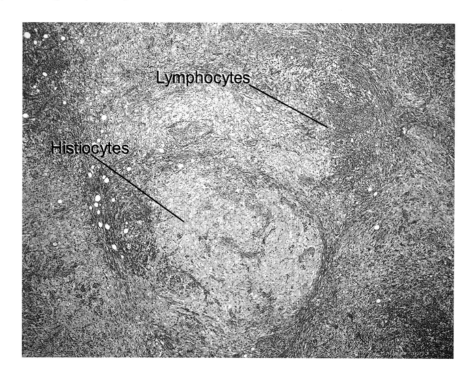

Fig. 10.24 Rosai–Dorfman disease

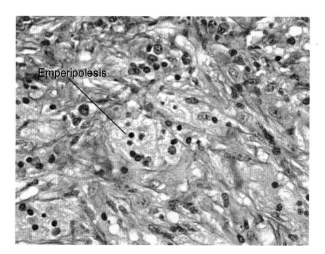

Fig. 10.25 Rosai–Dorfman disease emperipolesis

Langerhans cell histiocytosis (histiocytosis X)

Key Features

- Polymorphous infiltrate, including eosinophils with prominent edema and hemorrhage
- Reniform (kidney bean-shaped) nuclei
- Folliculotropism common in acute type
- S100 positive, CD1a positive, langerin (CD207) positive

The infiltrate can be a perivascular, bandlike, or periappendageal pattern. Variable eosinophils, lymphocytes, and sparse neutrophils accompany the characteristic large cells with lobulated, notched, or grooved nuclei that resemble kidney beans. Due to the edema, these cells appear to be "floating in the sea." Acute Langerhans cell histiocytosis is described in further detail in Chapter 15.

In the past, Langerhans cell histiocytosis was subclassified into Letterer–Siwe disease, Hand–Schüller–Christian disease, or eosinophilic granuloma, based on the clinical findings. Eosinophilic granuloma is typically localized to one site, such as bone or skin, whereas the other two affect several organ systems. Hand–Schüller–Christian disease is typically associated with the triad of diabetes insipidus, exophthalmos, and lytic bone lesions. Letterer–Siwe disease is more disseminated and involves multiple organs. Because many patients do not clearly fit into these categories, the prognosis is currently based on the patient's age, number of organs involved, and the degree of organ dysfunction. Children are most commonly affected, but adult cases have been observed. The scalp, ears, and intertriginous areas are preferred cutaneous sites.

Similar to Langerhans cells of normal skin, Birbeck granules, with the appearance of a tennis racket, are pathognomonic ultrastructural markers (see Appendix 2).

Congenital self-healing "reticulohistiocytosis" is a form of Langerhans cell histiocytosis that generally presents with one or several cutaneous nodules at or shortly after birth and resolves spontaneously.

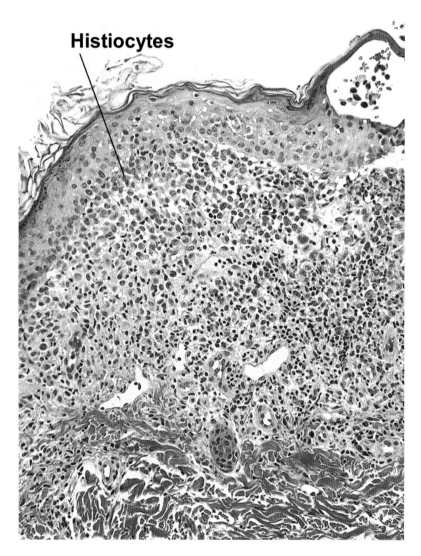

Histiocytes

Fig. 10.26 Langerhans cell histiocytosis

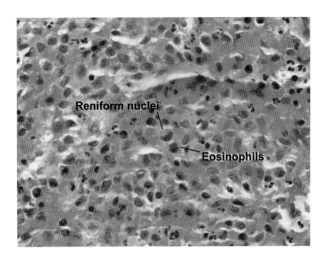

Fig. 10.27 Langerhans cell histiocytosis

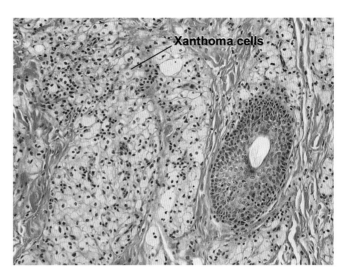

Fig. 10.28 Xanthelasma

Xanthomas

Xanthomas represent the accumulation of lipid in histiocytes, known as *foam cells* or *xanthoma cells*. Xanthomas can be subdivided by clinical morphology, anatomic location, and mode of development into tuberous, tendinous, eruptive, planar, and verruciform. Many are associated with inherited or acquired disorders of lipoprotein metabolism, but normolipemic planar xanthoma is related to plasma cell dyscrasia.

Planar xanthomas are further subdivided on the basis of their location into xanthelasma, intertriginous xanthomas, xanthoma striatum palmaris, and diffuse (generalized) plane xanthomas.

Intertriginous xanthomas are pathognomonic of homozygous familial hypercholesterolemia. Xanthoma striatum palmaris is characteristic of familial dysbetalipoproteinemia (type III) and, as the name describes, is identified in the palmar creases. The great majority of patients with diffuse plane xanthomas are normolipemic, and there is an association with IgG paraproteinemia and progression to myeloma.

Xanthelasma

Key Features

- Thin skin, many vellus follicles, and striated muscle suggest the eyelid location
- Foam cells form a band in the superficial or mid-dermis

Xanthelasma are the most common form of xanthoma and are characterized by periorbital yellowish plaques. Lipid levels are normal in around half of patients.

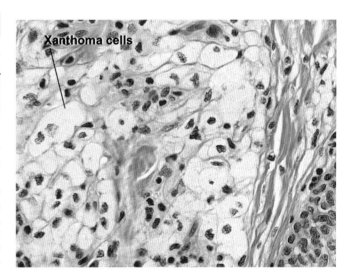

Fig. 10.29 Xanthelasma

Tuberous xanthoma

Key Features

- Fibrotic nodule with variable and occasionally sparse foam cells
- Cholesterol clefts may be found

Tuberous xanthomas are typically seen on the elbows, knees, and buttock in cases with an increase in chylomicron and very-low-density lipoprotein (VLDL) remnants. These lesions are most characteristic of familial dysbetalipoproteinemia (type II), but can also be seen in homozygous and heterozygous hypercholesterolemia, hepatic cholestasis, cerebrotendinous xanthoma, and β-sitosterolemia.

Tendinous xanthomas are histologically similar to tuberous xanthomas, except they occur in ligaments, fasciae, and tendons, especially the tendons of the hands and feet and the Achilles tendon. These lesions are most common with severe familial hypercholesterolemia.

Eruptive xanthoma

Key Features

- Foam cells and extracellular lipid
- Scattered lymphocytes and neutrophils, especially in early lesions

The lipid deposition in the dermis is so rapid in eruptive lesions that the phagocytic capacity of the histiocytes is overwhelmed, resulting in free or extracellular lipid.

Eruptive lesions are most common on the buttock and thigh as crops of yellow papules with a red halo. These lesions are associated with an increase in triglycerides, as in uncontrolled diabetes, hypothyroidism, after alcohol ingestion, and use of exogenous estrogens or retinoids. In the Frederickson classification of hyperlipidemias, they can be seen in type I (elevated chylomicrons), typically due to abnormal or deficient lipoprotein lipase or Apo C-II deficiency, type IV (elevated VLDLs), and type V (elevated chylomicrons and VLDLs).

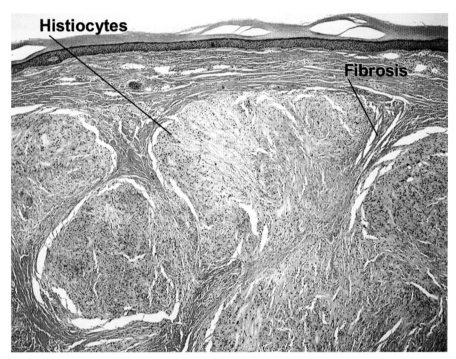

Fig. 10.30 Tuberous xanthoma

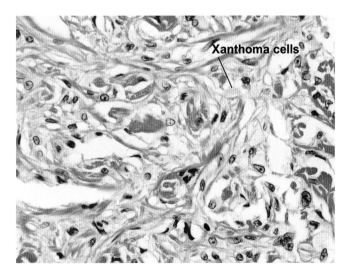

Fig. 10.31 Tuberous xanthoma

Differential Diagnosis

Histologically, eruptive xanthomas may be confused with granuloma annulare at scan. However, on close inspection, there is intracellular and extracellular lipid in the xanthoma rather than extracellular mucin of granuloma annulare. Gout may also be considered in the differential diagnosis, but the material deposited in gout is feathery and there are no foam cells.

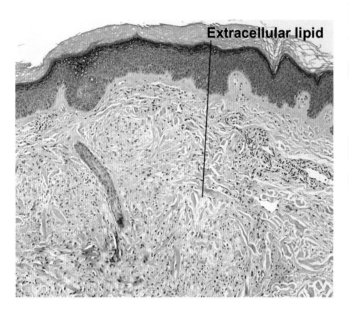

Fig. 10.32 Eruptive xanthoma

Verruciform xanthoma

Key Features

- Papillomatosis
- Foam cells in the dermal papillae
- Red to orange V-shaped wedges of parakeratosis with neutrophils

Verruciform xanthomas are not associated with increased serum lipids and may be due to degeneration of or damage to cells in the overlying epidermis. Oral lesions are common, although genital sites, extragenital skin, and nail beds may be involved.

Differential Diagnosis

The low-power appearance is that of verruca. Close inspection reveals the foamy histiocytes.

Gout

Key Features

- Palisaded granuloma surrounding amorphous, gray-blue material with a feathery appearance
- Uric acid crystals are doubly refractile with polarization if tissue is fixed in ethanol or incompletely fixed in formalin

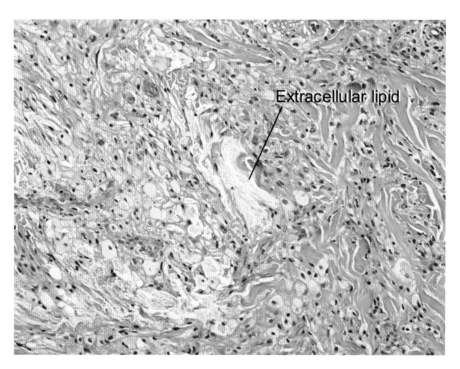

Fig. 10.33 Eruptive xanthoma

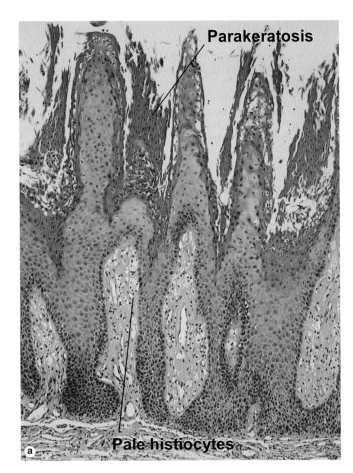

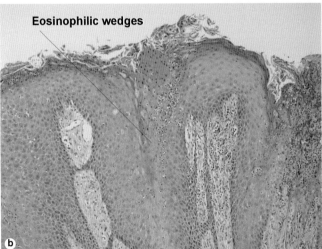

Fig. 10.34 Verruciform xanthoma: the red V-shaped zones of necrotic epithelium with neutrophils are like arrows pointing downward toward the inconspicuous xanthoma cells

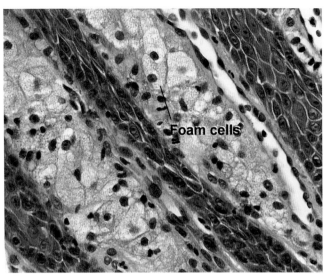

Fig. 10.35 Verruciform xanthoma

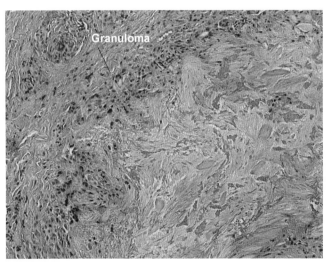

Fig. 10.36 Gout

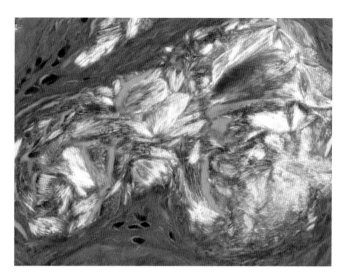

Fig. 10.37 Gout (polarized microscopy)

Foreign-body granuloma

Key Features

- Foreign-body giant cells typically have randomly distributed nuclei
- Polarizable foreign body may be present
- Caution: The presence of polarizable silica does not rule out the possibility of sarcoidosis

Any material foreign to the dermis or fat can elicit a granulomatous response, including keratin from a ruptured cyst, hemostatic agents, splinter, and cosmetic fillers (see Appendix 3).

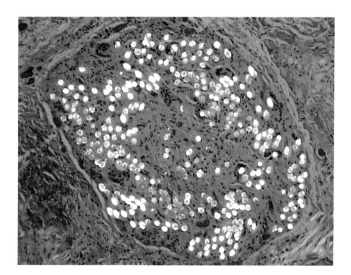

Fig. 10.38 Foreign-body granuloma to suture material (polarized microscopy)

Further reading

Beatty EC Jr. Rheumatic-like nodules occurring in nonrheumatic children. AMA Arch Pathol 1959;68(2):154–9.

de Oliveira FL, de Barros Silveira LK, Machado Ade M, et al. Hybrid clinical and histopathological pattern in annular lesions: an overlap between annular elastolytic giant cell granuloma and granuloma annulare? Case Rep Dermatol Med 2012;102915.

Hanno R, Needelman A, Eiferman RA, et al. Cutaneous sarcoidal granulomas and the development of systemic sarcoidosis. Arch Dermatol 1981;117(4):203–7.

Mitteldorf C, Tronnier M. Histologic features of granulomatous skin diseases. J Dtsch Dermatol Ges 2016;14(4):378–88.

Mohsin SK, Lee MW, Amin MB, et al. Cutaneous verruciform xanthoma: a report of five cases investigating the etiology and nature of xanthomatous cells. Am J Surg Pathol 1998;22(4):479–87.

O'Brien JP. Actinic granuloma. An annular connective tissue disorder affecting sun- and heat-damaged (elastotic) skin. Arch Dermatol 1975;111(4):460–6.

Silverman RA, Rabinowitz AD. Eosinophils in the cellular infiltrate of granuloma annulare. J Cutan Pathol 1985;12(1):13–17.

Walsh NM, Hanly JG, Tremaine R, et al. Cutaneous sarcoidosis and foreign bodies. Am J Dermatopathol 1993;15(3):203–7.

Wick MR. Granulomatous & histiocytic dermatitides. Semin Diagn Pathol 2017;34(3):301–11.

Inflammatory vascular diseases

Dirk M. Elston

Leukocytoclastic vasculitis (LCV)

Key Features

- Perivascular infiltrate with neutrophils
- Karyorrhexis (nuclear dust, leukocytoclasis)

- Expansion of the vessel wall
- Fibrin deposition within the vessel wall
- Erythrocyte extravasation

Clinical lesions of leukocytoclastic vasculitis are purpuric and often palpable. Vasculitis involving arterioles commonly produces livedo reticularis or stellate infarcts.

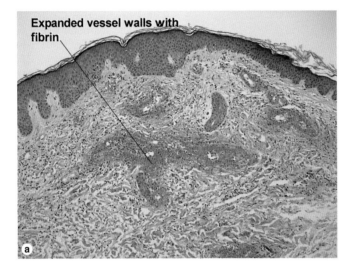

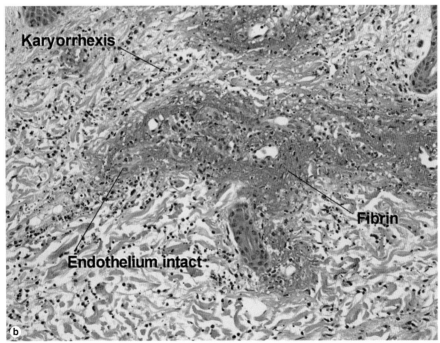

Fig. 11.1 Leukocytoclastic vasculitis

Classification of vasculitis

Vasculitis is classified by the type of inflammatory infiltrate, type of vessel involved, the presence or absence of endothelial necrosis, associated systemic findings, immunofluorescent patterns, and serologic findings. American College of Rheumatology (ACR) classification criteria are mostly clinical, with little emphasis on histologic findings. The Chapel Hill criteria include histologic features, especially vessel size. Because many entities demonstrate involvement of vessels of various sizes, any classification will have limitations.

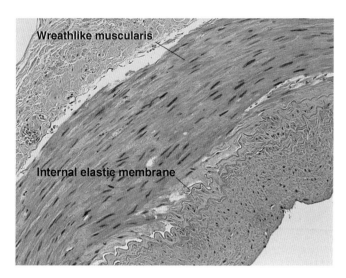

Fig. 11.2 Characteristic features of an artery

Large vessel vasculitis

When a large vessel is involved by vasculitis, it is critical to determine whether the involved vessel is an artery or a vein. Arteries are characteristically round, with a wreathlike muscularis and an internal elastic membrane. Veins are characteristically oval, with a bundled muscularis. They may have visible valves and lack an internal elastic membrane. So-called *arterialization* of veins occurs when they are subjected to elevated hydrostatic pressure. This phenomenon is occasionally noted in cutaneous vessels, but is best demonstrated in coronary artery bypass grafts. The grafted vein develops a prominent internal elastic membrane, but retains the bundled muscularis characteristic of a vein.

Giant cell arteritis (temporal arteritis)

Key Features

- Muscular artery with wreathlike muscularis and prominent internal elastic membrane
- Subendothelial granulomatous inflammation
- With progression, becomes transmural inflammation
- Incidental atherosclerotic changes (calcification, subintimal plaques) often present in the vessel

Temporal arteritis often involves the vessel in a focal, beaded fashion, so an adequate length of temporal artery (ideally 2 cm) should be submitted for examination.

Chapel Hill criteria

Granulomatous arteritis involving the major branches of the aorta, with a predilection for the extracranial branches of the carotid artery. The temporal artery is frequently involved. Patients are usually >50 years of age. Frequently associated with polymyalgia rheumatica.

American College of Rheumatology criteria

Age >50; new headache; abnormal temporal artery clinically; elevated sedimentation rate; positive temporal artery biopsy (three criteria give >93% sensitivity, >91% specificity).

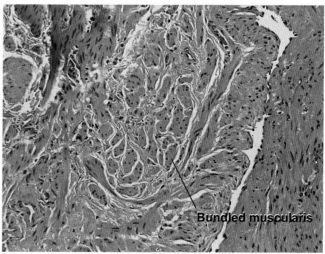

Fig. 11.3 Characteristic features of a vein

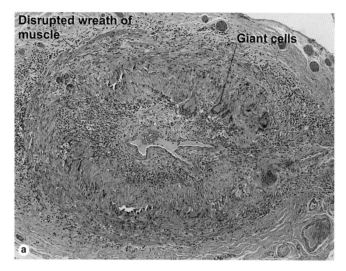

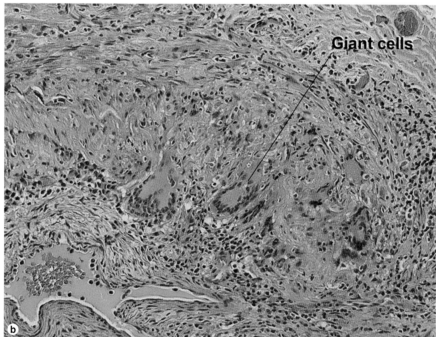

Fig. 11.4 Temporal arteritis

Takayasu arteritis

Key Features

- Granulomatous vasculitis involving large muscular arteries

Chapel Hill criteria

Granulomatous arteritis involving the aorta and its major branches. Usually <50 years of age.

American College of Rheumatology criteria

Age <40; claudication; decreased pulses; >10 mmHg difference in pressure between arms; bruits; abnormal arteriogram (three criteria give >90% sensitivity, >97% specificity).

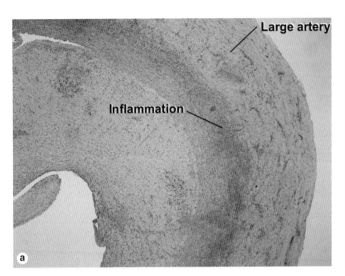

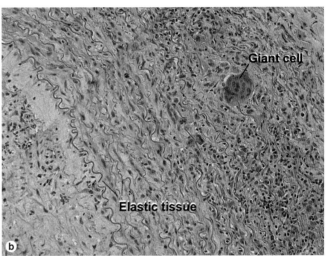

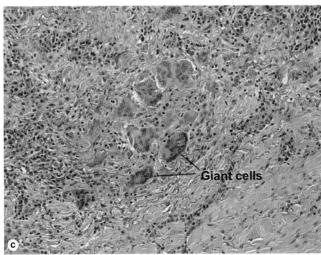

Fig. 11.5 Takayasu arteritis

Polyarteritis nodosa

Key Features

- Large artery involved, typically in the deep dermis or subcutaneous tissue
- Often involves branch points of vessels
- Acute phase is neutrophilic with karyorrhexis
- Chronic phase may demonstrate a granulomatous component
- Fat necrosis is common

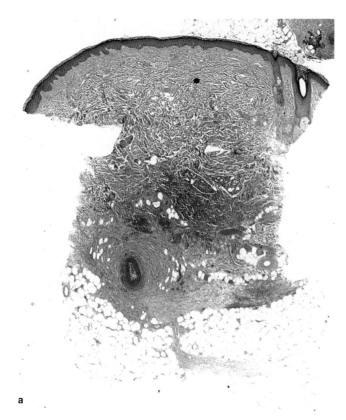

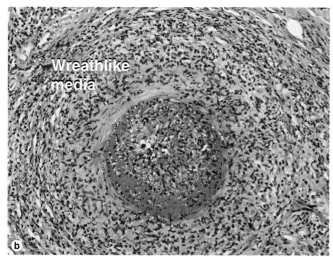

Fig. 11.6 Polyarteritis nodosa

Polyarteritis nodosa commonly presents with livedo reticularis and subcutaneous erythematous or hyperpigmented nodules. The biopsy typically demonstrates neutrophilic vasculitis involving an artery within the subcutaneous fat. Surrounding lobular necrosis is present.

Chapel Hill criteria

Necrotizing inflammation involving medium or small arteries without glomerulonephritis or vasculitis in arterioles, capillaries, or venules.

American College of Rheumatology criteria

Weight loss >4 kg; livedo reticularis; testicular pain or tenderness; myalgia/myopathy or muscle tenderness; neuropathy; hypertension (diastolic >90); renal impairment; hepatitis B infection; abnormal arteriogram; biopsy of an artery with neutrophilic inflammation (three criteria give >82% sensitivity, >86% specificity).

Thrombophlebitis

Key Features

- Vasculitis involving an oval vessel with bundled muscularis
- Vessel lacks an internal elastic membrane and may contain valves
- Thrombus present within vessel

Thromboangiitis obliterans (Buerger disease)

Key Features

- Endarteritis
- Prominent neutrophilic inflammation involving the thrombus

Buerger disease is a rare disease typically seen in male smokers. It is characterized by a combination of acute inflammation and thrombosis of large distal-extremity vessels.

American College of Rheumatology criteria

Age >50; history of smoking; distal peripheral vascular obstructive disease (below knee or elbow); and three additional criteria, such as thrombophlebitis saltans/migrans; involvement of upper extremity; characteristic angiography.

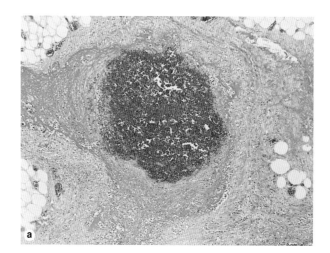

Fig. 11.7 Buerger disease

continued

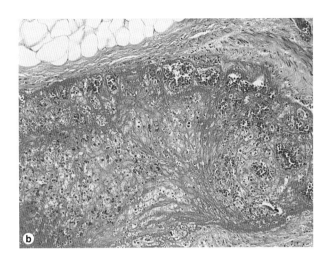

Fig. 11.7, cont'd

Medium vessel vasculitis

Key Features

- Involves a mix of vessel sizes (postcapillary venules *plus* larger, deeper vessels)
- Endothelial necrosis is common
- Often antineutrophil cytoplasmic antibody (ANCA) associated
- The most common causes include:
  - Granulomatosis with polyangiitis (formerly Wegener's granulomatosis) (commonly c-ANCA/antiproteinase 3)
  - Churg–Strauss syndrome (commonly p-ANCA/antimyeloperoxidase)
  - Microscopic polyangiitis (commonly p-ANCA/antimyeloperoxidase)
  - Septic vasculitis
  - Rheumatoid vasculitis
- This group of five disorders is sometimes referred to as the *big 5* because the vessels include those bigger than the postcapillary venule and the patients are often in bigger trouble.

These diseases are characterized by leukocytoclastic vasculitis involving vessels larger than the postcapillary venule. The endothelium is frequently necrotic. The biopsy demonstrates a superficial and deep perivascular infiltrate with neutrophils, karyorrhexis, expansion of the vessel wall, fibrin deposition within the vessel wall, and erythrocyte extravasation.

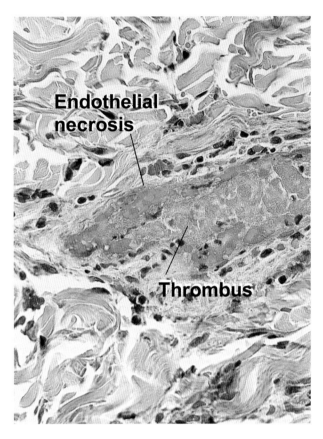

Fig. 11.8 "Big 5" pattern of vasculitis

Granulomatosis with polyangiitis (formerly Wegener's granulomatosis)

Key Features

- Leukocytoclastic vasculitis (LCV) involving a mix of vessel sizes (postcapillary venule plus larger, deeper vessels)
- Endothelial necrosis is common
- May involve skin, upper respiratory tract, kidneys
- LCV evolves into stellate abscess (palisaded granuloma with central neutrophils)
- Giant cells present in the granuloma

Granulomatosis with polyangiitis (formerly Wegener's granulomatosis) commonly involves the upper airway. The skin of the nose may become necrotic. Skin lesions may occur in other locations, especially the extremities. The histologic pattern is that of a "big 5" vasculitic disorder. Individual vasculitic foci may evolve into stellate abscesses (palisaded granulomas with a central stellate collection of neutrophils). Multinucleate giant cells are present in the granulomas. Granulomatous vasculitis may be present in medium-sized vessels.

Chapel Hill criteria

Granulomatous inflammation of the respiratory tract; necrotizing vasculitis of small to medium vessels; necrotizing glomerulonephritis common.

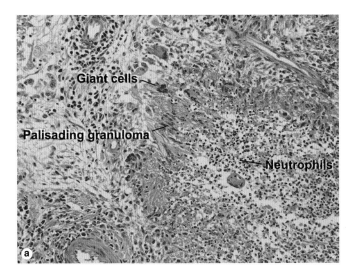

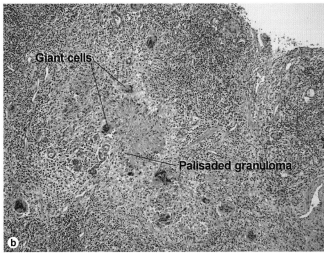

Fig. 11.9 Granulomatosis with polyangiitis (formerly Wegener's granulomatosis), palisading granuloma with stellate abscess

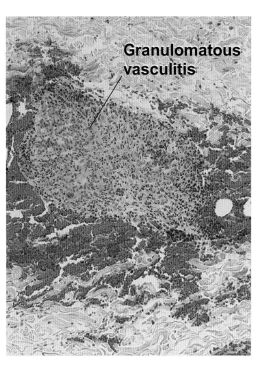

Fig. 11.10 Granulomatosis with polyangiitis (formerly Wegener's granulomatosis), granulomatous vasculitis

American College of Rheumatology criteria

Nasal or oral inflammation; chest x-ray with nodules; infiltrate or cavities; microscopic hematuria or red cell casts; granulomatous inflammation on biopsy (two criteria give >88% sensitivity, >92% specificity).

Differential Diagnosis

Palisaded granulomatous dermatitis with stellate abscess formation may be seen in Granulomatosis with polyangiitis (formerly Wegener's granulomatosis) (giant cells peripherally, neutrophils centrally), Churg–Strauss syndrome (epithelioid cells peripherally, eosinophils centrally), atypical mycobacterial infection, sporotrichosis, nocardiosis, cat scratch disease, lymphogranuloma venereum, and tularemia.

Eosinophilic granulomatosis with polyangiitis (Churg-Strauss syndrome)

Key Features

- Leukocytoclastic vasculitis involving a mix of vessel sizes (postcapillary venule plus larger, deeper vessels)
- Endothelial necrosis is common
- Asthma common
- May involve skin and kidneys
- LCV may produce stellate abscesses (palisaded granuloma with central eosinophils)
- Granuloma composed of epithelioid cells without giant cells

Churg–Strauss syndrome is a vasculitic disorder that commonly presents with a prodrome of asthma. Some cases have been induced by leukotriene inhibitors.

The histologic pattern is that of a "big 5" vasculitic disorder. Palisaded granulomas with central stellate abscesses are commonly seen. Unlike those of Granulomatosis with polyangiitis (formerly Wegener's granulomatosis), these rarely contain multinucleated giant cells and the central abscess is composed of eosinophils rather than neutrophils. Flame figures (eosinophil granules adherent to collagen fibers) similar to those of Well syndrome may be present.

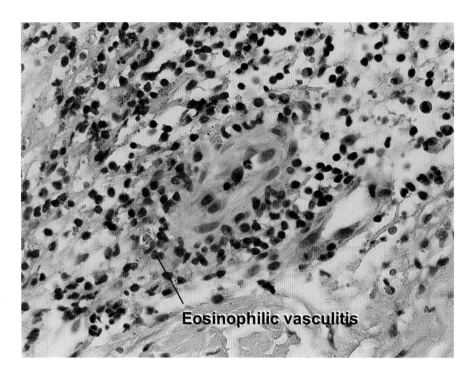

Fig. 11.11 Churg–Strauss syndrome, vasculitis with eosinophils

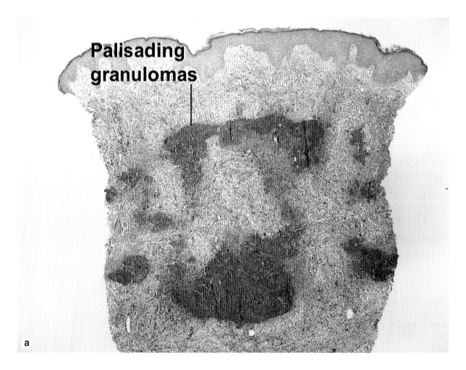

Fig. 11.12 Churg–Strauss syndrome, palisading granuloma with stellate abscess

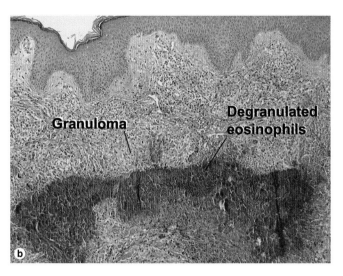

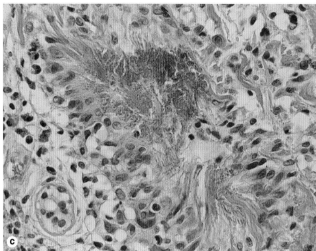

Fig. 11.12, cont'd

Chapel Hill criteria

Eosinophil-rich and granulomatous inflammation involving respiratory tract; necrotizing vasculitis of small to medium vessels; associated asthma and peripheral eosinophilia.

American College of Rheumatology criteria

Asthma; eosinophilia (>10%); neuropathy; pulmonary infiltrates; paranasal sinus involvement; extravascular eosinophils in tissue (four criteria give >85% sensitivity, >99% specificity).

Microscopic polyangiitis

Key Features

- Leukocytoclastic vasculitis involving a mix of vessel sizes (postcapillary venules plus larger, deeper vessels)
- Endothelial necrosis is common

The histologic pattern is that of a "big 5" vasculitic disorder. Endothelial necrosis is a prominent feature. The histologic pattern, ANCA positivity, and systemic involvement define the syndrome.

Chapel Hill criteria

Necrotizing vasculitis; few or no immune deposits; small to medium vessels involved; necrotizing arteriolitis may be present; necrotizing glomerulonephritis and pulmonary capillaritis common.

Rheumatoid vasculitis

Key Features

- Leukocytoclastic vasculitis involving a mix of vessel sizes (postcapillary venules plus larger, deeper vessels)
- Endothelial necrosis is common

The histologic pattern resembles that of the other "big 5" vasculitides. The vasculitis is associated with a rheumatoid factor and rheumatoid arthritis. Unlike most other connective tissue disease–associated vasculitis, rheumatoid vasculitis commonly ulcerates and scars.

Septic vasculitis

Key Features

- Vasculitis involves a mix of vessel sizes (postcapillary venules plus larger, deeper vessels)
- Endothelial necrosis is common
- "Dirty" necrosis with ample neutrophilic debris

Septic vasculitis is typically associated with dirty necrosis of arterioles. Because of the arteriolar involvement, livedo reticularis and stellate infarcts are commonly seen clinically.

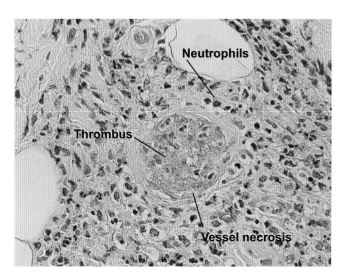

Fig. 11.13 Septic vasculitis

Small vessel leukocytoclastic vasculitis

Key Features

- Involves principally postcapillary venules
- Endothelial necrosis is rare
- Rarely ANCA associated
- The most common causes include:
  - Drug induced
  - Most connective tissue diseases (other than rheumatoid vasculitis)
  - Mixed cryoglobulin disease
  - Serum sickness
  - Henoch–Schönlein purpura

- This group of five disorders is sometimes referred to as the *little 5* because only the postcapillary venule is involved

The biopsy demonstrates a superficial perivascular infiltrate with neutrophils, karyorrhexis, expansion of the vessel wall, fibrin deposition within the vessel wall, and erythrocyte extravasation. The vasculitis involves primarily the postcapillary venules, although an occasional perforating vessel may be involved. These perforating vessels connect the subpapillary and deep plexus and are vertically oriented. Endothelial necrosis is exceedingly rare. Direct immunofluorescence may be helpful, especially in the case of Henoch–Schönlein purpura. A urinalysis should routinely be performed to look for signs of active renal involvement.

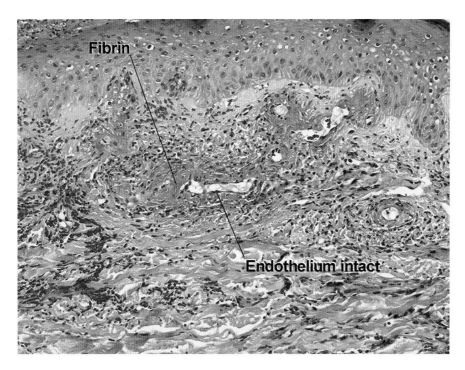

Fibrin

Endothelium intact

Fig. 11.14 "Little 5" pattern of leukocytoclastic vasculitis

Henoch–Schönlein purpura

Key Features

- "Little 5" pattern of LCV
- IgA in vessels on direct immunofluorescence (DIF)
- Typically children
- Extensor involvement with large mottled patches of purpura
- Bone, joint, gut, and renal involvement

Henoch–Schönlein purpura is the most common IgA vasculitis. The clinical features and DIF pattern are distinctive, but the hematoxylin and eosin (H&E) findings are like that of the other "little 5" disorders.

Chapel Hill criteria

Vasculitis with IgA dominant deposits; small to medium vessels; involves skin, gut, and glomeruli; associated with arthralgia or arthritis.

American College of Rheumatology criteria

Palpable purpura; age <20; bowel pain; vessel wall neutrophils on biopsy (two criteria give 87% sensitivity, 88% specificity).

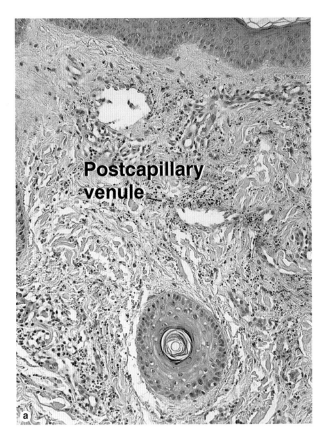

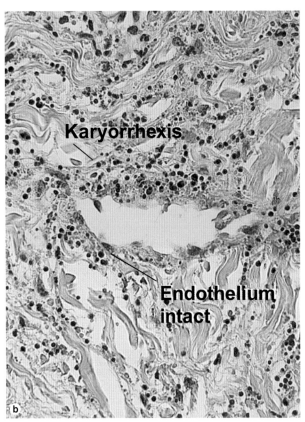

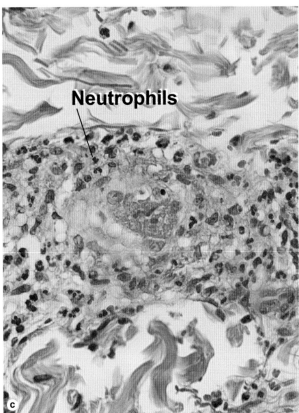

Fig. 11.15 Henoch–Schönlein purpura, "little 5" pattern of leukocytoclastic vasculitis

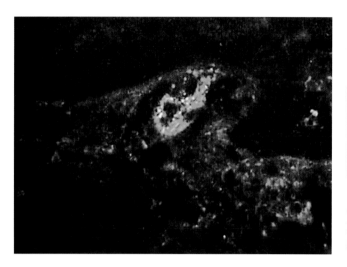

Fig. 11.16 Henoch–Schönlein purpura, IgA deposition in vessels (DIF)

Mixed cryoglobulin disease

Key Features

- "Little 5" pattern of LCV
- Cryoglobulins present

Mixed cryoglobulin disease is often associated with chronic infection, especially with hepatitis C. The H&E findings are like that of the other "little 5" disorders.

Chapel Hill criteria

Vasculitis of small to medium vessels; cryoglobulin deposits; skin and glomeruli often involved.

Drug-induced and idiopathic leukocytoclastic vasculitis (idiopathic leukocytoclastic angiitis)

Key Features

- "Little 5" pattern of LCV

We use the term *idiopathic leukocytoclastic vasculitis here* for cases with no known cause. The ACR criteria lump drug-induced vasculitis into this category. The histologic features of both fall into the "little 5" pattern.

> **PEARL**
>
> Most drug-induced vasculitis presents with a "little 5 pattern". Exceptions: A "big 5" pattern may be seen with montelukast, propothiouracil, methimazole, hydralazine, and minocycline.

Chapel Hill criteria

Isolated leukocytoclastic angiitis without systemic vasculitis or glomerulonephritis.

American College of Rheumatology criteria

Age >16; implicated drug; palpable purpura; cutaneous eruption; positive biopsy (three criteria give 71% sensitivity, >83% specificity).

Unique forms of vasculitis

Granuloma faciale

Key Features

- Typically facial skin (sebaceous follicles, *Demodex* mites)
- Grenz zone
- LCV with eosinophils
- Onion-skin fibrosis in chronic cases
- "Granuloma" in the name *only*—not on the slide

Granuloma faciale presents clinically as reddish-brown macules or plaques with patulous follicular openings. Histologically, it is a chronic leukocytoclastic vasculitis with eosinophils. Over time, onion-skin fibrosis develops around vessels. A grenz (border) zone commonly separates the infiltrate from the adjacent follicular epithelium. Despite the name, there are no granulomas in the tissue.

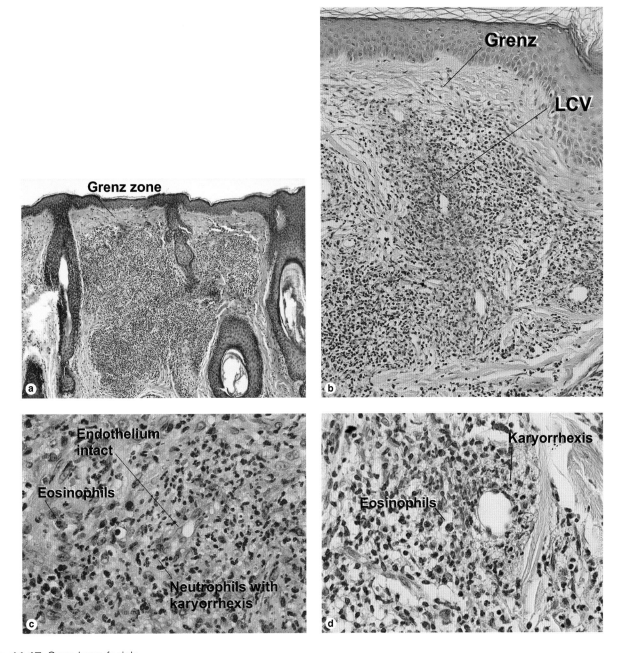

Fig. 11.17 Granuloma faciale

Erythema elevatum diutinum

Key Features

- Not facial skin
- LCV ± eosinophils
- Onion-skin fibrosis

Erythema elevatum diutinum (EED) presents with red-to-orange plaques on extensor surfaces. Like granuloma faciale, EED represents a chronic fibrosing form of leukocytoclastic vasculitis. It is distinguished histologically by a nonfacial location and greater fibrosis. EED has been associated with chronic streptococcal infection, HIV infection, and IgA gammopathy. The histologic changes are similar to those of granuloma faciale, but the surrounding skin has features of acral skin. Extracellular cholesterol clefts deposit in some chronic cases as a result of years of erythrocyte extravasation.

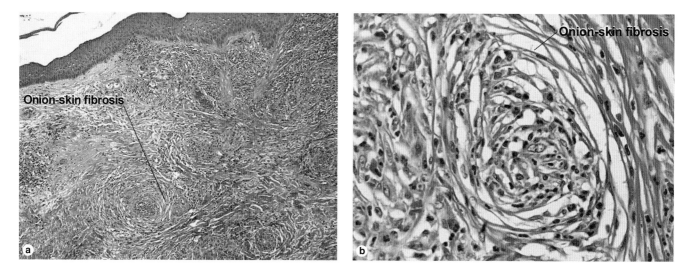

Fig. 11.18 Erythema elevatum diutinum

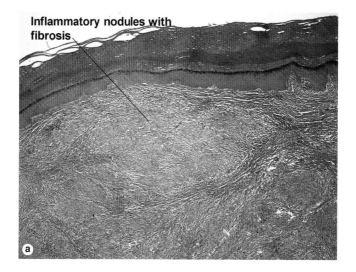

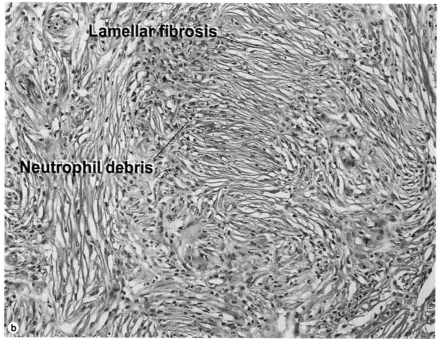

Fig. 11.19 Erythema elevatum diutinum with extensive fibrosis

Kawasaki disease

Key Features

- Diagnosis is made clinically
- Coronary arteritis presents histologically

Chapel Hill criteria

Involves large, medium, and small arteries, with associated mucocutaneous lymph node syndrome; coronary arteries often involved; usually affects children.

Incidental vasculitis

Key Features

- Not associated with immune complex disease
- Occurs in ulcers and adjacent to suppurative folliculitis
- May mimic "big 5" or "little 5" pattern

Leukocytoclastic vasculitis is frequently seen as an incidental finding in the base of a chronic ulcer or adjacent to a focus of suppurative folliculitis. Focal incidental leukocytoclastic vasculitis also occurs in Sweet syndrome, bowel bypass syndrome, pyoderma gangrenosum, and neutrophilic dermatosis of the dorsal hands.

Neutrophilic dermatoses

Sweet syndrome (acute febrile neutrophilic dermatosis)

Key Features

- Marked papillary dermal edema
- Nodular and diffuse infiltrate of neutrophils with karyorrhexis
- Focal LCV is common

Sweet syndrome is a distinct syndrome characterized by bouts of red, hot, tender erythematous plaques; fever; and peripheral leukocytosis. Most cases follow bouts of upper respiratory infection in predisposed individuals. About 10% of patients have an associated myeloproliferative disorder. The most striking histologic features of Sweet syndrome are the nodular and diffuse infiltrates of neutrophils, karyorrhexis, and marked papillary dermal edema. In the presence of these findings and a characteristic clinical presentation, the presence of focal leukocytoclastic vasculitis does not alter the diagnosis of Sweet syndrome.

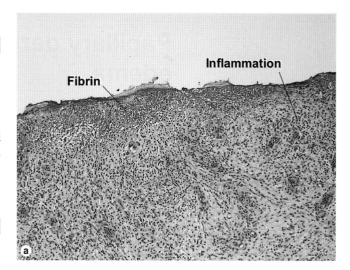
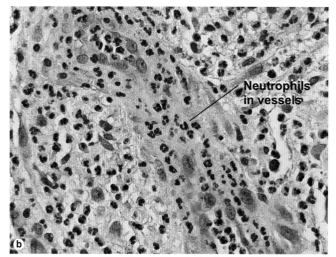
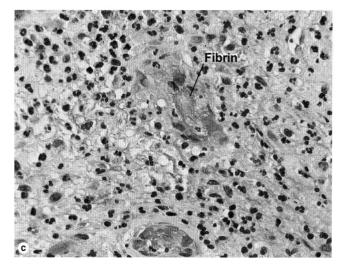

Fig. 11.20 Incidental leukocytoclastic vasculitis in the base of a chronic ulcer

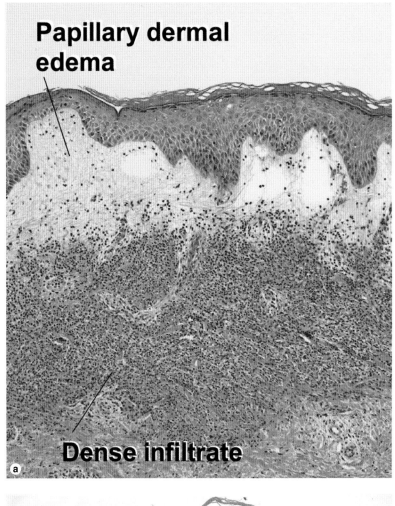

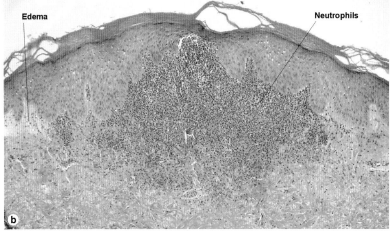

Fig. 11.21 (A) Sweet syndrome. **(B)** Pustular dermatosis of the dorsal hands

Other neutrophilic dermatoses

Key Features

- Look like Sweet syndrome
- Marked papillary dermal edema
- Nodular and diffuse infiltrate of neutrophils with karyorrhexis
- Focal LCV is common

Neutrophilic dermatosis of the dorsal hands, pyoderma gangrenosum, bowel-bypass syndrome, and the autoinflammatory syndromes such as familial Mediterranean fever and Muckle–Wells syndrome have a similar appearance to the lesions of Sweet syndrome. Ulcerative lesions typically demonstrate more prominent foci of leukocytoclastic vasculitis. *Erythema marginatum* is a superficial gyrate erythema characterized by a superficial perivascular neutrophilic infiltrate. The papillary dermal edema is less prominent.

Pyoderma gangrenosum

Key Features

Early lesions
- Superative folliculitis or neutrophilic dermatitis

Late lesions
- Ulceration with epidermal necrosis and mixed infiltrate

Urticaria

Key Features

Early lesions of urticaria
- Superficial dermal vessels filled with neutrophils

Late lesions of urticaria
- Perivascular and interstitial polymorphous infiltrate
- Superficial dermal vessels often still contain neutrophils within the lumen
- Diapedesis of neutrophils through the vessel wall into the surrounding dermis

- Distinct absence of karyorrhexis
- No fibrin in vessel walls
- No expansion of vessel walls
- Interstitial neutrophils, eosinophils, and mononuclear cells

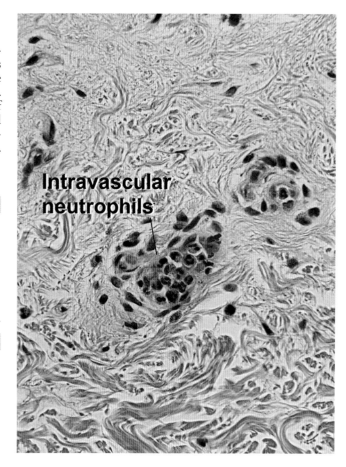

Fig. 11.22 Acute stage of a wheal

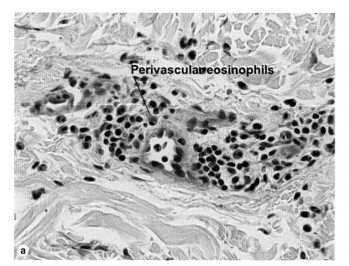

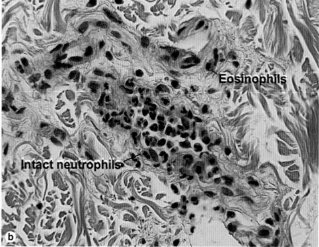

Fig. 11.23 Chronic stage of an urticarial wheal

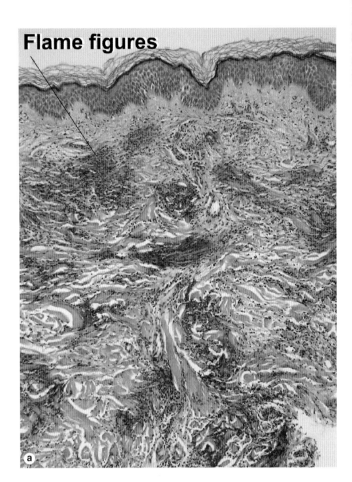

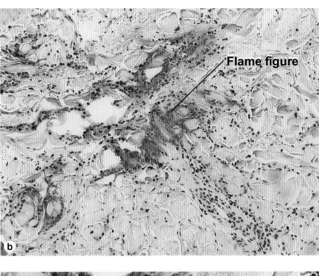

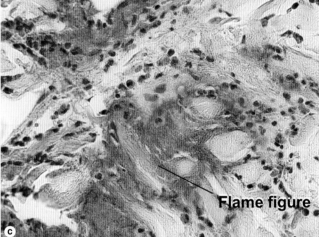

Fig. 11.24 Wells syndrome

The edema of an urticarial wheal is not visible histologically. Instead, the only significant finding in acute lesions of urticaria is intravascular margination of neutrophils. With time, the neutrophils travel through the vessel wall into the surrounding dermis and are joined by eosinophils and mononuclear cells. In contrast to leukocytoclastic vasculitis, karyorrhexis is absent, the vessels walls are not expanded, and no fibrin is seen in the vessel walls. Erythrocyte extravasation is uncommon.

Wells syndrome (eosinophilic cellulitis)

Key Features

- Flame figures (eosinophil degranulation onto collagen)

Wells syndrome is characterized by recurrent erythematous plaques that demonstrate flame figures histologically. Some cases may represent a distinct entity, but most represent exaggerated arthropod reactions.

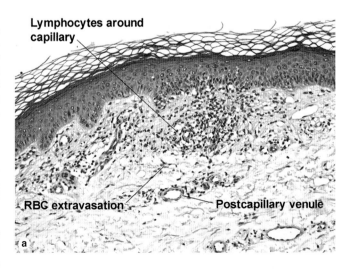

Fig. 11.25 (A) Pigmenting purpuric eruption.

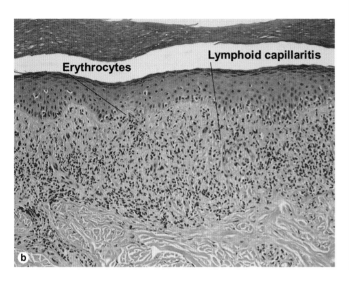

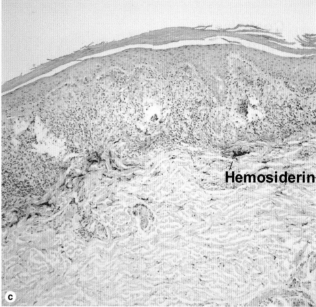

Fig. 11.25, cont'd (B and C) Lichen aureus

Perivascular lymphoid infiltrates

Pigmenting purpuric eruption

Key Features

- Inflammation purely lymphoid
- Surrounds capillaries (centered above the level of the postcapillary venule)
- Erythrocyte extravasation
- Hemosiderin deposits over time

All types of pigmenting purpura represent forms of chronic lymphocytic capillaritis. Clinical variants include thumbprint hemosiderosis with cayenne pepper spots (Schamberg disease), annular telangiectatic purpura (Majocchi purpura), lichenoid purpura (Gougerot–Blum purpura), and eczematous purpura (pigmenting purpura of Doucas and Kapetanakis). In all forms, an iron stain (Perl's, Prussian blue, ferricyanide, Gomori iron) can be used to demonstrate hemosiderin. Lichen aureus is a localized form of pigmenting purpura related to an underlying incompetent perforator valve.

Gyrate erythemas

Key Features

- Dense "coat-sleeve" perivascular lymphoid infiltrate
- Vessels are intact

Superficial gyrate erythemas include erythema marginatum (discussed under the neutrophilic disorders) and erythema centrifugum. Erythema annulare centrifugum is characterized clinically by an expanding erythematous ring with a characteristic trailing scale. Histologically, the erythematous ring corresponds to a focus of superficial perivascular coat-sleeve lymphoid infiltrate. Trailing behind this is a small spongiotic focus, and trailing behind that is a small focus of parakeratosis. The infiltrate, spongiotic, and parakeratotic foci line up at about a 45-degree angle. Deep gyrate erythemas lack epidermal changes and are characterized by a dense superficial and deep coat-sleeve perivascular lymphoid infiltrate.

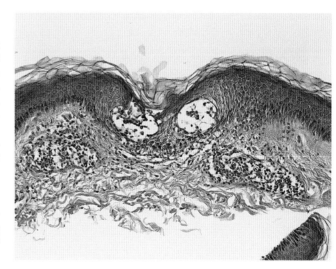

Fig. 11.26 Erythema annulare centrifugum

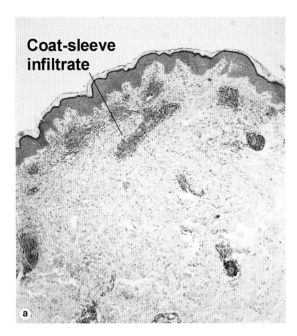

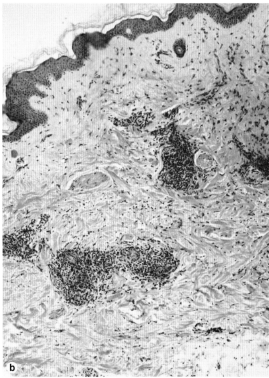

Fig. 11.27 Deep gyrate erythema

Tumid lupus erythematosus

Key Features

- Perivascular lymphoid inflammation
- Lymphocytes in eccrine coil
- Dermal mucin

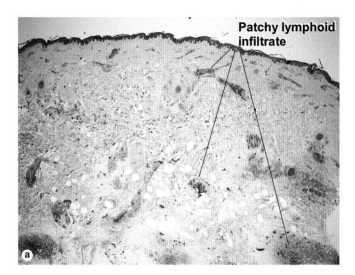

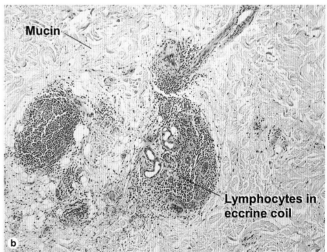

Fig. 11.28 Tumid lupus erythematosus

Polymorphous light eruption

Key Features

- Perivascular lymphoid inflammation
- Papillary dermal edema
- ± Spongiosis

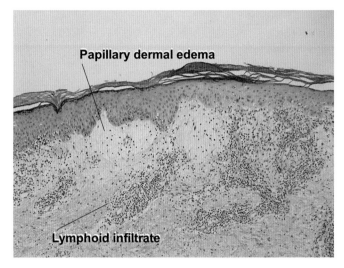

Fig. 11.29 Polymorphous light eruption

Morbilliform drug eruptions

Key Features

- Evidence of an acute process (basket-weave corneum, papillary dermal edema, dilated superficial vessels, neutrophils in vessels, red cell extravasation)
- Mild vacuolar interface commonly present

Features that suggest a drug eruption include presence of a polymorphous infiltrate, as well as combinations of findings not corresponding to any well-defined disease.

Features that weigh against a diagnosis of a morbilliform drug eruption include signs of chronicity (acanthosis, hyperkeratosis, papillary dermal fibrosis, macrophages in dermis).

Lymphoid vasculitis

Key Features

- Perivascular lymphoid infiltrate with damage to the vessel wall

True lymphoid vasculitis may be seen in Degos disease, insect bites, rickettsial disease, pityriasis lichenoides, and perniosis.

Degos disease (malignant atrophic papulosis)

Key Features

- Red papules that develop ivory white atrophic centers
- Bowel perforation and stroke
- Wedge-shaped superficial and deep perivascular lymphoid infiltrate with vascular damage
- Over time, central epidermal depression and atrophy, avascular necrosis of dermal structures, and marked dermal mucinosis

Degos disease is a distinct clinical picture that may be a manifestation of lupus erythematosus.

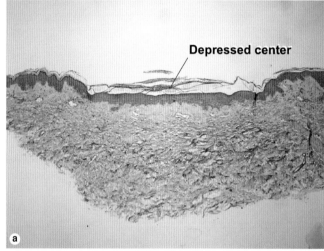

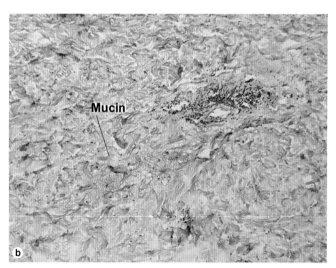

Fig. 11.30 Degos disease

Insect bite

Key Features

- Dense, wedge-shaped perivascular lymphoid infiltrate
- Eosinophils
- Variable vascular damage
- Variable atypical lymphocytes
- Focal leukocytoclastic vasculitis may be present
- Papillary dermal edema may be prominent

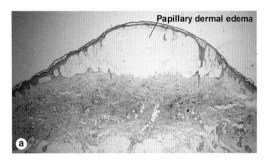

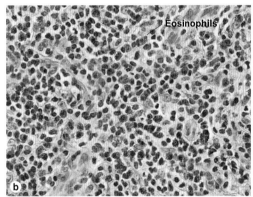

Fig. 11.31 Insect bite

Perniosis

Key Features

- Superficial and deep perivascular lymphoid infiltrate
- Fluffy edema and expansion of vessel walls without fibrin
- Acral skin

The so-called *fluffy edema* of perniosis is often more prominent in deeper dermal vessels. The vessel wall is expanded, and white space surrounds lymphocyte nuclei within the vessel wall.

Occlusive vascular diseases

Type I cryoglobulinemia

Key Features

- Vessels occluded by pink, jellylike substance
- Erythrocyte extravasation

Type I, monoclonal cryoglobulinemia is a manifestation of plasma cell dyscrasia. The intravascular deposits have an appearance resembling dark pink to red jelly.

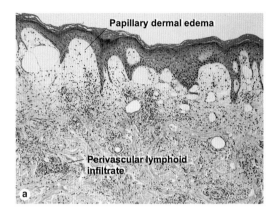

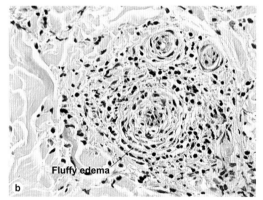

Fig. 11.32 Perniosis

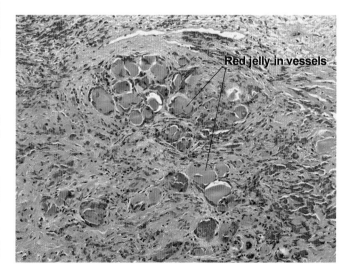

Fig. 11.33 Type I cryoglobulinemia

Cholesterol embolization

Key Features

- Arteriole containing cholesterol clefts

Cholesterol embolization typically occurs after catheterization or anticoagulation. Spontaneous embolization may also occur. The patient presents with livedo reticularis, dark mottled toes, and worsening renal function.

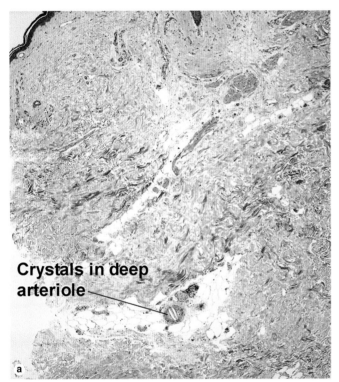

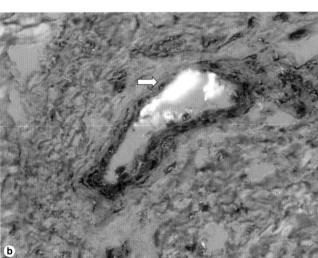

Fig. 11.34 Cholesterol embolization (**B**: frozen section, polarized microscopy)

Livedoid vasculopathy (Segmental hyalinizing vasculopathy)

Key Features

- Hyalinized vessel walls
- Thrombi
- Cannon-ball tufting of vessels often present in superficial dermis (stasis change)

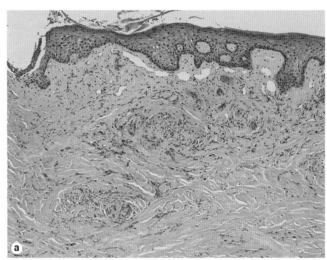

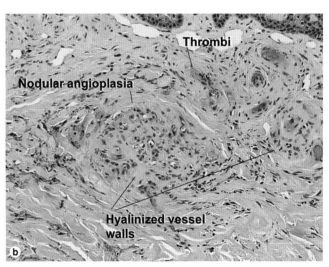

Fig. 11.35 Livedoid vasculopathy (Segmental hyalinizing vasculopathy)

continued

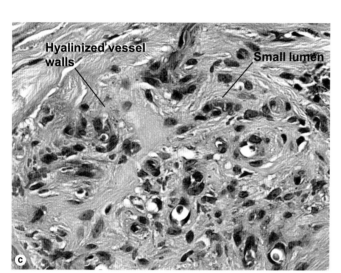

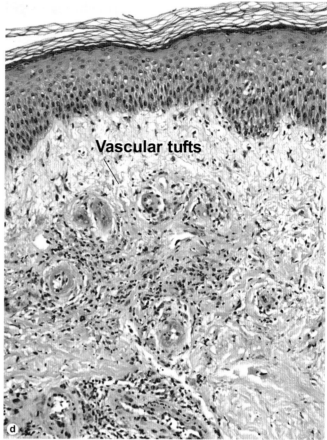

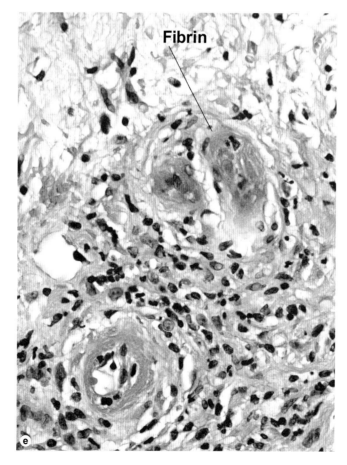

Fig. 11.35, cont'd

Collagenous vasculopathy

Key Features

- Irregular dilated vessels in superficial dermis
- Collagenous cuffs
- Progressive telangiectasia initially on the lower extremities, becoming generalized

Stasis change

Key Features

- Cannon-ball tufting of vessels often present in superficial dermis (stasis change)
- Erythrocyte extravasation
- Dermal hemosiderin
- Small thrombi may be present

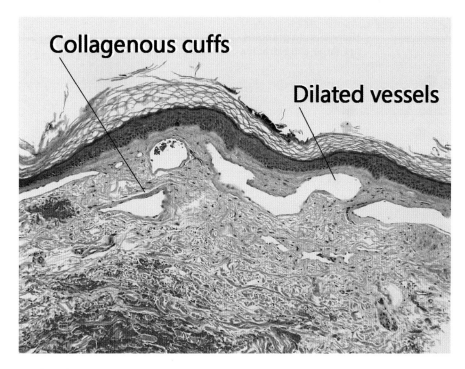

Fig. 11.36 Collagenous vasculopathy

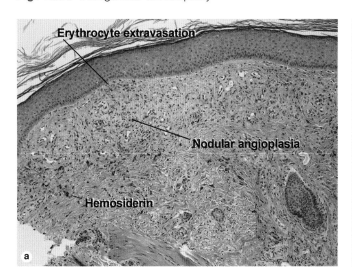

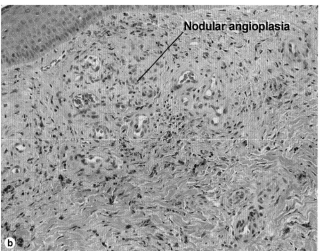

Fig. 11.37 Stasis change

continued

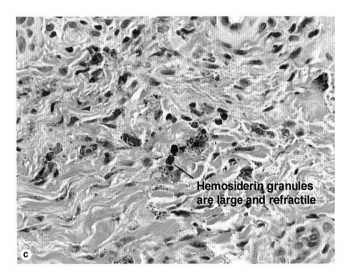

Fig. 11.37, cont'd

Coagulopathy

Key Features

- Thrombi in vessels

Purpura fulminans, antiphospholipid syndrome, and acquired deficiencies or inherited mutations affecting protein C, protein S, antithrombin III, factor V Leiden, and prothrombin all result in vascular thrombi with variable purpura and necrosis. Coumadin and heparin necrosis are included in this group. Segmental hyalinizing vasculopathy also fits within this group and may present with ulceration or atrophie blanche. Levamisole-induced necrosis may have both thrombi and vasculitis.

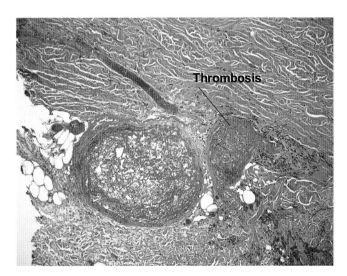

Fig. 11.38 Coumadin necrosis

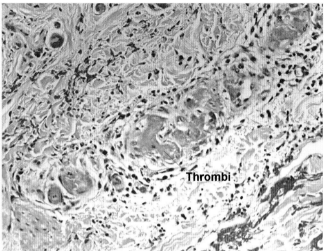

Fig. 11.39 Levamisole-induced necrosis

Noninflammatory purpura

Scurvy

Key Features

- Follicular hyperkeratosis
- Corkscrew hairs
- Perifollicular hemorrhage

Solar ("senile") purpura (Bateman or actinic purpura)

Key Features

- Solar elastosis
- Erythrocyte extravasation

Other noninflammatory purpura

Key Features

- Erythrocyte extravasation

Ecchymoses and thrombocytopenic purpura present with erythrocyte extravasation in the absence of inflammation.

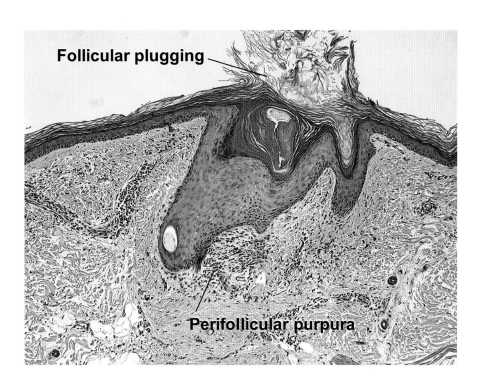

Fig. 11.40 Scurvy

Further reading

Barut K, Sahin S, Kasapcopur O. Pediatric vasculitis. Curr Opin Rheumatol 2016;28(1):29–38.

Carlson JA, Ng BT, Chen KR. Cutaneous vasculitis update: diagnostic criteria, classification, epidemiology, etiology, pathogenesis, evaluation and prognosis. Am J Dermatopathol 2005;27(6):504–28.

Lazarus B, John GT, O'Callaghan C, et al. Recent advances in anti-neutrophil cytoplasmic antibody-associated vasculitis. Indian J Nephrol 2016;26(2):86–96.

Lionaki S, Blyth ER, Hogan SL, et al. Classification of antineutrophil cytoplasmic autoantibody vasculitides: the role of antineutrophil cytoplasmic autoantibody specificity for myeloperoxidase or proteinase 3 in disease recognition and prognosis. Arthritis Rheum 2012;64(10):3452–62.

Ozen S. Problems in classifying vasculitis in children. Pediatr Nephrol 2005;20(9):1214–18.

Pagnoux C, Guillevin L. Cardiac involvement in small and medium-sized vessel vasculitides. Lupus 2005;14(9): 718–22.

Watts RA, Scott DG. ANCA vasculitis: to lump or split? Why we should study MPA and GPA separately. Rheumatology (Oxford) 2012;51(12):2115–17.

Yazici H, Yazici Y. Diagnosis and/or classification of vasculitis: different? Curr Opin Rheumatol 2016;28(1):3–7.

Genodermatoses

Tammie Ferringer

Pseudoxanthoma elasticum

Key Features

- Curled and frayed, calcified elastic fibers in the reticular dermis (pink or blue squiggles)
- Elastic tissue (Verhoeff–Van Gieson) and calcium (Von Kossa) stains highlight the distorted elastic fibers

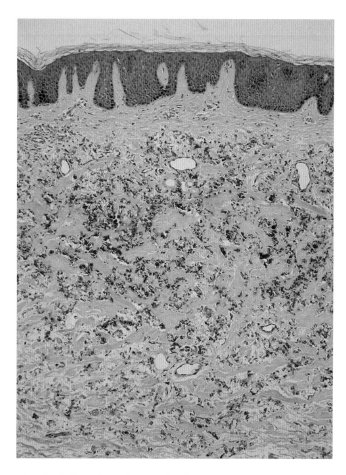

Fig. 12.1 Pseudoxanthoma elasticum

Pseudoxanthoma elasticum is an autosomal-recessive and, less commonly, autosomal-dominant disorder due to a mutation in the *ABCC6* transporter gene. It results in calcification of the elastic fibers of the skin, eyes, and artery walls. The skin changes become apparent around the second decade and simulate "plucked chicken skin" in the flexural areas. Biopsy of a scar may reveal the elastic tissue abnormalities in a patient with no cutaneous lesions. Eye changes include angioid streaks and retinal hemorrhage that may cause blindness. The vascular changes may lead to hypertension, stroke, myocardial infarction, mitral valve prolapse, and gastrointestinal hemorrhage.

Similar histologic findings can also be seen after topical exposure to calcium salts. Periumbilical perforating pseudoxanthoma elasticum (perforating calcific elastosis) affects multiparous black women but is limited to an isolated area. Patients on long-term penicillamine for Wilson disease may develop altered elastic fibers with overlapping features of pseudoxanthoma elasticum and elastosis perforans serpiginosa. The penicillamine-induced, altered elastic fibers have small lateral buds arranged perpendicularly to the primary elastic fiber resembling the twigs on a bramble bush but do not calcify.

Differential Diagnosis

Angioid streaks due to rupture in Bruch membrane are associated with other disorders. The mnemonic "PEPSI LiTe" is helpful in remembering the associated diseases:

- *P*aget disease of bone
- *E*hlers–Danlos syndrome
- *P*seudoxanthoma elasticum
- *S*ickle cell anemia
- *I*ncreased phosphate
- *L*ead poisoning
- *T*halassemia

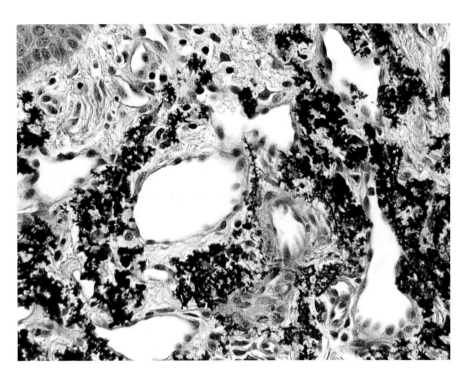

Fig. 12.2 "Bramble bush" elastic fibers induced by penicillamine

Ichthyosis vulgaris

Key Features

- Compact orthohyperkeratosis with paradoxically diminished or absent granular layer

In most other conditions, hyperorthokeratosis is associated with a prominent granular layer and parakeratosis is associated with a diminished or absent granular layer. Ichthyosis vulgaris (in which there is little to no granular layer despite hyperkeratosis) and axillary granular parakeratosis (in which there is a granular layer despite the presence of parakeratosis) are exceptions to this rule.

Ichthyosis vulgaris is an autosomal-dominant disorder with retention of the stratum corneum (rather than hyperproliferation) resulting in hyperkeratosis. There is a deficiency in profilaggrin resulting in inadequate keratohyaline granule synthesis. There are fine brown to transparent scales that spare the flexures. Accentuation of the palmoplantar creases, keratosis pilaris, and coexisting atopic dermatitis may be present.

Acquired ichthyosis in association with malignancy, especially Hodgkin lymphoma, may clinically and histologically mimic ichthyosis vulgaris. Acquired ichthyosis may also occur with niacin therapy.

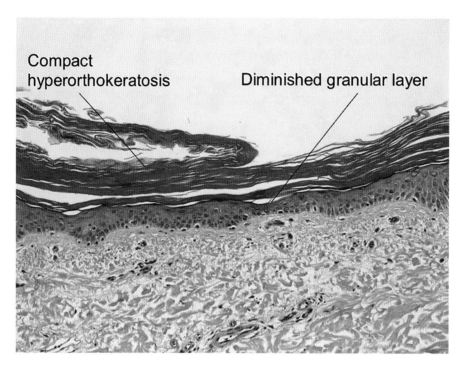

Fig. 12.3 Ichthyosis vulgaris

Incontinentia pigmenti (Bloch–Sulzberger syndrome)

Key Features

Vesicular stage
- Eosinophilic spongiosis (spongiosis resulting in intraepidermal vesicles with prominent exocytosis of eosinophils)
- Occasional dyskeratotic cells may be present

Verrucous stage
- Hyperkeratosis and papillomatosis with few eosinophils and little spongiosis
- Prominent dyskeratosis in whorls and clusters

Pigmented stage
- Pigment incontinence
- Hypopigmented lesions reveal normal to decreased melanocytes with or without dermal fibrosis

This X-linked dominant disorder is typically lethal in males. A mutation in the *NEMO* gene leads to defective nuclear factor kappa-B (NF-κB) activation. There is evolution through overlapping stages. At birth or soon after, linear vesicular lesions evolve into verrucous lesions weeks to months later. At 3–6 months of age there are streaks and whorls of hyperpigmentation that do not correlate with the areas of prior vesicles. The pattern has been likened to marble cake. Hypopigmentation may replace the hyperpigmentation decades later. Other cutaneous findings include alopecia and nail dystrophy. Ocular, dental (peg teeth), skeletal, and neurologic abnormalities may be present.

Differential Diagnosis

The microscopic differential for spongiosis with eosinophils ("eosinophilic spongiosis") can be remembered by the mnemonic "HAAPPIE." The dyskeratotic cells help distinguish incontinentia pigmenti from the other conditions.

- *H*erpes gestationis
- *A*rthropod bite/*A*llergic contact dermatitis
- *P*emphigus
- *P*emphigoid
- *I*ncontinentia pigmenti
- *E*rythema toxicum neonatorum

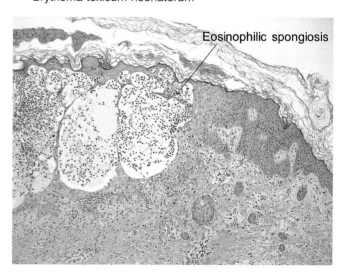

Fig. 12.4 Incontinentia pigmenti, vesicular stage

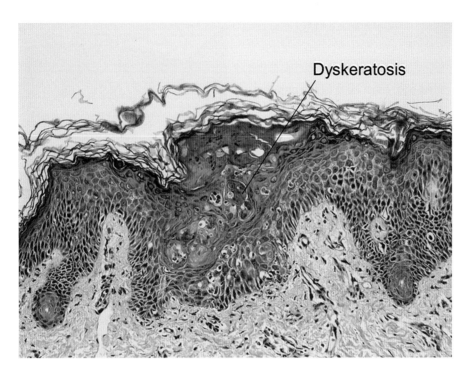

Fig. 12.5 Incontinentia pigmenti, verrucous stage

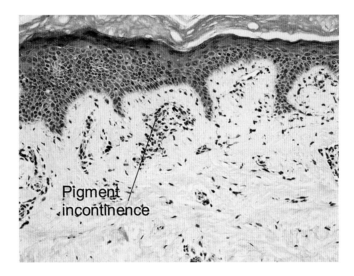

Fig. 12.6 Incontinentia pigmenti, pigmented stage

Mastocytosis

Key Features

- Uniformly spaced "fried-egg" mast cells fill the papillary dermis and extend into the reticular dermis in nodular lesions
- Subepidermal bullae, basal layer hyperpigmentation, and scattered eosinophils may be present
- Subtle increase in perivascular, spindle-shaped, hyperchromatic mast cells in telangiectasia macularis eruptiva perstans (TMEP)

Mastocytosis comprises a spectrum of diseases. A solitary mastocytoma may occur in childhood with a tendency to spontaneous involution. Urticaria pigmentosa is a sporadic rather than inherited disorder characterized by multiple tan macules, papules, or nodules. There is a congenital or early-onset form that is rarely associated with systemic disease and typically clears by puberty. In contrast, adult-onset urticaria pigmentosa persists and can be associated with systemic involvement, especially bone marrow. The majority of lesions urticate with stroking (Darier sign). Mutations in *c-kit* have been found in sporadic adult cases and in children with extensive or persistent disease, but not in typical pediatric urticaria pigmentosa. TMEP is a rare adult form of mastocytosis with erythema, telangiectasia, and faint tan macules on the trunk and extremities, rarely with a Darier sign.

In macular and TMEP lesions, the mast cells are limited to a superficial perivascular infiltrate. The mast cells may have small round nuclei with ample cytoplasm and resemble fried eggs, or they may be spindle shaped and simulate large hyperchromatic fibroblasts. The presence of more than five perivascular mast cells around each vessel is suggestive of mastocytosis. Special stains are recommended for identification. Mast cells are red with Leder stain (ASD-chloroacetate esterase) and the granules stain metachromatically with toluidine blue and Giemsa methods. Immunohistochemistry for CD117 (the *c-kit*–encoded tyrosine kinase receptor) and mast cell tryptase also identifies mast cells. Lesions degranulated by stroking (Darier sign) may show no intracellular granules with Giemsa staining. A Leder stain is preferred in this setting.

Multiple or solitary nodular lesions reveal closely packed, uniformly spaced, round to cuboidal mast cells that fill the papillary dermis and may extend into the reticular dermis and subcutaneous tissue. These mast cells may be visibly granular and may have a "fried-egg" appearance with a central nucleus and eosinophilic to pale gray cytoplasm. A scattering of eosinophils is usually present, and basal hyperpigmentation may be identified. These lesions can be distinguished from Langerhans cell histiocytosis by the absence of epidermal involvement, folliculotropism, and reniform nuclei and with special stains. The cuboidal cells may resemble nevus cells, but mast cell lesions lack junctional and dermal nesting and lack the nuclear pseudoinclusions typical of melanocytes.

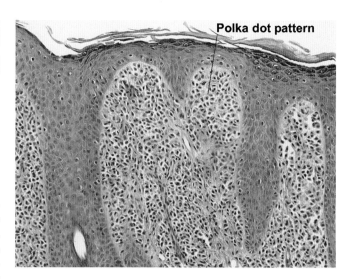

Fig. 12.7 Mastocytoma

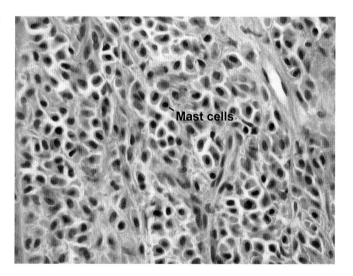

Fig. 12.8 Mastocytoma

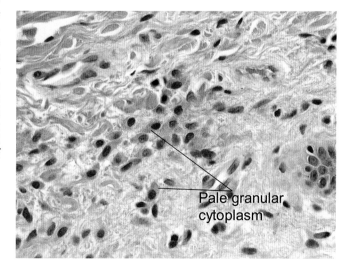

Fig. 12.9 Mast cells

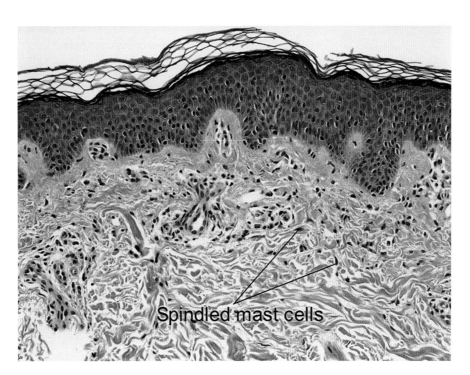

Fig. 12.10 Telangiectasia macularis eruptiva perstans

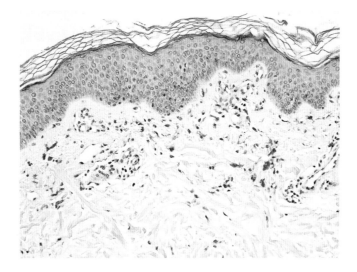

Fig. 12.11 Telangiectasia macularis eruptive perstans (Leder stain)

Epidermolytic ichthyosis (bullous congenital ichthyosiform erythroderma)

Key Features

- Compact hyperorthokeratosis
- Granular and vacuolar degeneration of the upper layers of the epidermis
- Red and blue clumped keratohyaline granules and vacuoles (granular layer "chewed up")

Epidermolytic hyperkeratosis is a histologic pattern that can be seen in several clinical settings, including palmoplantar keratoderma, solitary epidermolytic acanthoma, and epidermolytic ichthyosis. Not uncommonly, epidermolytic hyperkeratosis is an incidental finding in biopsies of another lesion such as a dysplastic nevus.

Epidermolytic ichthyosis is an autosomal-dominant condition characterized by widespread blistering and erythema at birth that evolve into generalized furrowed hyperkeratosis with accentuation in the flexures. There is a wide morphologic spectrum. Mutations in keratin genes (*K1* and *K10*) have been identified. This generalized disorder has been reported in the offspring of patients with linear epidermal nevi that histologically reveal epidermolytic hyperkeratosis, suggesting that these "epidermal nevi" represent mosaicism for the trait.

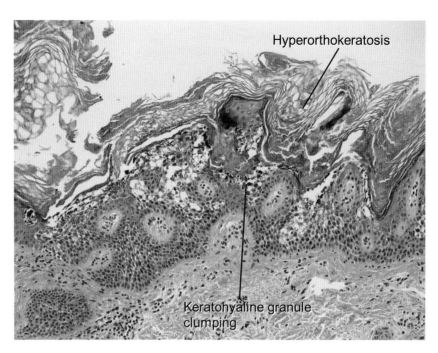

Fig. 12.12 Epidermolytic hyperkeratosis

Lipoid proteinosis (hyalinosis cutis et mucosae, Urbach–Wiethe disease)

Key Features

- Eosinophilic hyaline deposits around blood vessels, sweat glands, and in thick bundles perpendicular to the surface
- Onion-skin concentric pattern around vessels and adnexal structures

- Much deeper and more extensive than in erythropoietic protoporphyria (EPP)

Lipoid proteinosis is an autosomal-recessive disorder resulting in hoarseness, pitted scars, beaded nodules along the eyelids, verrucous lesions, and seizures due to calcifications of the hippocampus. The material is periodic acid–Schiff-positive and diastase-resistant reduplicated basement membrane (type IV collagen). Stains for amyloid and mucin are unpredictable.

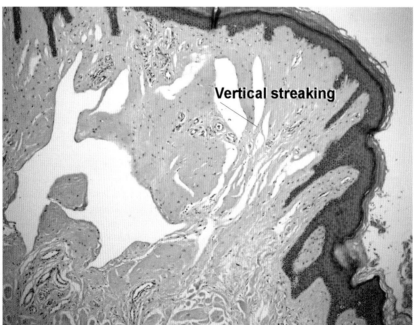

Fig. 12.13 Lipoid proteinosis

Goltz syndrome (focal dermal hypoplasia, Goltz–Gorlin syndrome)

Key Features

- Narrow Blaschko segments involved
- In early lesions, the fat is perivascular and subepidermal
- In older, more polypoid lesions, fat replaces most of the dermis

This X-linked dominant condition is also associated with orogenital raspberry-like papillomas, hypodontia, ectrodactyly, and ocular defects. It is due to a mutation in the *PORCN* gene.

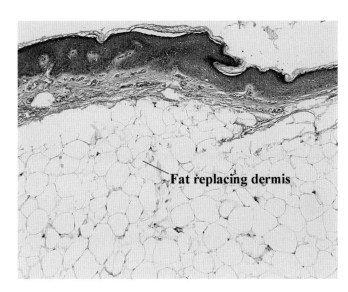

Fig. 12.14 Goltz syndrome

Dowling–Degos disease (reticulated pigmented anomaly of the flexures)

Key Features

- Resembles multiple foci of reticulated seborrheic keratosis "hanging off" hair follicles
- Comedo-like, dilated, keratin-filled follicular infundibula

Dowling–Degos disease is an autosomal-dominant disorder due to mutation in the keratin 5 gene. Onset of the reticulated pigmentation occurs in the third to fourth decade involving the axillae and groin.

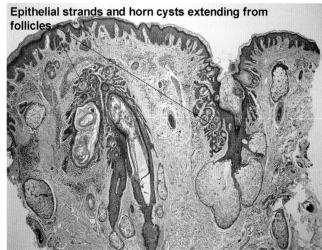

Epithelial strands and horn cysts extending from follicles

Fig. 12.15 Dowling–Degos disease

Galli–Galli disease

Key Features

- Similar to Dowling–Degos disease, but with foci of acantholysis

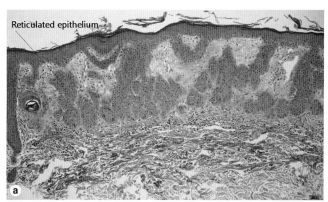

Reticulated epithelium

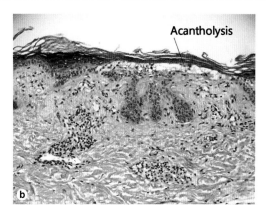

Acantholysis

Fig. 12.16 Galli–Galli disease

Table 12.1 Key features of genodermatoses

Syndrome	Inheritance	Mutation	Noncutaneous features	Cutaneous features	Pathology of cutaneous features	Elsewhere in text
Birt–Hogg–Dubé syndrome	AD	Folliculin	Chromophobe renal carcinoma, renal oncocytoma, pulmonary cysts, spontaneous pneumothorax	Multiple fibrofolliculomas and/or trichodiscomas	Fibrofolliculoma: fibrous orb with epithelial strands radiating from a central follicle-like structure. Trichodiscoma: fibrous orb without identified epithelial strands, likely fibrofolliculoma cut in a different plane of section	Pilar and sebaceous neoplasms (Ch. 4)
Brooke–Spiegler syndrome	AD	*CYLD*		Multiple trichoepitheliomas spiradenomas, and cylindromas	Trichoepithelioma: basaloid islands and papillary mesenchymal bodies in a fibroblast-rich stroma without retraction. Cylindroma: islands of basaloid cells with little cytoplasm outlined by eosinophilic membrane in a jigsaw-puzzle pattern. Spiradenoma: large islands of blue cells with little cytoplasm peppered by lymphocytes	Pilar and sebaceous neoplasms (Ch. 4) and sweat gland neoplasms (Ch. 5)
Cowden syndrome (multiple hamartoma syndrome)	AD	*PTEN*	Hamartomatous polyps of the colon, breast, endometrial, and thyroid cancer; macrocephaly; Lhermitte–Duclos disease	Multiple facial tricholemmomas, cobblestone oral mucosal papules, acral keratoses, palmoplantar keratoses, sclerotic fibroma	Tricholemmoma: pale lobule hanging down from the epidermis that is outlined by thick eosinophilic basement membrane. Sclerotic fibroma: hypocellular hyalinized collagen in curved or parallel strands giving a storiform or whorled appearance	Pilar and sebaceous neoplasms (Ch. 4) and fibrous tumors (Ch. 20

Table 12.1 Key features of genodermatoses—cont'd

Syndrome	Inheritance	Mutation	Noncutaneous features	Cutaneous features	Pathology of cutaneous features	Elsewhere in text
Darier disease (keratosis follicularis)	AD	*ATP2A2*		Greasy yellow-brown crusted and hyperkeratotic papules in seborrheic areas, cobblestone of the mucosa, palmoplantar pits, acrokeratosis verruciformis of Hopf on dorsal hands, nails with "V" nicking and longitudinal red and white streaks	Acantholysis in the lower epidermis with suprabasilar clefting and dyskeratosis	Blistering diseases (Ch. 9)
Epidermolytic ichthyosis (bullous congenital ichthyosiform erythroderma)	AD	*K1* and *K10*		Blistering and erythema at birth evolving to furrowed hyperkeratosis, especially in flexures	Compact hyperorthokeratosis with clumping and fragmentation of the granular layer (epidermolytic hyperkeratosis)	Genodermatoses (Ch. 12)
Epidermodysplasia verruciformis	AR (most)	*EVER1* and *EVER2*		Multiple red-brown, flat, wartlike papules on the trunk and extremities with increased squamous cell carcinoma in sun-exposed areas in the twenties and thirties	Flat, wartlike lesions: acanthotic with basket-weave stratum corneum and swollen, large, steel-blue cells with perinuclear halo	Viral infections, helminths, and arthropods (Ch. 19)
Epidermolysis bullosa simplex	AD	*K5* and *K14*		Blister formation with minimal trauma, especially of hands and feet	Appears to be a cell-poor subepidermal blister but occurs due to basal cell cytolysis and cleavage within the basal cells, leaving wispy remnants of basal cells at the floor of the blister	

continued

Table 12.1 Key features of genodermatoses—cont'd

Syndrome	Inheritance	Mutation	Noncutaneous features	Cutaneous features	Pathology of cutaneous features	Elsewhere in text
Erythropoietic protoporphyria	AD (most)	Ferrochelatase	Increased protoporphyrins in feces and blood, cholelithiasis and hepatic failure	Photosensitivity with erythema, edema, and burning pain with exposure; with time waxy thickening of the face and knuckles, erosions, and shallow scars on the face	Hyalin cuffs around postcapillary venules in patients without significant solar elastosis	Metabolic disorders (Ch. 14)
Fabry disease (angiokeratoma corporis diffusum)	XR	Alpha-galactosidase-A	Acroparesthesias, corneal opacity, renal failure, cardiac or cerebrovascular pathology	Angiokeratomas in bathing trunk distribution, hypohidrosis	Hyperkeratosis and acanthosis with ectatic vessels in the dermal papillae	Vascular tumo (Ch. 23)
Gardner syndrome (familial adenomatous polyposis)	AD	APC	Gastrointestinal polyps and adenocarcinoma, osteomas, supernumerary or unerupted teeth	Epidermoid cysts, lipomas, Gardner fibroma, desmoid tumor	Epidermoid cysts with focal pilomatrical features: shadow cells and/or basaloid matrical cells in cyst wall. Gardner fibroma: tumor of thick hypocellular collagen bundles. Desmoid tumor: spindle cells with hyalinized or myxoid collagenous stroma that infiltrates skeletal muscle and fat	Benign tumor and cysts of t epidermis (Ch 2) and fibrous tumors (Ch. 2
Goltz syndrome (focal dermal hypoplasia)	XD	PORCN	Osteopathia striata, coloboma, lobster claw deformity	Linear, red-brown, raised or depressed macules of thin skin following lines of Blaschko	Dermis replaced by adipose tissue	Genodermatos (Ch. 12) and tumors of fat, muscle, cartilage, and bone (Ch. 21

ble 12.1 Key features of genodermatoses—cont'd

yndrome	Inheritance	Mutation	Noncutaneous features	Cutaneous features	Pathology of cutaneous features	Elsewhere in text
orlin syndrome evoid basal cell rcinoma ndrome)	AD	*PTCH*	Odontogenic keratocysts, medulloblastoma, calcification of the falx, bifid ribs, ovarian fibromas, macrocephaly, frontal bossing, pectus deformity	Palmar pits, basal cell carcinomas	Basal cell carcinoma: blue islands with peripheral palisade and retraction artifact in a fibromyxoid stroma	Malignant tumors of the epidermis (Ch. 3)
ailey–Hailey sease (familial enign mphigus)	AD	*ATP2C1*		Erosive erythematous plaques with crust involving the axilla, neck, and genital area	Acantholysis at all levels of an acanthotic epidermis resembling a "dilapidated brick wall"	Blistering diseases (Ch. 9)
thyosis lgaris	AD	Profilaggrin		Fine brown scales that spare the flexures	Compact hyperorthokeratosis with paradoxically reduced or absent granular layer	Genodermatoses (Ch. 12)
continentia gmenti (Bloch– lzberger ndrome)	XD	*NEMO*	Ocular, dental (peg teeth), skeletal, and neurologic abnormalities	Linear vesicles in the neonatal period evolving to verrucous lesions and then hyperpigementation or hypopigmentation	Vesicles are due to eosinophilic spongiosis with dyskeratosis. Verrucous lesions are hyperkeratotic and papillomatous with dyskeratosis. Pigmented stage is due to pigment incontinence	Genodermatoses (Ch. 12)
oid proteinosis yalinosis cutis mucosae, bach–Wiethe sease)	AR	*ECM1*	Hoarseness, seizures, cobblestone oral mucosa, bean-shaped suprasellar calcifications of the temporal lobe	Pitted scars, beaded nodules along the eyelids, verrucous lesions	Onion-skin, eosinophilic deposits around blood vessels, sweat glands, and thick perpendicular bundles in the papillary dermis	Genodermatoses (Ch. 12) and metabolic disorders (Ch. 14)

continued

Table 12.1 Key features of genodermatoses—cont'd

Syndrome	Inheritance	Mutation	Noncutaneous features	Cutaneous features	Pathology of cutaneous features	Elsewhere in text
Multiple endocrine neoplasia, type 1 (Wermer syndrome)	AD	MEN1	Endocrine tumors, including parathyroid, pituitary, adrenocortical, and gastrinoma	Multiple angiofibromas, collagenomas, lipomas	Angiofibromas: concentric perivascular and periadnexal fibrosis with stellate fibroblasts. Collagenomas (connective tissue nevi): increased dense sclerotic mass of broad collagenous bundles with diminished elastic	Fibrous tumors (Ch. 20) and alterations in collagen and elastin (Ch. 13
Muir–Torre syndrome	AD	MSH2, MLH1, MSH6 and PMS2	Colorectal, breast, and genitourinary cancers	Keratoacanthomas, sebaceous adenoma, sebaceous epithelioma, sebaceous carcinoma	Sebaceous tumors: basaloid tumors with variable amounts of clear sebocytes with scalloped nuclei and multivacuolated cytoplasm. Keratoacanthoma: crateriform glassy squamous proliferation with elastin trapping, neutrophilic microabscesses, and eosinophils	Pilar and sebaceous neoplasms (Ch. 4) malignant tumors of the epidermis (Ch. 3)
Neurofibromatosis (von Recklinghausen disease)	AD	Neurofibromin	Lisch nodules of the iris, optic nerve glioma, sphenoid dysplasia	Café-au-lait macules, axillary freckling, and numerous neurofibromas, often including plexiform neurofibroma	Neurofibroma: pale myxoid stroma with haphazard, small, comma-shaped nuclei	Neural tumors (Ch. 22)
Porphyria cutanea tarda	AD	Uroporphyrinogen decarboxylase	Liver function abnormalities	Blisters, erosions, and milia on the dorsal hands and photoexposed sites, hypertrichosis, hyperpigmentation, sclerodermoid plaques	Subepidermal pauciinflammatory blister with festooning of dermal papillae, caterpillar bodies of the overlying epidermis, and perivascular hyaline material	Blistering diseases (Ch.

able 12.1 Key features of genodermatoses—cont'd

yndrome	Inheritance	Mutation	Noncutaneous features	Cutaneous features	Pathology of cutaneous features	Elsewhere in text
seudoxanthoma asticum	AR	*ABCC6*	Angioid streaks, hypertension, stroke, gastrointestinal hemorrhage	"Plucked chicken skin" in flexures	Curled and frayed calcified elastic fibers (pink or blue squiggles)	Genodermatoses (Ch. 12)
eed syndrome nultiple utaneous and erine omyomatosis)	AD	Fumarate hydratase	Uterine leiomyomas, renal cell carcinoma	Multiple cutaneous leiomyomas	Piloleiomyomas are circumscribed dermal nodules composed of bundles of smooth muscle fibers with cigar-shaped nuclei and a perinuclear vacuole	Tumors of fat, muscle, cartilage, and bone (Ch. 21)
ombo syndrome	AD		Vasodilation with cyanosis	Vermiculate atrophoderma, milia, hypotrichosis, trichoepitheliomas, and basal cell carcinomas	Trichoepitheliomas: basaloid islands and papillary mesenchymal bodies in a fibroblast-rich stroma without retraction. Basal cell carcinoma: blue islands with peripheral palisade and retraction artifact in a fibromyxoid stroma	Pilar and sebaceous neoplasms (Ch. 4) and malignant tumors of the epidermis (Ch. 3)
berous :lerosis	AD	Tuberin (*TSC2*) and hamartin (*TSC1*)	Retinal nodular hamartomas, cortical tuber, subependymal nodule, subependymal giant cell astrocytoma, epilepsy, mental retardation, cardiac rhabdomyoma, lymphangiomyomatosis, renal angiomyolipoma	Adenoma sebaceum (angiofibromas), periungual fibromas, shagreen patch, hypopigmented ash leaf macules	Angiofibromas: concentric perivascular and periadnexal fibrosis with stellate fibroblasts. Shagreen patches (connective tissue nevi): increased dense sclerotic mass of broad collagenous bundles with diminished elastic	Fibrous tumors (Ch. 20) and alterations in collagen and elastin (Ch. 13)
hite sponge evus	AD	*K4* and *K13*		Diffuse, white-gray, spongy, folded plaques on the buccal, labial, and other mucosal sites	Vacuolation of mucosal epithelium with dense perinuclear eosinophilic condensation	Viral infections, helminths, and arthropods (Ch. 19)

D, autosomal dominant; *AR,* autosomal recessive; *XD,* X-linked dominant; *XR,* X-linked recessive.

Further reading

Bolognia JL, Braverman I. Pseudoxanthoma-elasticum-like skin changes induced by penicillamine. Dermatology 1992;184(1):12–18.

Eng AM, Bryant J. Clinical pathologic observations in pseudoxanthoma elasticum. Int J Dermatol 1975;14(8):586–605.

Lebwohl M, Phelps RG, Yannuzzi L, et al. Diagnosis of pseudoxanthoma elasticum by scar biopsy in patients without characteristic skin lesions. N Engl J Med 1987;317(6):347–50.

Meyrick Thomas RH, Kirby JD. Elastosis perforans serpiginosa and pseudoxanthoma elasticum-like skin change due to D-penicillamine. Clin Exp Dermatol 1985;10(4):386–91.

Shukla SA, Veerappan R, Whittimore JS, et al. Mast cell ultrastructure and staining in tissue. Methods Mol Biol 2006;315:63–76.

Sybert VP, Dale BA, Holbrook KA. Ichthyosis vulgaris: identification of a defect in synthesis of filaggrin correlated with an absence of keratohyaline granules. J Invest Dermatol 1985;84(3):191–4.

Alterations in collagen and elastin

Tammie Ferringer

Lichen sclerosus (et atrophicus)

Key Features

- Red (compact stratum corneum)
- White (papillary dermal pallor)
- Blue (lymphoid band beneath zone of pallor)
- Synonymous with balanitis xerotica obliterans on the glans penis

Lichen sclerosus may involve skin or mucosa. Follicular plugging is common, and the plugs may resemble comedones clinically. The epidermis is commonly atrophic, and the rete pattern is effaced; however, scratching may produce pseudoepitheliomatous hyperplasia, especially in vulvar lesions. Squamous cell carcinoma rarely develops in long-standing genital lesions of lichen sclerosus and must be distinguished from pseudoepitheliomatous hyperplasia. Papillary dermal edema may produce a subepidermal bulla. Vacuolar interface dermatitis and pigment incontinence are common. Epidermotropic lymphocytes may be hyperchromatic and may mimic mycosis fungoides. The differential diagnosis also includes radiation dermatitis (Table 13.1) and morphea.

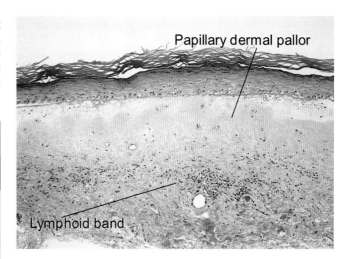

Papillary dermal pallor

Lymphoid band

Fig. 13.1 Lichen sclerosus

Chronic radiation dermatitis

Key Features

- Papillary dermal pallor without vacuolar change or lymphoid band
- Large stellate radiation fibroblasts
- Radiation elastosis
- Loss of adnexa
- Dilated ectatic vessels superficially

There is typically hyperkeratosis and epidermal atrophy with effaced rete that may alternate with hyperplasia. Stellate cells with large nuclei are usually present (radiation fibroblasts). The eccrine glands are atrophic and the pilosebaceous structures are absent; however, the arrector pili muscle may survive. The dermal collagen is hyalinized. Radiation elastosis may resemble solar elastosis but extends into follicular fibrous tracts. The superficial blood vessels are dilated, whereas the deeper vessels have thick walls.

Table 13.1 Features of lichen sclerosus and chronic radiation dermatitis

Feature	Lichen sclerosus	Chronic radiation dermatitis
Compact, red stratum corneum	Yes	Yes
Superficial dermal pallor	Yes	Yes
Epidermal atrophy	Variable	Variable
Follicular plugging	Common	Rare
Vacuolar interface dermatitis	Yes	No
Lymphoid band	Yes	No
Pigment incontinence	Common	Usually absent
Superficial dermal vessels	Normal to slight dilatation	Widely ectatic
Radiation elastosis	No	Yes
Adnexal structures	Present	Absent
Large, stellate fibroblasts	No	Yes
Deep dermis	Normal	Sclerotic
Shape of punch biopsy	Tapered	Square

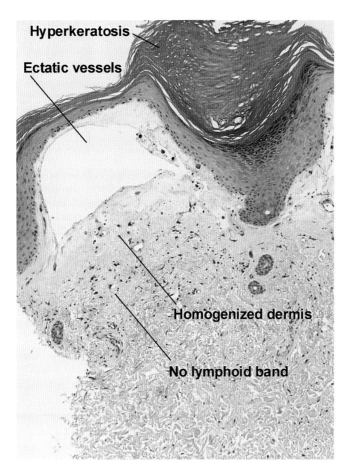

Fig. 13.2 Chronic radiation dermatitis

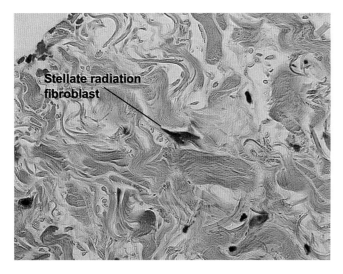

Fig. 13.3 Chronic radiation dermatitis

The severity of radiation damage varies with the total dose, its fractionation, and the depth of penetration. Acute radiodermatitis occurs within weeks of irradiation and presents as erythema and edema followed by hyperpigmentation. Although typically diagnosed clinically, there is vacuolization and sparse degenerated keratinocytes similar to a phototoxic eruption. Chronic changes arise months to years after the initial exposure. There is atrophy, fragility, telangiectasias, altered pigmentation, and alopecia. Nonmelanoma skin cancers can develop years later and may behave in an aggressive manner with increased risk of metastasis, especially with squamous cell carcinoma.

Morphea/scleroderma

Key Features

- Rectangular punch
- Thick, closely packed, hyalinized collagen bundles in the lower dermis
- Loss of adventitial fat resulting in "trapped" eccrine glands
- Sparse, deep lymphoplasmacytic infiltrate
- Reduced number of CD34+ interstitial cells in the dermis
- Superficial dermal pallor may be present, but the vacuolar interface dermatitis and lymphoid band of lichen sclerosus are lacking

Scleroderma encompasses a group of diseases. Localized cutaneous disease may present as morphea or linear scleroderma (including *en coup de sabre*). In addition to cutaneous lesions, Raynaud phenomenon and variable organ involvement characterize diffuse systemic scleroderma and limited systemic scleroderma (CREST). Although the histologic features are similar, morphea is usually more inflammatory and lacks the intimal thickening and luminal obliteration of vessels seen in systemic scleroderma.

There is controversy concerning the relationship of lichen sclerosus and morphea. Some regard lichen sclerosus as a superficial expression of morphea, explaining the lichen sclerosus–like changes in the papillary dermis overlying some lesions of morphea. However, lesions of morphea with superficial pallor do not demonstrate a superficial lymphoid band, vacuolar interface dermatitis, or follicular plugging. Deep dermal sclerosis is always present.

The sclerotic process in linear scleroderma and deep morphea (morphea profunda) extends into the subcutaneous fat and possibly fascia and bone. Unlike chronic radiation dermatitis, radiation elastosis is absent and radiation fibroblasts are not identified. Elastic fibers in morphea are often brightly eosinophilic.

Other disorders with dermal sclerosis include sclerodermoid graft-versus-host disease (GvHD), porphyria cutanea tarda, vinyl chloride exposure, and reactions to bleomycin. There are conflicting data regarding the relationship with *Borrelia burgdorferi* infection and morphea and lichen sclerosus. A relationship has been found in some studies in Europe; however, other studies, especially those in North America, have failed to show an association.

Differential Diagnosis

Typical punch biopsies exhibit a tapered or cone-shaped outline. However, a thickened or sclerotic dermis can result in a square or rectangular biopsy. This can be seen in:

- Morphea/scleroderma
- Chronic GvHD
- Chronic radiodermatitis
- Scar
- Normal skin of the back
- Connective tissue nevi
- Scleredema

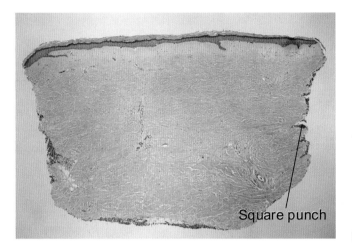

Square punch

Fig. 13.4 Morphea

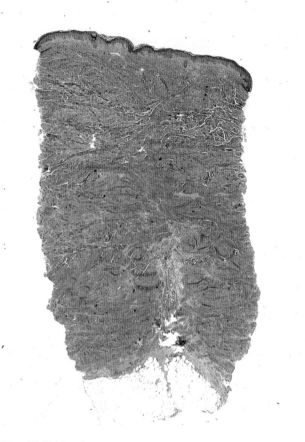

Fig. 13.6 Morphea

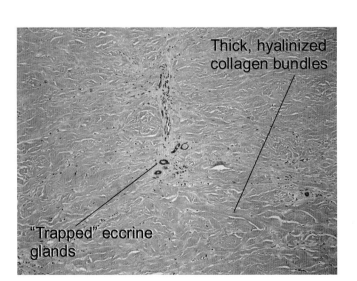

Thick, hyalinized collagen bundles

"Trapped" eccrine glands

Fig. 13.5 Morphea

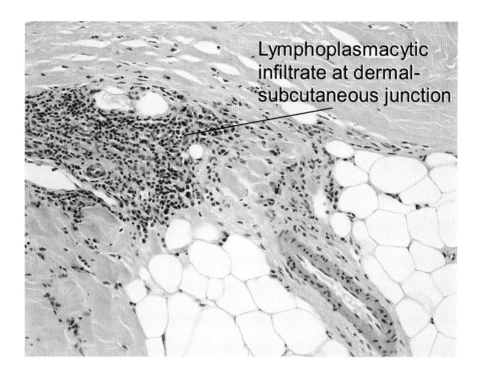

Fig. 13.7 Morphea

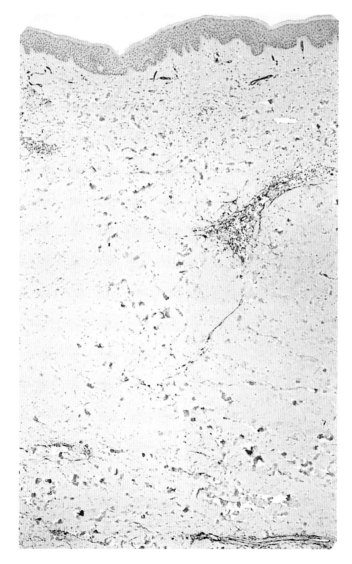

Fig. 13.8 Morphea, CD34 revealing loss of interstitial reactivity

Sclerodermoid graft-versus-host disease

Key Features

- Minimal basal vacuolization
- Dermis is thickened and sclerotic
- Adnexal structures are destroyed

Dermal sclerosis begins in the papillary dermis and may extend into the subcutaneous tissue. In the chronic phase of GvHD, an early lichenoid stage and a later sclerotic stage can be distinguished. Each stage can occur without the other. Unlike radiation dermatitis, vascular ectasia and radiation fibroblasts are not identified. Clinically, the skin often has a corrugated appearance.

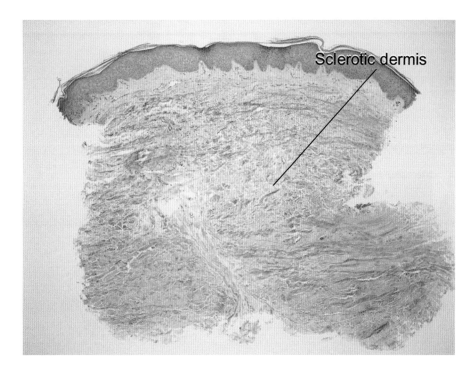

Sclerotic dermis

Fig. 13.9 Sclerodermoid graft-versus-host disease

Eosinophilic fasciitis (Shulman syndrome)

Key Features

- Thick eosinophilic fascia due to fibrosis and hyalinization of collagen
- Variable infiltrate of lymphocytes, plasma cells, and occasional eosinophils

Eosinophilic fasciitis is a scleroderma-like disorder of the fascia that can be distinguished by the sudden onset of painful edema and progressive induration, typically involving an extremity or extremities after strenuous exercise. The condition is named for its association with peripheral eosinophilia. Eosinophils may be found in the tissue but are not required, and are typically absent. The fibrosis and hyalinization involve the fascia and deep subcutaneous septa. In many cases, the overlying adipose tissue shows no significant changes. A deep incisional biopsy to include fascia is required for diagnosis.

Scleroderma with fascial involvement may appear similar histologically, but can be distinguished clinically. Similar changes are described in eosinophilia–myalgia syndrome secondary to L-tryptophan ingestion, although there is greater dermal involvement in eosinophilia–myalgia syndrome and the late stage is characterized by dermal mucinosis.

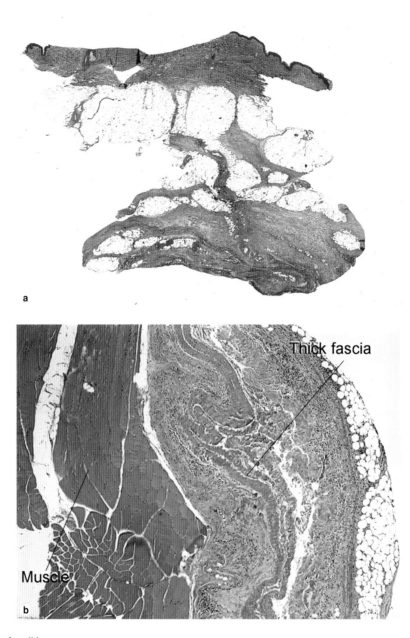

Fig. 13.10 Eosinophilic fasciitis

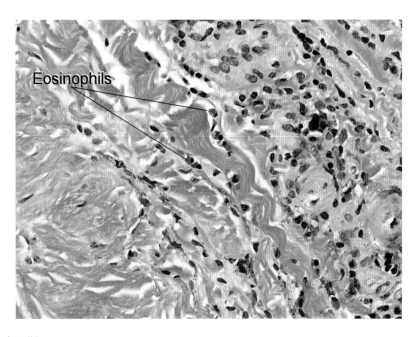

Fig. 13.11 Eosinophilic fasciitis

Elastosis perforans serpiginosa

Key Features

- Tortuous channel through an acanthotic epidermis with extrusion of altered elastic fibers
- Large, bulky, red elastic fibers

The papules of elastosis perforans serpiginosa coalesce in an arcuate or serpiginous pattern, most commonly on the neck, face, or upper extremity. Elastic tissue stains reveal increased abnormal, thickened elastic fibers in the dermis in the vicinity of the channel.

Patients on long-term penicillamine for Wilson disease may develop altered elastic fibers with overlapping features of pseudoxanthoma elasticum and elastosis perforans serpiginosa. The penicillamine-induced, altered elastic fibers have small lateral buds arranged perpendicularly to the primary elastic fiber, resembling the twigs on a bramble bush, but do not calcify.

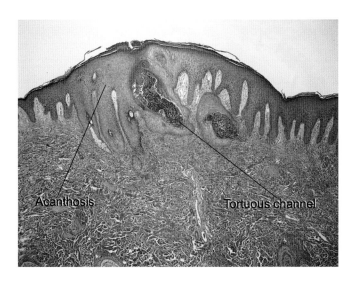

Fig. 13.12 Elastosis perforans serpiginosa

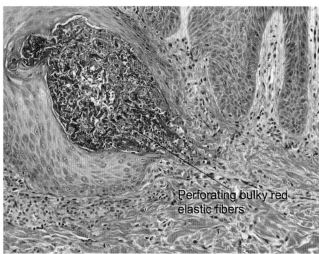

Fig. 13.13 Elastosis perforans serpiginosa

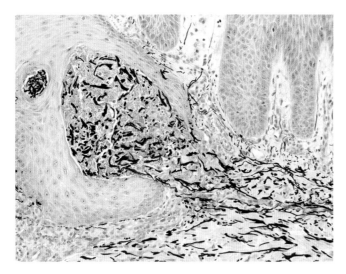

Fig. 13.14 Elastosis perforans serpiginosa (elastic tissue stain)

Elastosis perforans serpiginosa–associated disorders

The mnemonic "RAP MOPED" is helpful in remembering the associated diseases.

- Rothmund–Thompson syndrome
- Acrogeria
- Penicillamine
- Marfan syndrome
- Osteogenesis imperfecta
- Pseudoxanthoma elasticum
- Ehlers–Danlos syndrome
- Down syndrome

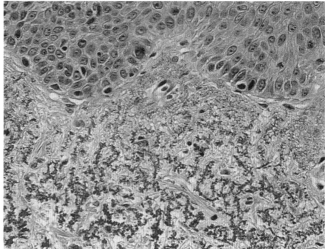

Fig. 13.15 Penicillamine-induced altered elastic fibers

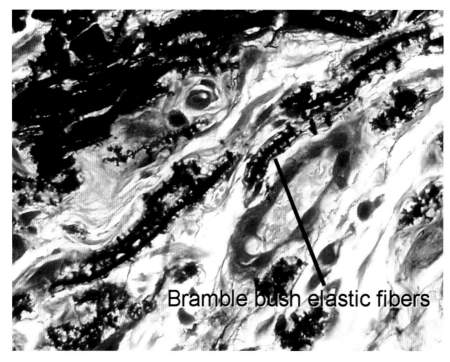

Bramble bush elastic fibers

Fig. 13.16 Penicillamine-induced altered elastic fibers (Verhoeff–van Gieson)

Reactive perforating collagenosis

Key Features

- Broad channel
- Vertical extrusion of degenerated basophilic collagen bundles
- Masson trichrome stain distinguishes the extruded collagen from elastic tissue

The primary lesion is a small papule with a hyperkeratotic central umbilication. Classic, true reactive perforating collagenosis is an inherited genodermatosis, most often in an autosomal-dominant pattern. These lesions occur in children and are precipitated by minor trauma.

An adult-acquired form has been described in association with diabetes and chronic renal failure. This form, known as *acquired perforating dermatosis* or *perforating disorder of renal disease*, encompasses features of Kyrle disease and perforating folliculitis.

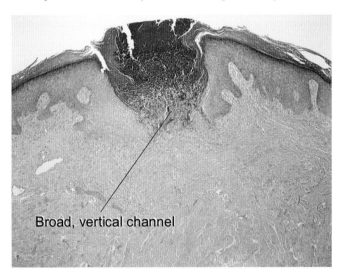

Fig. 13.17 Reactive perforating collagenosis

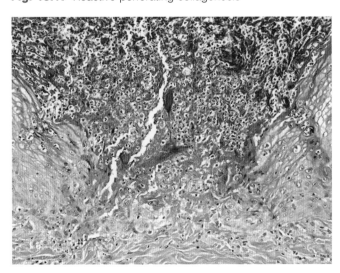

Fig. 13.18 Reactive perforating collagenosis

Scar and keloid

Scar

Key Features

- Fibroblasts with east–west orientation
- Blood vessels with north–south orientation
- Loss of elastic tissue
- Epidermis is often effaced (see Chapter 20)

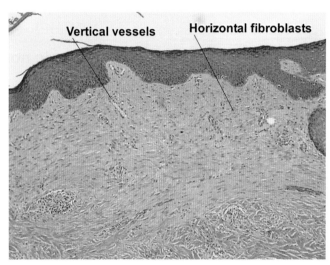

Fig. 13.19 Scar

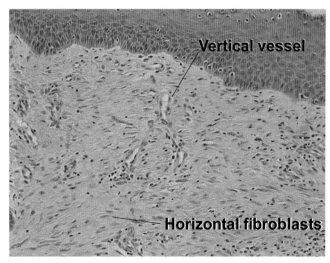

Fig. 13.20 Scar

Hypertrophic scar

Key Features

- Nodules or whorls of thickened collagen and fibroblasts

Keloid

Key Features

- Background of hypertrophic scar
- Broad, hyalinized, eosinophilic "bubble gum" collagen fibers

Keloids clinically differ from hypertrophic scars by extending beyond the confines of the original wound. Elastic fibers and adnexal structures are diminished or absent in both scars and keloids. Recent surgical scars may also contain signs of Monsel's solution, gelfoam, or aluminum chloride (see Appendix 3).

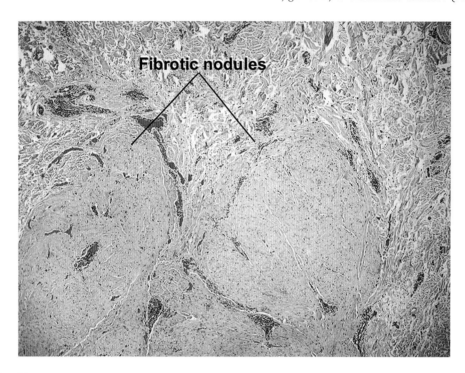

Fig. 13.21 Hypertrophic scar

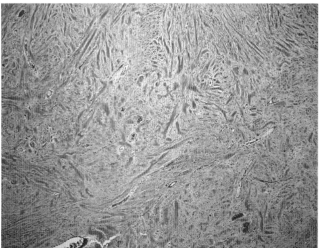

Fig. 13.22 Keloid

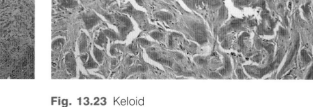

Fig. 13.23 Keloid

Acne keloidalis nuchae

Key Features

- Hypertrophic scar (not keloid)
- Suppurative folliculitis with hair shafts free in the dermis
- Plasma cell infiltrate

The plasma cell infiltrate is related to the predominance on the posterior neck. Plasma cells are typically a component of the inflammatory infiltrate on the face, occipital scalp/posterior neck, axillae, breast, genital area, and shins. Hair shafts free in the dermis are surrounded by microabscesses and/or giant cells.

PEARL

There is no mycosis in mycosis fungoides, no granuloma in granuloma faciale, and no keloid in acne keloidalis.

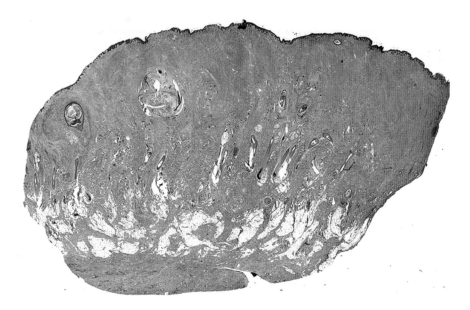

Fig. 13.24 Acne keloidalis nuchae

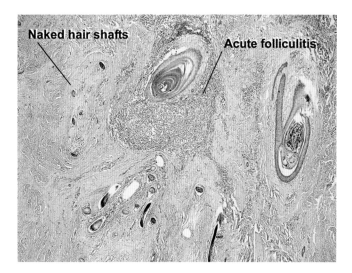

Fig. 13.25 Acne keloidalis nuchae

Favre–Racouchot syndrome (nodular elastosis with cysts and comedones)

Key Features

- Dilated, keratin-filled follicles
- Small cysts
- Solar elastosis

This solar degeneration condition presents with yellowish plaques lateral to the eyes that are studded with cysts and multiple open comedones. Smoking may act in conjunction with the solar damage to create this syndrome. Solar elastosis is a bluish, amorphous material that is primarily sun-damaged elastic and/or collagen fibers.

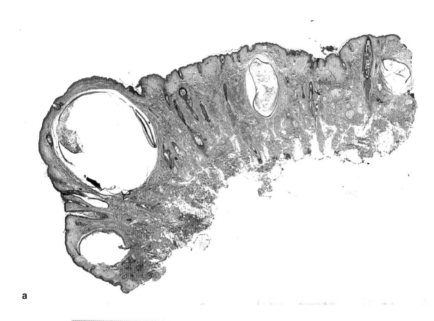

a

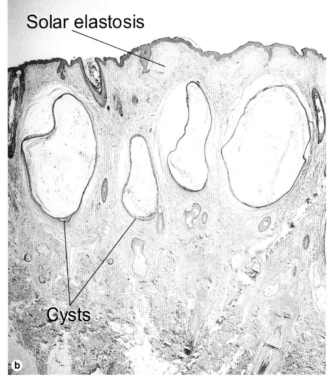

b

Fig. 13.26 Favre–Racouchot syndrome

Chondrodermatitis nodularis helicis

Key Features

- Ulcer or erosion with adjacent acanthosis overlying a zone of fibrin
- Fibrin is flanked on either side by granulation tissue

Depending on the depth of the biopsy, cartilage may be present but is not required for diagnosis. Collagen degeneration occurs from a combination of pressure, poor vascularity, and solar damage.

Acrodermatitis chronica atrophicans

Key Features

- Early lesions show a diffuse lymphoplasmacytic infiltrate resembling "polka dots"
- Late lesions show epidermal and dermal atrophy with attenuated, wispy collagen fibers

Borrelial spirochetes may be found with silver stains. This is a late manifestation of infection by *Borrelia*. It is most frequently reported in Europe, where *B. afzelii* is endemic.

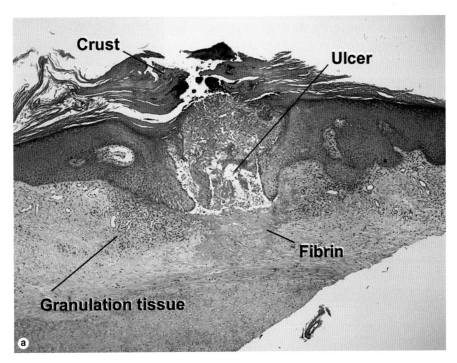

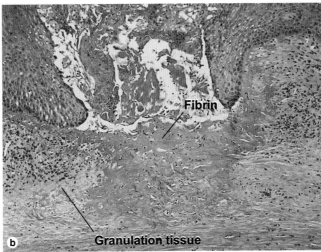

Fig. 13.27 Chondrodermatitis nodularis helicis

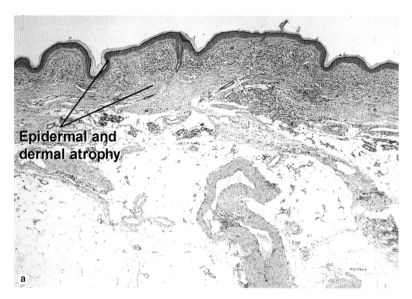

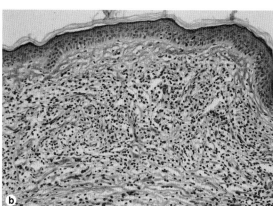

Fig. 13.28 Acrodermatitis chronica atrophicans

Ochronosis

Key Features

- Glassy, yellow-brown (ochre-colored), banana-shaped deposits in the dermis

The inherited form, also known as *alkaptonuria*, is an autosomal-recessive disorder due to homogentisic acid oxidase deficiency. Exogenous ochronosis occurs as a result of application of hydroquinone or contact with phenol (carbolic acid).

Colloid milium

Key Features

- Pale pink, fissured deposits that fill and expand the dermal papillae

The adult type develops in the setting of severe sun damage on the face, neck, and dorsal hands. This material represents the final product of severe solar degeneration but can stain weakly with amyloid stains (crystal violet, Congo red, thioflavin T). However, it fails to react with pagoda red. The juvenile form develops on the head and neck before the development of sun damage. This type is Congo red negative but positive with antikeratin antibodies, confirming the origin of the material from degenerated keratinocytes.

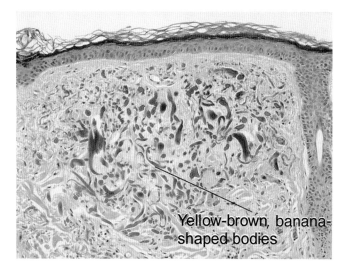

Fig. 13.29 Ochronosis

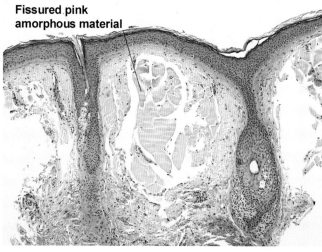

Fig. 13.30 Colloid milium

Anetoderma

Key Features

- Essentially normal hematoxylin and eosin (H&E)–stained sections
- Elastic fibers are sparse to absent in the superficial and middermis with elastic tissue stains (Verhoeff–van Gieson)

These oval lesions have an atrophic or wrinkled surface and bulge outward or are slightly depressed and herniate inward with pressure. The upper trunk and upper arms of young adults are typically affected. Primary lesions have been reported with clinical inflammation (Jadassohn–Pellizzari type) and without (Schweninger–Buzzi type) a preceding inflammatory stage. Clinically inflamed lesions may have a perivascular and sometimes interstitial infiltrate, but established lesions look like normal skin on H&E-stained sections and reveal minimal to no elastic fibers with special stains. Secondary anetoderma can occur from various processes, including syphilis, other infectious processes, granulomatous diseases, lupus, and lymphoma.

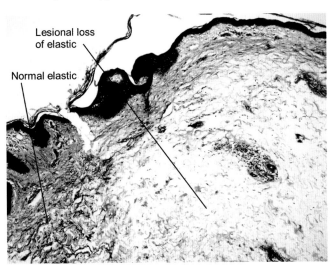

Lesional loss of elastic

Normal elastic

Fig. 13.31 Anetoderma (Verhoeff–van Gieson)

Atrophoderma

Key Features

- H&E-stained features are subtle unless compared with normal adjacent skin
- Dermal thickness is reduced in comparison to normal adjacent skin
- Collagen shows varying degrees of homogenization

Lesions typically are sharply demarcated, gray-brown, atrophic, round to oval, depressed areas with a "cliff-drop" border. Some have suggested that atrophoderma is an atrophic abortive variant of morphea. In contrast to morphea, there is no violaceous border or induration, and lesions tend to be chronic. A superficial perivascular and interstitial inflammatory infiltrate consisting of lymphocytes and histiocytes can be seen. Elastic fibers appear normal.

Connective tissue nevus

Key Features

- Collagenoma: thickened dermis due to broad haphazard bundles of collagen that are less well packed than normal collagen and widely spaced elastic fibers likely due to a dilution phenomenon
- Elastoma: H&E-stained sections show a normal or slightly thickened dermis but accumulation of broad, branching, and interlacing elastic fibers in the mid and lower dermis with elastic tissue stains

Connective tissue nevi are hamartomas of the extracellular connective tissue, whether it is collagen, elastic, or glycosaminoglycans that is present in abnormal amounts. Collagenomas can be inherited in an autosomal-dominant pattern or associated with Proteus syndrome and tuberous sclerosis (shagreen patches). They present as skin-colored papules, nodules, or plaques. Elastomas are associated with Buschke–Ollendorff syndrome.

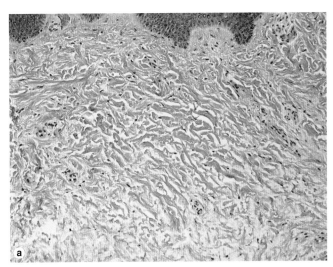

a

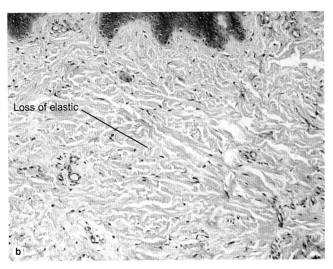

Loss of elastic

b

Fig. 13.32 (A and B) Collagenoma. **(B)** Elastic stain (Verhoeff–van Gieson)

Aplasia cutis congenita

Key Features

- Epidermis is absent or thin
- Appendages are absent or rudimentary

Aplasia cutis is due to congenital absence of skin. It may present as an ulceration, membranous lesion, or atrophic scarring, most commonly on the vertex of the scalp. It may be associated with limb defects (Adams–Oliver syndrome), mental retardation, epidermal nevi, epidermolysis bullosa (Bart syndrome), chromosomal abnormalities, fetus papyraceus, or focal dermal hypoplasia.

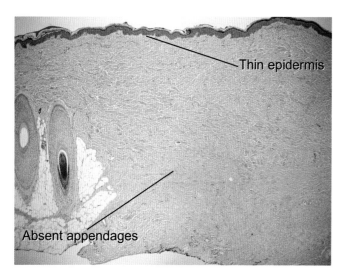

Fig. 13.33 Aplasia cutis congenita

Further reading

Aberer E, Klade H, Hobisch G. A clinical, histological, and immunohistochemical comparison of acrodermatitis chronica atrophicans and morphea. Am J Dermatopathol 1991;13(4):334–41.

Aiba S, Tabata N, Ohtani H, et al. CD34+ spindle-shaped cells selectively disappear from the skin lesion of scleroderma. Arch Dermatol 1994;130(5):593–7.

Blackburn WR, Cosman B. Histologic basis of keloid and hypertrophic scar differentiation. Clinicopathologic correlation. Arch Pathol 1966;82(1):65–71.

Fretzin DF, Beal DW, Jao W. Light and ultrastructural study of reactive perforating collagenosis. Arch Dermatol 1980;116(9):1054–8.

Gebhart W, Bardach H. The "lumpy-bumpy" elastic fiber. A marker for long-term administration of penicillamine. Am J Dermatopathol 1981;3(1):33–9.

Graham JH, Marques AS. Colloid milium: a histochemical study. J Invest Dermatol 1967;49(5):497–507.

Handfield-Jones SE, Atherton DJ, Black MM, et al. Juvenile colloid milium: clinical, histological and ultrastructural features. J Cutan Pathol 1992;19(5):434–8.

Kazlouskaya V, Malhotra S, Lambe J, et al. The utility of elastic Verhoeff-Van Gieson staining in dermatopathology. J Cutan Pathol 2013;40(2):211–25.

Rahbari H. Histochemical differentiation of localized morphea-scleroderma and lichen sclerosus et atrophicus. J Cutan Pathol 1989;16(6):342–7.

Santos-Alarcón S, López-López OF, Flores-Terry MÁ, et al. Collagen anomalies as clues for diagnosis: part 1. Am J Dermatopathology 2017;39(8):559–86.

Uitto J, Santa Cruz DJ, Bauer EA, et al. Morphea and lichen sclerosus et atrophicus. Clinical and histopathologic studies in patients with combined features. J Am Acad Dermatol 1980;3(3):271–9.

Wienecke R, Schlupen EM, Zochling N, et al. Staining of amyloid with cotton dyes. Arch Dermatol 1984;120(9):1184–5.

Metabolic disorders

Tammie Ferringer

Mucinoses

The mucinoses are a group of disorders characterized by mucin deposition in the dermis. The mucin is typically non–sulfated acid mucopolysaccharide (hyaluronic acid) that appears as wispy, faint blue threads on routine sections. It can be better appreciated with colloidal iron, Alcian blue, and toluidine blue staining.

Scleredema (of Buschke)

Key Features

- Thickened dermis
- Widened spaces with mucin between normal collagen bundles
- The mucin is most prominent in the deep dermis
- No inflammatory infiltrate or increased fibroblasts

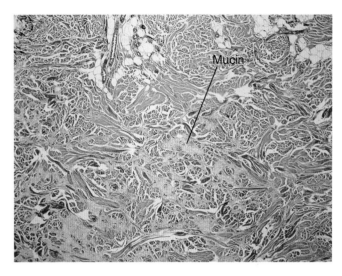

Fig. 14.2 Scleredema

- The histologic features can be subtle and mimic normal skin at scan, but there is increased space between collagen fibers in the deep dermis

Scleredema most often occurs in the setting of insulin-dependent, adult-onset diabetes on the upper back, an area that normally displays a thick dermis. Scleredema can also occur suddenly after a streptococcal infection or in association with a monoclonal gammopathy.

Pretibial myxedema

Key Features

- Large amounts of mucin throughout the dermis
- Collagen bundles separated by mucin and reduced to thin wisps

Pretibial myxedema is found in patients with Graves disease, especially those with exophthalmos. It may not develop until after correction of the hyperthyroidism.

Differential Diagnosis

The mucin deposition in pretibial myxedema involves the full thickness of the dermis, whereas the mucin in stasis is restricted to the papillary dermis. Nodular angioplasia and hemosiderin deposition are also features of stasis. Scleredema lacks attenuation of collagen fibers.

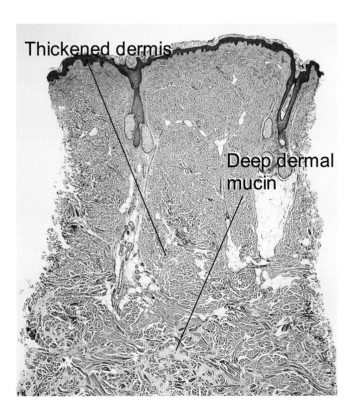

Fig. 14.1 Scleredema

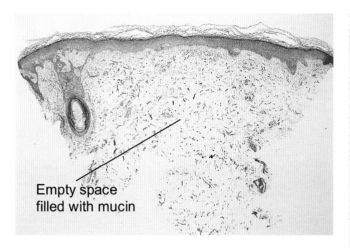

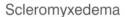

Fig. 14.3 Pretibial myxedema

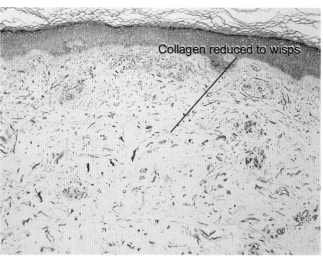

Fig. 14.4 Pretibial myxedema

Scleromyxedema

Key Features

- Increase in dermal fibroblasts, fine collagen fibers, and interstitial mucin

Papular mucinosis (lichen myxedematosus) is composed of linear arrays of waxy papules. Scleromyxedema is a variant in which the papules coalesce with diffuse sclerosis of the skin. An immunoglobulin (Ig) G lambda gammopathy is associated with scleromyxedema and many cases of papular mucinosis.

Differential Diagnosis

Histologically, scleromyxedema resembles nephrogenic systemic fibrosis. The clinical setting varies in that nephrogenic systemic fibrosis occurs in patients with renal failure with involvement of the distal extremities, whereas scleromyxedema is associated with IgG paraproteinemia and typically involves the face.

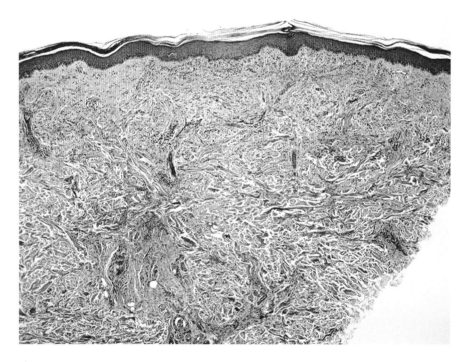

Fig. 14.5 Scleromyxedema

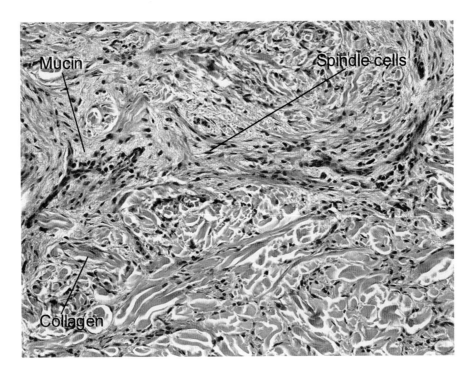

Fig. 14.6 Scleromyxedema

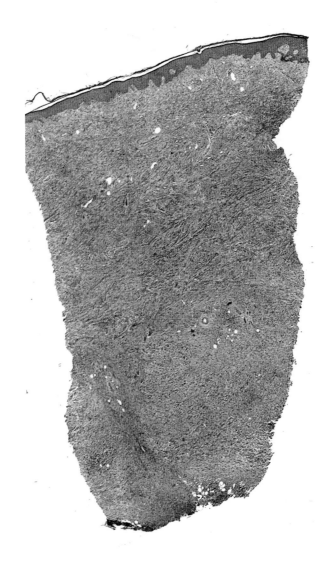

Fig. 14.7 Nephrogenic systemic fibrosis

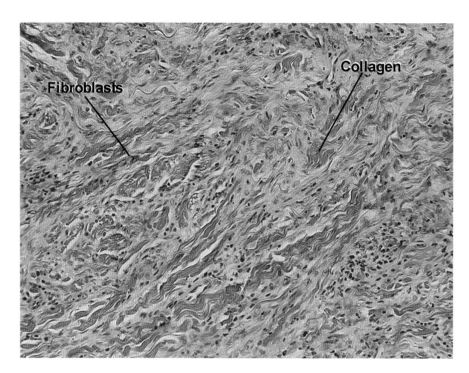

Fig. 14.8 Nephrogenic systemic fibrosis

Tumid lupus

Key Features

- Interface damage is subtle or absent
- Superficial and deep perivascular and periadnexal lymphocytic infiltrate
- Infiltrate typically involves the eccrine coil
- Abundant mucin is present in the reticular dermis

Reticular erythematous mucinosis is indistinguishable histologically from tumid lupus. Many consider it a variant of tumid lupus.

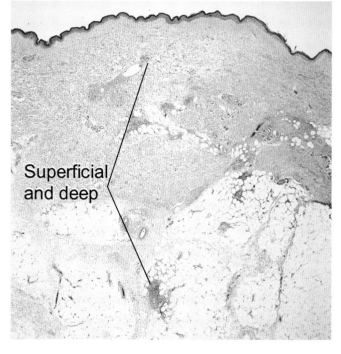

Fig. 14.9 Tumid lupus

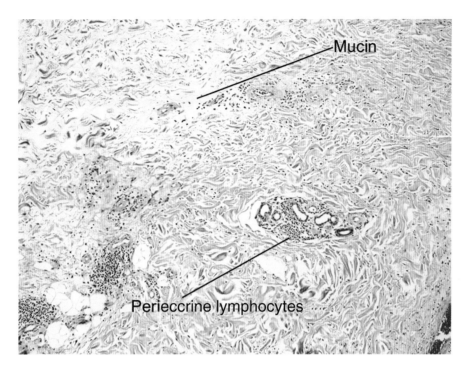

Fig. 14.10 Tumid lupus

Focal mucinosis

- Dome-shaped papule containing a pool of mucin

Digital myxoid cyst resembles focal mucinosis, but on acral skin.

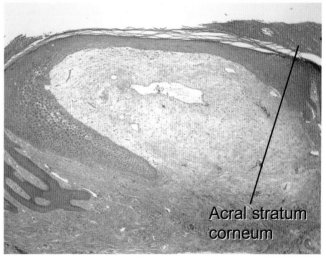

Fig. 14.12 Digital myxoid cyst

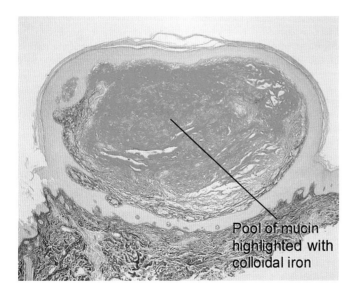

Fig. 14.11 Focal mucinosis (colloidal iron)

Amyloidosis

Primary systemic amyloidosis is due to deposition of light chains. Skin lesions may occur, but in those with no obvious lesions, a blind biopsy of salivary glands or abdominal fat can be examined for the presence of amyloid. Light-chain–derived nodular cutaneous amyloidosis is produced locally by plasma cells and may or may not be associated with systemic amyloidosis. Secondary systemic amyloidosis lacks clinical skin lesions, but may demonstrate amyloid deposits in minor salivary glands or abdominal fat. Epidermal (keratin)-derived forms of amyloidosis include macular and lichen amyloidosis. Amyloid is brick red with Congo red stain and apple green with polarization. The cotton dye pagoda red is most specific for amyloid. Staining with thioflavin T is very sensitive but requires examination with a fluorescent microscope, resulting in yellow-green fluorescence of amyloid deposits. Crystal violet is a metachromatic stain that is highly sensitive for epidermal-derived amyloid.

The clinical types of amyloidosis and their associated amyloid protein are listed in Table 14.1. In addition to the specific fibrillar component, amyloid P, a nonfibrillar glycoprotein, binds to all types of amyloid fibrils. Antisera to these proteins can be used immunohistochemically to identify the amyloid deposition.

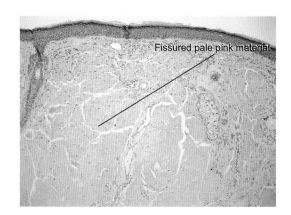

Fig. 14.13 Nodular amyloid

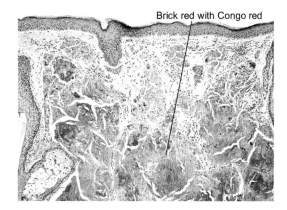

Fig. 14.14 Nodular amyloid (Congo red)

Table 14.1 Clinical types of amyloidosis and their associated amyloid protein

Clinical type	Amyloid fibril protein	Precursor substance
Localized cutaneous		
Macular	AK	Altered keratin
Lichenoid	AK	Altered keratin
Nodular	AL (Aλ and Aκ)	Immunoglobulin light chain
Systemic		
Primary/myeloma-associated	AL (Aλ and Aκ)	Immunoglobulin light chain
Secondary	AA	Serum amyloid A
Familial Mediterranean fever	AA	Serum amyloid A
Muckle–Wells syndrome	AA	Serum amyloid A
Familial amyloid polyneuropathy	Prealbumin (transthyretin)	
Hemodialysis-associated	β2-microglobulin	

Macular amyloid

Key Features

- Sparse pink deposits in the papillary dermis
- Amyloid is outlined by a fine network of melanophages

Macular amyloid is a keratin-derived deposition produced by chronic scratching. Clinically, there is mottled hyperpigmentation of the interscapular area. This sparse deposition can be easily overlooked and may mimic normal skin.

Differential Diagnosis

At scan, some biopsies mimic normal skin and require closer inspection or clinical history to determine the diagnosis. Joe English's mnemonic "I vacuum dog pus" includes many of these subtle histologic entities:

- *I*chthyosis vulgaris
- *V*itiligo
- *A*rgyria
- *C*andida
- *U*rticaria
- *U*rticaria pigmentosa (especially telangiectasia macularis eruptiva perstans)
- *M*acular amyloid
- *D*ermatophyte

Nodular amyloidosis

Key Features

- Large, fissured, pale pink masses
- Plasma cells usually prominent

Nodular amyloid consists of light chains (AL) and may be a purely cutaneous lesion or occur in association with primary systemic amyloidosis. Lesions may be a manifestation of a localized plasmacytoma.

- *Onchocerciasis* (microfilaria)
- *Gold* (chrysiasis)
- *Pseudoxanthoma* elasticum and psoriasis (guttate)
- *Ulerythema* ophryogenes
- *Seborrheic* dermatitis and scleredema

Alternatively, what initially appears to be normal skin at scan can be approached systematically, starting in the stratum corneum looking for organisms, then moving deeper to look for absence of a granular layer; followed by the epidermal pattern; alteration in pigmentation; deposition in the dermal papillae, perivascular, or interstitial infiltrate; and down to the eccrine glands looking for silver granules.

Lichen amyloid

Key Features

- Hyperkeratosis and acanthosis
- Pink amorphous deposits in the papillary dermis outlined by a network of melanophages

Lichen amyloid is a keratin-derived deposition that histologically resembles macular amyloid with superimposed changes of lichen simplex chronicus. Clinically, it presents as intensely pruritic papules in rows, usually on the anterior shins.

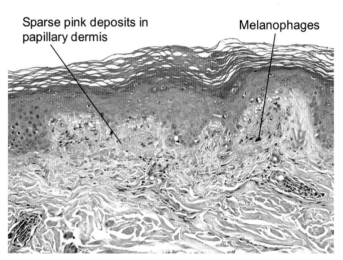

Fig. 14.15 Macular amyloid

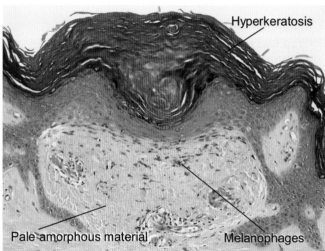

Fig. 14.16 Lichen amyloid

Cutaneous calcification

The cutaneous deposition of calcium—calcinosis cutis—has been divided into dystrophic, metastatic, and idiopathic forms. Dystrophic calcium deposition occurs in the presence of normal calcium levels, with the deposits forming in damaged tissue as in dermatomyositis, scleroderma, or in scars. Scrotal calcinosis represents calcified epidermoid cysts. Metastatic calcifications occur in normal tissue and are associated with elevated serum calcium or phosphate or both. Calciphylaxis is a unique form of metastatic calcification. Subepidermal calcified nodules are of unknown pathogenesis and belong to the category of idiopathic calcifications. Calcium typically appears basophilic on hematoxylin and eosin-stained sections and stains black with von Kossa's silver stain and red with alizarin red.

Calciphylaxis

Key Features

- Calcified small vessels in the subcutaneous fat
- Necrosis

Calciphylaxis occurs most frequently in the setting of chronic renal failure and/or hyperparathyroidism, usually in patients with diabetes.

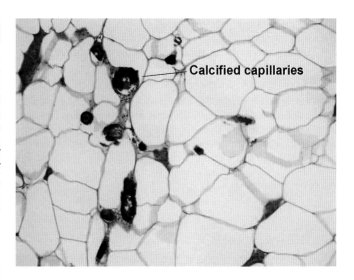

Fig. 14.17 Calciphylaxis

Subepidermal calcified nodule

Key Features

- Pseudoepitheliomatous hyperplasia with transepidermal elimination of calcium

This is an idiopathic process most common on the chin of a child or heel of a newborn.

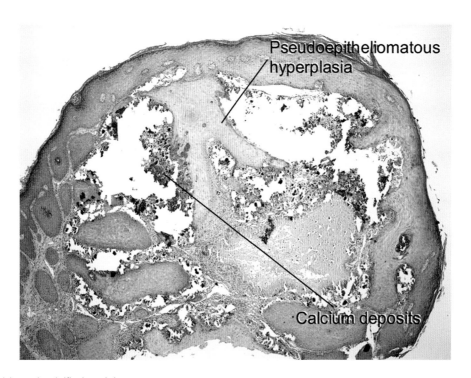

Fig. 14.18 Subepidermal calcified nodule

Scrotal calcinosis

Key Features

- Amorphous masses of calcium
- Smooth muscles scattered through the dermis indicate genital site

Although considered "idiopathic" by some, the condition appears to represent calcification of epidermoid cysts.

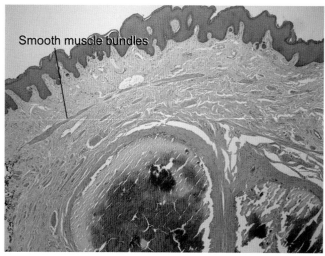

Fig. 14.20 Scrotal calcinosis

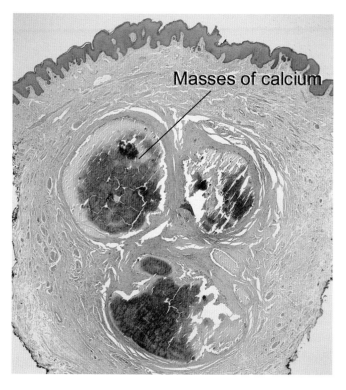

Fig. 14.19 Scrotal calcinosis

Gout

Key Features

- Palisaded granuloma surrounding amorphous gray material with a feathery appearance

Formalin fixation destroys the uric acid crystals, leaving feathery clefts. Brown crystals that are doubly refractile with polarization are present if the tissue was fixed in ethanol or was incompletely fixed in formalin.

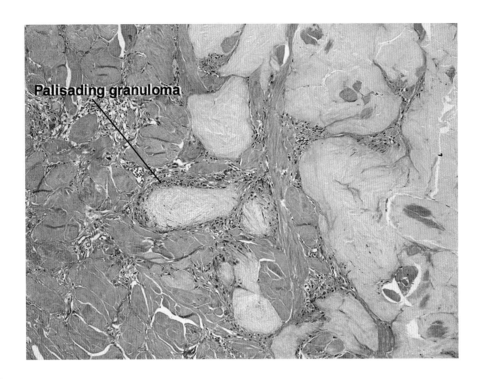

Fig. 14.21 Gout

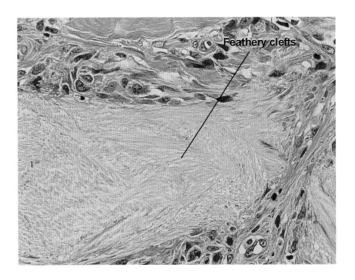

Fig. 14.22 Gout

Erythropoietic protoporphyria (EPP)

Key Features

- Hyaline cuff (reduplicated basement membrane) around postcapillary venules
- No solar elastosis is present because patients avoid the burning sensation associated with sun exposure

EPP is associated with a deficiency of ferrochelatase. It is the only disorder of porphyrin metabolism with normal urine porphyrins (EPP stands for *empty pee pee*). There are increased protoporphyrins in the feces and blood.

Differential Diagnosis

The hyaline material in EPP affects the superficial vessels, whereas lipoid proteinosis involves the superficial and deeper vessels as well as eccrine glands. Porphyria cutanea tarda demonstrates much smaller hyaline cuffs around superficial vessels, as well as solar elastosis in the surrounding skin. It often also demonstrates caterpillar bodies, subepidermal bullae, and festooning.

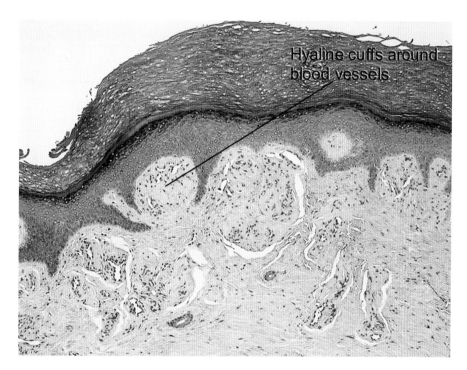

Fig. 14.23 Erythropoietic protoporphyria (EPP)

Colloid milium

Key Features

- Pale pink, fissured deposits that fill and expand the dermal papillae

The adult type develops in the setting of severe sun damage on the face, neck, and dorsal hands. This material represents the final product of severe solar degeneration but can stain weakly with amyloid stains (crystal violet, Congo red, thioflavin T). However, it fails to react with pagoda red. The juvenile form develops on the head and neck before the development of sun damage. This type is Congo red negative but positive with antikeratin antibodies, confirming the origin of the material from degenerated keratinocytes.

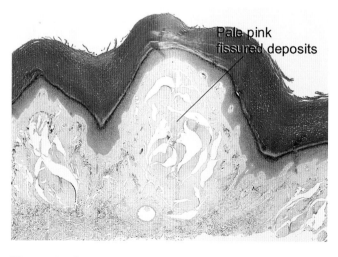

Fig. 14.24 Colloid milium

Mucocele

Key Features

- Pseudocystic space containing mucin
- Muciphages and granulation tissue surround the space

Mucoceles occur due to disruption in the excretory duct of minor salivary glands with mucin extravasation into the connective tissue. The lower labial and buccal mucosa are most commonly affected. Involvement of the floor of the mouth is referred to as *ranula*.

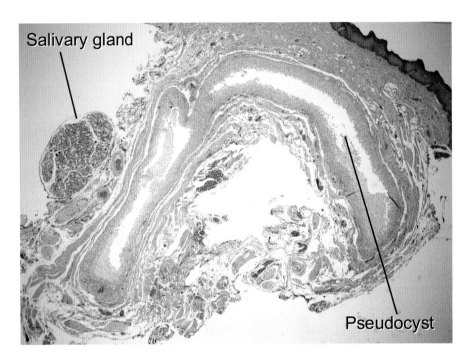

Fig. 14.25 Mucocele

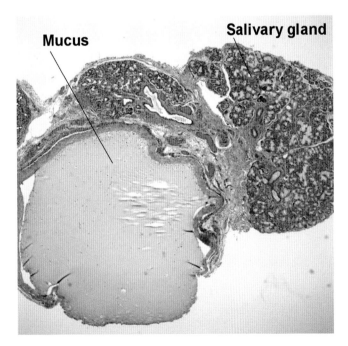

Fig. 14.26 Mucocele

Oxalosis

Key Features

- Yellow-brown, radially arranged, refractile, needle-shaped crystals
- Vascular involvement and thrombi may be seen, especially in primary disease

Primary oxalosis is an autosomal-recessive disorder associated with overproduction of serum oxalate. These patients present with recurrent calcium oxalate stones and renal failure. Vascular deposition of oxalate produces livedo reticularis, acrocyanosis, distal gangrene, and ulcerations.

Secondary oxalosis occurs with ethylene glycol poisoning, excessive intake of ascorbic acid, pyridoxine deficiency, various intestinal diseases, repeated oral antibiotic use leading to elimination of oxalate-degrading bacteria in the intestine, and chronic hemodialysis. Skin manifestations in patients with secondary oxalosis occur as the result of extravascular deposition.

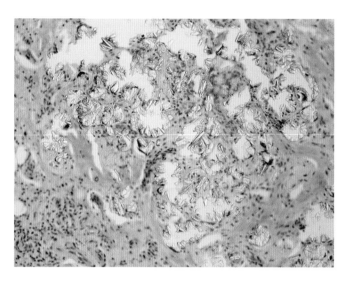

Fig. 14.27 Oxalosis

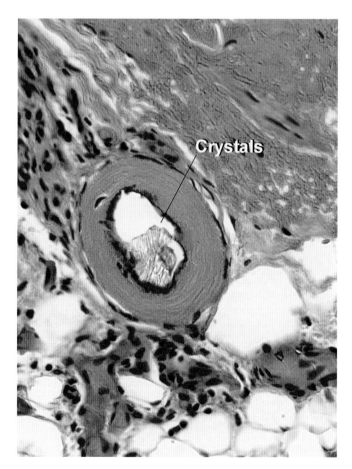

Fig. 14.28 Oxalosis

Further reading

Blackmon JA, Jeffy BG, Malone JC, et al. Oxalosis involving the skin: case report and literature review. Arch Dermatol 2011;147(11):1302–5.

Girardi M, Kay J, Elston DM, et al. Nephrogenic systemic fibrosis: clinicopathological definition and workup recommendations. J Am Acad Dermatol 2011;65(6): 1095–1106.e7.

Hashimoto K, Nakayama H, Chimenti S, et al. Juvenile colloid milium: Immunohistochemical and ultrastructural studies. J Cutan Pathol 1989;16(3):164–74.

Kövary PM, Vakilzadeh F, Macher E, et al. Monoclonal gammopathy in scleredema. Observations in three cases. Arch Dermatol 1981;117(9):536–9.

Kucher C, Xu X, Pasha T, et al. Histopathologic comparison of nephrogenic fibrosing dermopathy and scleromyxedema. J Cutan Pathol 2005;32(7):484–90.

Markova A, Lester J, Wang J, et al. Diagnosis of common dermopathies in dialysis patients: a review and update. Semin Dial 2012;25(4):408–18.

Masuda C, Mohri S, Nakajima H. Histopathological and immunohistochemical study of amyloidosis cutis nodularis atrophicans – comparison with systemic amyloidosis. Br J Dermatol 1988;119(1):33–43.

Saad AG, Zaatari GS. Scrotal calcinosis: is it idiopathic? Urology 2001;57(2):365.

Yanagihara M, Mehregan AH, Mehregan DR. Staining of amyloid with cotton dyes. Arch Dermatol 1984;120(9):1184–5.

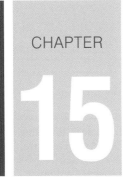

15

Disorders of skin appendages

Dirk M. Elston

Noninflammatory alopecia

Transverse (horizontal) sections are generally best for evaluation of noninflammatory alopecia. Vertical sections may be used if serial ribbons of sections are cut from the block. A combination of vertical and transverse sections is always acceptable.

Pattern alopecia (androgenetic balding)

Key Features

- Miniaturization of follicular units
- Variability in diameter of follicles (anisotrichosis)
- In vertical sections, hairs extend to variable depths in proportion to their diameter
- Decreased anagen/telogen ratio
- Many fibrous tract remnants with normal diameter and vascularity

The essential histologic finding in pattern alopecia is progressive miniaturization of the follicular unit. This occurs predominantly in the central scalp and in an asynchronous fashion. The biopsy will demonstrate variability in hair diameter. Focal spongiotic infundibulofolliculitis is common (mild seborrheic folliculitis). In long-standing cases, solar elastosis as well as elastotic degeneration of the fibrous tract remnants may be seen. Advanced-pattern alopecia demonstrates a marked increase in vellus hairs (hair shaft diameter < inner root sheath diameter). Large sebaceous glands may be present, especially in males.

Telogen effluvium

Key Features

- Many telogen hairs

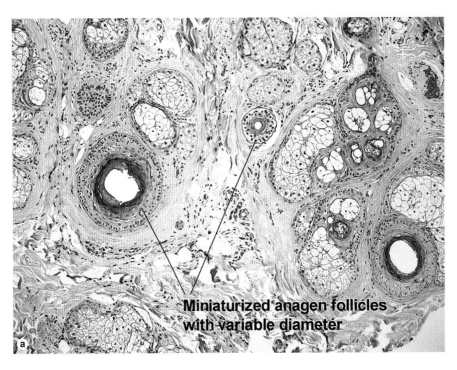

Miniaturized anagen follicles with variable diameter

Fig. 15.1 (A and B) Pattern alopecia.

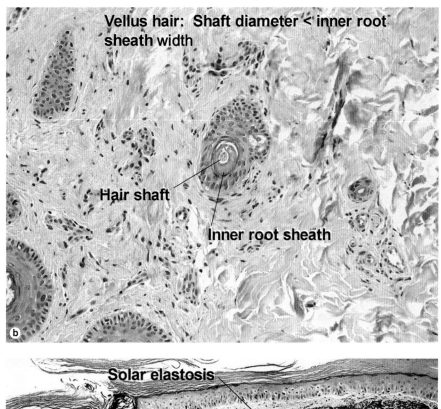

Vellus hair: Shaft diameter < inner root sheath width

Hair shaft

Inner root sheath

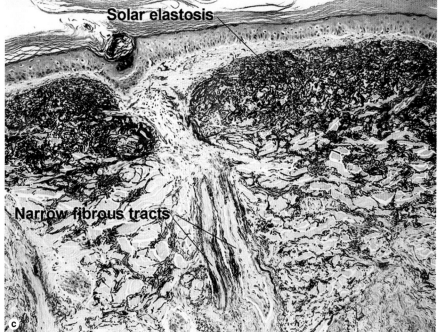

Solar elastosis

Narrow fibrous tracts

Fig. 15.1, cont'd (C) Solar elastosis and narrow fibrous tract remnants in pattern alopecia (Verhoeff–van Gieson stain).

Continued

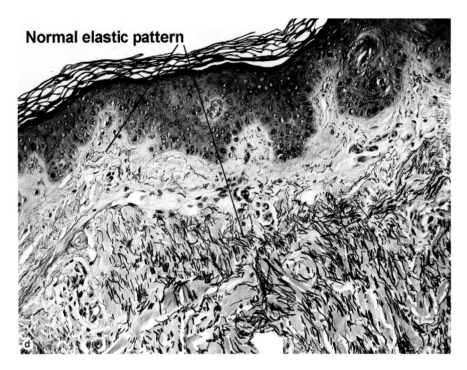

Fig. 15.1, cont'd (D) Normal elastic tissue pattern for comparison (Verhoeff–van Gieson stain)

Telogen effluvium has many telogen hairs. Telogen effluvium caused by premature interruption of anagen growth (such as by a febrile illness or crash diet) lacks the miniaturization of pattern alopecia. The shortened anagen cycle of pattern alopecia results in an altered anagen/telogen ratio, but not to the extent seen after febrile illness or crash dieting.

Trichotillomania (trichotillosis)

Key Features

- Empty anagen follicles
- Many catagen hairs characterized by apoptotic keratinocytes (Fig. 15.3C)
- Melanin casts within the follicular canal
- Trichomalacia

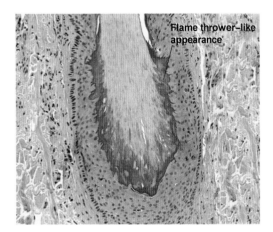

Fig. 15.2 Telogen effluvium: telogen hair

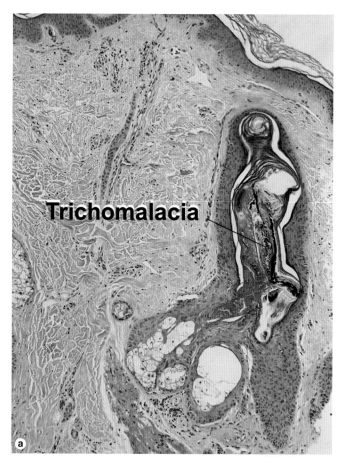

Trichomalacia

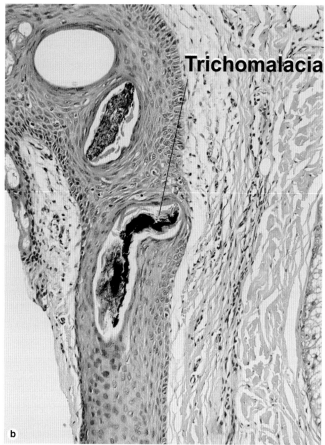

Trichomalacia

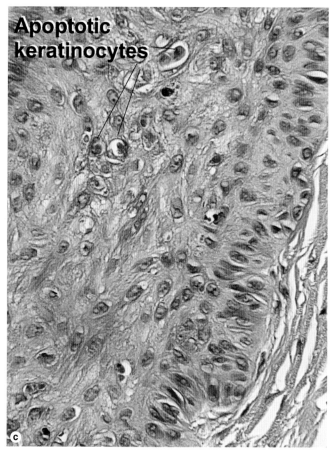

Apoptotic keratinocytes

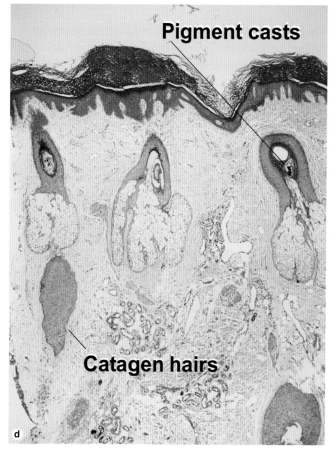

Pigment casts

Catagen hairs

Fig. 15.3 Trichotillomania

Continued

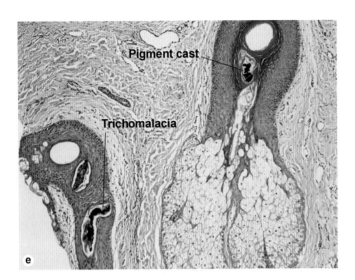

Fig. 15.3, cont'd

Traction alopecia

Key Features

- Resembles trichotillomania histologically

Inflammatory nonscarring alopecia

Either vertical or transverse (horizontal) sections may be used, but serial ribbons of sections should always be cut from the block. A combination of vertical and transverse sections is always acceptable.

Alopecia areata

Key Features

- Lymphoid inflammation at the level of the hair bulb
- Lymphocytes within fibrous tract remnants
- Eosinophils within fibrous tract remnants
- Melanin within fibrous tract remnants
- Follicular miniaturization
- Decreased anagen/telogen ratio
- Increase in catagen hairs
- Melanin casts within the follicular channel
- Dilation of follicular infundibula

The lymphocytes appear to target melanocytes within the hair bulb. White hairs are spared. The inflammation results in damage to the hair matrix, tapered hair shafts with fracture, and miniaturization of the follicular unit.

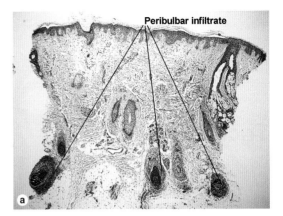

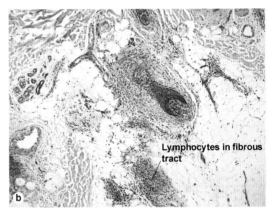

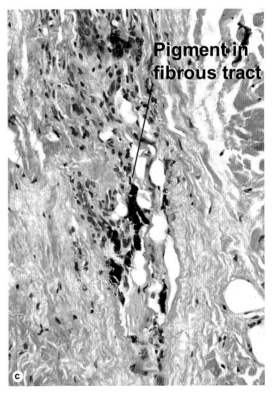

Fig. 15.4 Alopecia areata

Differential Diagnosis

Pattern alopecia

- Shares follicular miniaturization, decreased anagen/telogen ratio, and many fibrous tract remnants
- Lacks catagen hairs, melanin casts in follicular channels, lymphoid inflammation at the level of the hair bulb, lymphocytes within fibrous tract remnants, eosinophils within fibrous tract remnants, and melanin within fibrous tract remnants

Trichotillomania

- Shares catagen hairs and melanin casts in follicular channels
- Lacks follicular miniaturization, lymphoid inflammation at the level of the hair bulb, lymphocytes within fibrous tract remnants, eosinophils within fibrous tract remnants, and melanin within fibrous tract remnants

Table 15.1 Comparison between alopecia areata, pattern alopecia, and trichotillomania

Characteristic	Alopecia areata	Pattern alopecia	Trichotillomania
Miniaturization	Yes	Yes	No
Anagen/telogen ratio	Decreased	Decreased	Variable
Fibrous tract remnants	Increased	Increased	Normal
Catagen hairs	Common	Rare	Common
Pigment in hair canal	Common	No	Common
Pigment in fibrous tract	Common	No	No
Lymphs around bulb	Common	No	No
Lymphs in fibrous tracts	Common	No	No
Eosinophils in fibrous tracts	Common	No	No

Syphilitic alopecia

Key Features

- May be identical to alopecia areata
- May contain plasma cells (lacking in about one third of cases)

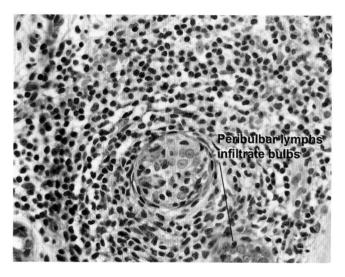

Fig. 15.5 Syphilitic alopecia

Alopecia mucinosa

Key Features

- Mucin within follicular epithelium
- Variable surrounding lymphoid infiltrate
- May be associated with mycosis fungoides (cutaneous T-cell lymphoma)

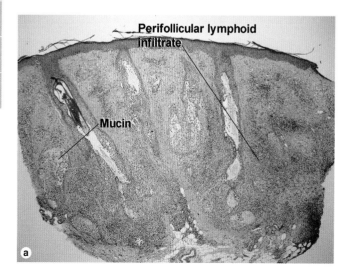

Fig. 15.6 Alopecia mucinosa

continued

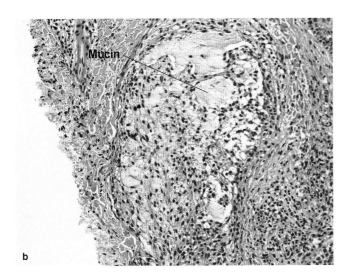

Fig. 15.6, cont'd

Folliculotropic mycosis fungoides (cutaneous T-cell lymphoma)

Key Features

- Large, hyperchromatic, angulated lymphocytes within the follicular epithelium
- Lymphocytes tend to line up along the epithelial side of the dermal–epidermal junction
- Dark lymphocytes are surrounded by a white space (lump of coal on a pillow), but little surrounding spongiosis

Papillary dermal fibrosis is often prominent. Immunostaining may demonstrate deletion of pan-T markers such as CD7, and gene rearrangements can often be demonstrated.

Tinea capitis and Majocchi fungal folliculitis

Key Features

- Mixed inflammatory infiltrate, neutrophils present, eosinophils variable
- Fungal spores within or surrounding hair shaft

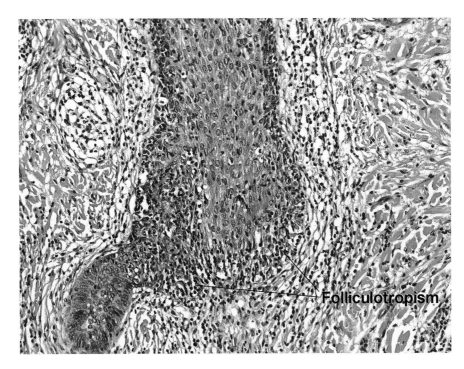

Fig. 15.7 Folliculotropic mycosis fungoides

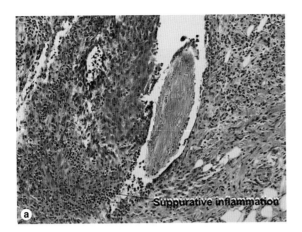

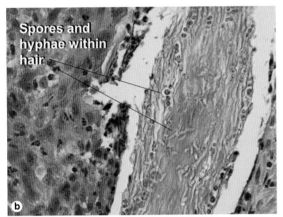

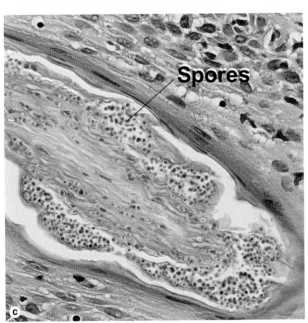

Fig. 15.8 Majocchi granuloma

Acne vulgaris

Key Features

- Infundibulum filled with laminated keratin and debris
- Suppurative inflammation may be present

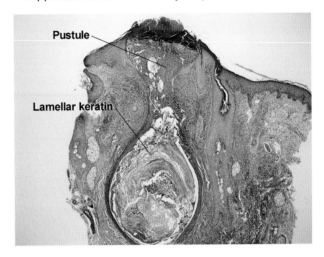

Fig. 15.9 Acne

Cicatricial alopecia

Serial vertical sections are generally superior to transverse (horizontal) sections in the setting of cicatricial alopecia, although the combination of vertical and transverse sections is better than either alone.

Lupus erythematosus

Key Features

- Lymphoid infiltrate at the level of the isthmus
- Interface change may be vacuolar or lichenoid
- Compact hyperkeratosis
- Follicular hyperkeratosis
- Basement membrane zone thickening
- Melanin pigment incontinence (melanoderma) underlying the dermal–epidermal junction
- Vertical columns of lymphocytes
- Perivascular lymphoid aggregates
- Lymphoid aggregates within the eccrine coil
- Dermal mucin between collagen bundles
- Underlying lupus panniculitis may be present
- Direct immunofluorescence (DIF): continuous granular band of immunoglobulin (Ig) G/A/M and C3 (full house) at the follicular basement membrane zone (see Chapter 7)

The features of discoid lupus erythematosus appear in a time-dependent fashion. Biopsies of early patches will show only perifollicular mucinous fibrosis and focal interface change. DIF will usually be negative at this stage. The biopsy should always be taken from an active lesion, of at least 3 months' duration. Burnt-out patches demonstrate scarring throughout the dermis in elastic tissue-stained sections.

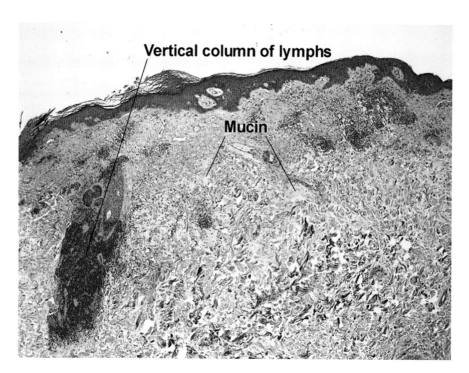

Fig. 15.10 Lupus erythematosus

Lichen planopilaris (LPP)

Key Features

- Lymphoid infiltrate at the level of the infundibulum
- Lichenoid interface dermatitis
- Entire fibrous tract remnant may be filled with Civatte bodies
- DIF: shaggy linear fibrin and cytoid bodies

As with lupus erythematosus, the features of LPP appear in a time-dependent fashion. Biopsies of early patches will show only perifollicular mucinous fibrosis and focal lymphoid inflammation. These changes are most notable about the infundibulum, whereas lupus erythematosus affects the isthmus preferentially. DIF will usually be negative in the early stages, but will often show shaggy linear fibrin and cytoid bodies in more advanced lesions. Burnt-out patches demonstrate wedge-shaped scars at the level of the infundibulum.

Table 15.2 Characteristics of discoid lupus erythematosus versus lichen planopilaris

Characteristic	Discoid lupus erythematosus	Lichen planopilaris
Hyperkeratosis	Yes	Yes
Interface dermatitis	Vacuolar or lichenoid	Lichenoid
Pigment incontinence	Yes	Yes
Lymphoid infiltrate	Centered at isthmus	Centered at the infundibulum
Basement membrane zone thickening	Common	No
Dermal mucin	Common	No
Lymphocytes in eccrine coil	Common	No
Lobular panniculitis with fibrin	Sometimes	No
Direct immunofluorescence	"Full house" common in established lesions, may have cytoid bodies	Negative or shaggy fibrin and cytoid bodies
Scar in late lesions	Throughout dermis	Superficial wedges

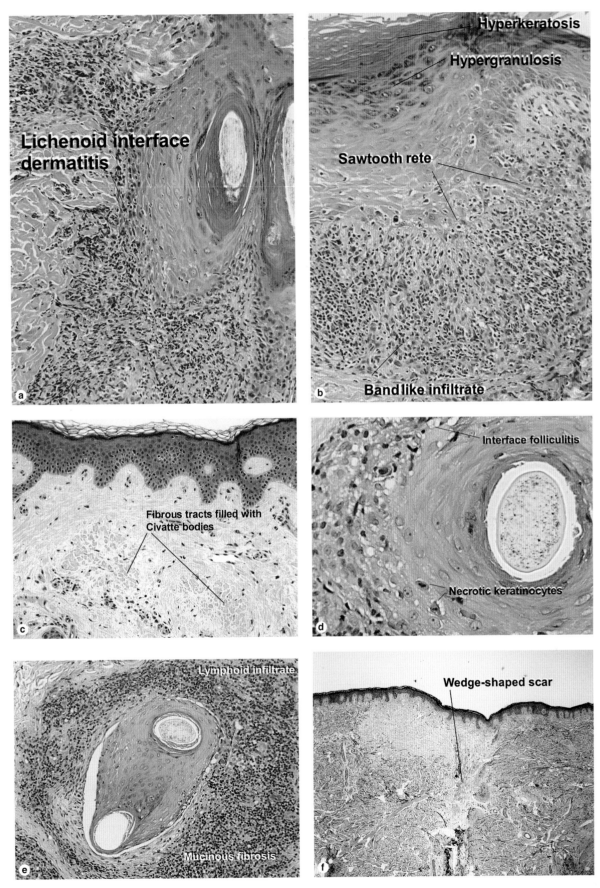

Fig. 15.11 (A–E) Lichen planopilaris. **(F)** Wedge-shaped scar characteristic of lichen planopilaris (Verhoeff–van Gieson stain)

Idiopathic pseudopelade

Key Features

- Shrunken, deep red dermis
- Broad "tree trunk" fibrous tract remnants
- Preserved elastic sheath
- Thick, elastic fibers in dermis

Most patients with ivory white scarring and spared terminal hairs have LPP. About 10% of patients with the same clinical features but lack follicular spines and have a unique histology distinct from other forms of alopecia. The dermis is shrunken and deeply eosinophilic with loss of the spaces between collagen bundles. This appearance has been likened to a sweater shrunken in the dryer. Fibrous tract remnants are broad and hyalinized, but the surrounding elastic sheath is intact. Hair granulomas may be noted in fibrous tract remnants. Elastic fibers in the surrounding dermis are thick and "recoiled" because of the contraction of the dermis.

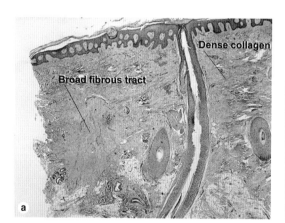

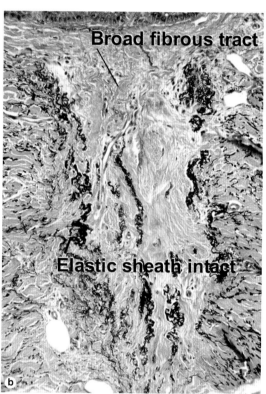

Fig. 15.12 (A) Idiopathic pseudopelade. **(B)** Idiopathic pseudopelade (Verhoeff–van Gieson stain)

Central centrifugal cicatricial alopecia (CCCA)

Key Features

- Central alopecia
- Mixed etiologies (including idiopathic pseudopelade, LPP, late-stage folliculitis decalvans)

Dissecting cellulitis

Key Features

- Clinically similar to nodulocystic acne
- Deep dermal and subcutaneous abscesses, sinus tracts, and granulation tissue

Folliculitis decalvans

Key Features

- Suppurative folliculitis
- Wedge-shaped scar with elastic stain (similar to LPP)
- "Six-pack" tufting of hairs

Patients with folliculitis decalvans present with recurrent crops of epilating follicular pustules. The histologic changes resemble those of a staphylococcal folliculitis. *Staphylococci* are sometimes cultured, and patients respond to prolonged courses of antistaphylococcal therapy.

Patients with acne keloidalis and progressive alopecia usually demonstrate overlap with folliculitis decalvans.

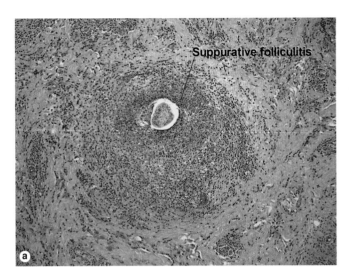
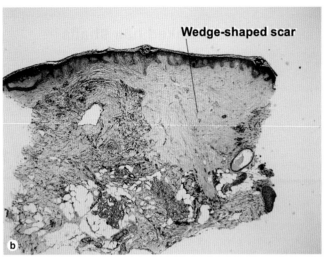

Fig. 15.13 (A) Folliculitis decalvans. **(B)** Wedge-shaped scar of folliculitis decalvans (Verhoeff–van Gieson stain)

Acne keloidalis

See Chapter 13, page 245.

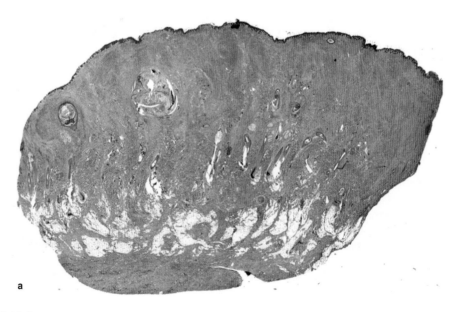

Fig. 15.14 Acne keloidalis

continued

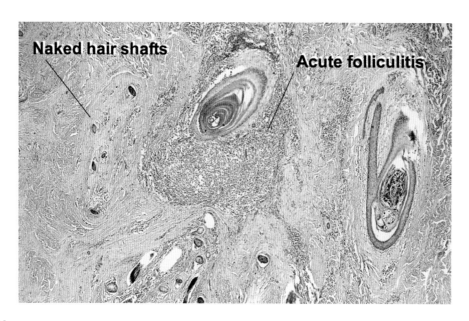

Fig. 15.14, cont'd

Acute Langerhans cell histiocytosis (histiocytosis X)

Key Features

- Perifollicular epithelioid histiocytes at the level of the infundibulum
- Overlying inflammatory crust common above the infundibulum
- Surrounding edema and erythrocyte extravasation

- Scattered eosinophils common
- Histiocytes stain with S100, CD-1a, peanut agglutinin, and langerin
- Electron microscopy: Birbeck granules

At scanning power, acute Langerhans cell histiocytosis has the appearance of a folliculitis at the level of the infundibulum. Instead of lymphocytes, the cells surrounding the follicle are histiocytes with ample cytoplasm and an eccentric, pale gray, vesicular nucleus. Kidney-shaped nuclei may be present. The surrounding dermis is pale and edematous with erythrocyte extravasation.

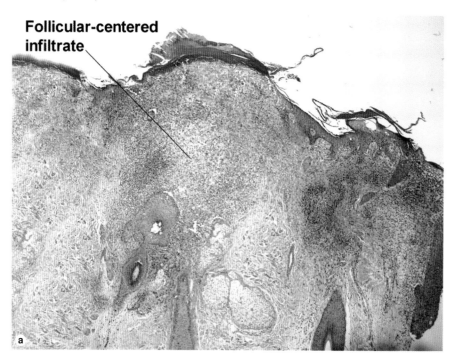

Fig. 15.15 Acute Langerhans cell histiocytosis

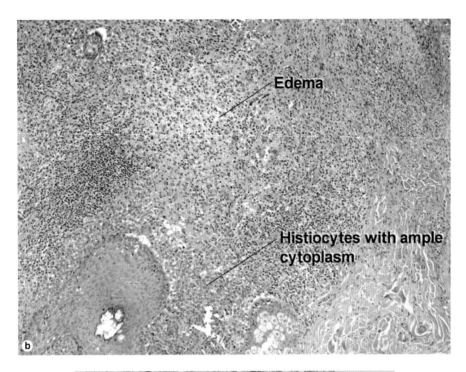

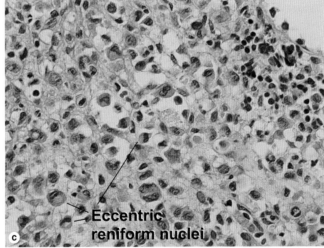

Fig. 15.15, cont'd

Miliaria

Key Features

• Spongiosis, pustule, or superficial subcorneal blister associated with the acrosyringium

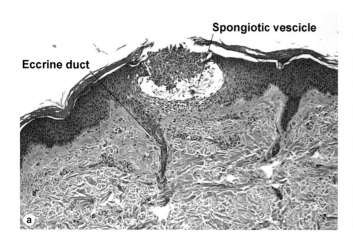

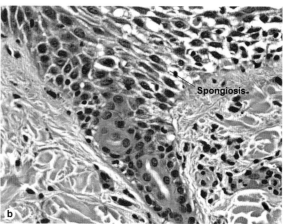

Fig. 15.16 Miliaria

Neutrophilic eccrine hidradenitis

Key Features

• Neutrophils within eccrine coil

Neutrophilic eccrine hidradenitis is commonly noted during induction chemotherapy for leukemia. It has also been reported prior to the diagnosis of leukemia, suggesting that it may occur as a paraneoplastic syndrome. In children, idiopathic eccrine hidradenitis may occur on the soles. *Pseudomonas* has been cultured from some of these patients.

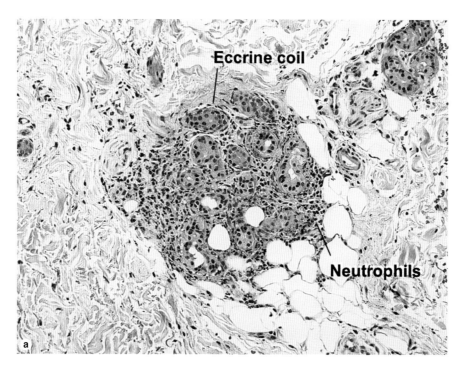

Fig. 15.17 Neutrophilic eccrine hidradenitis

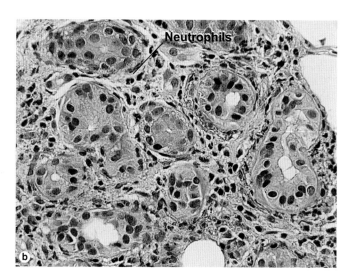

Fig. 15.17, cont'd

Hidradenitis suppurativa

Key Features

- Skin has features of axillary or anogenital skin
- Apocrine glands often present
- Suppurative folliculitis with abscess formation
- Sinus tracts with suppurative and granulomatous inflammation
- Granulation tissue
- Inflammation "spills over" to involve apocrine glands

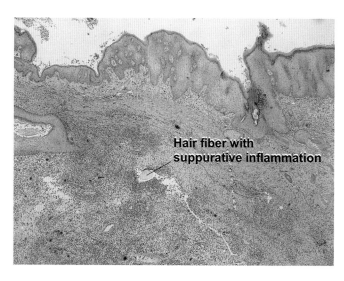

Fig. 15.18 Hidradenitis suppurativa

Pseudocyst of the auricle

Key Features

- Degeneration of cartilage creating a central cavity

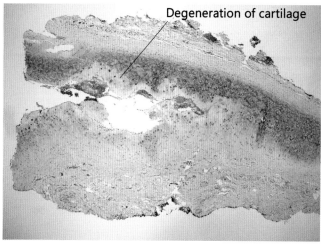

Fig. 15.19 Pseudocyst of the auricle

Relapsing polychondritis

Key Features

- Cartilage with neutrophilic infiltrate in the surrounding perichondrium
- DIF: continuous granular band of IgG/A/M and C3 (full house) in the perichondrium

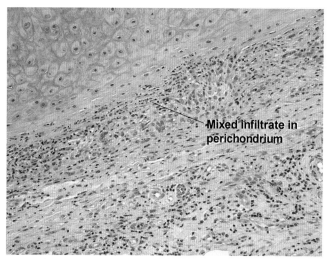

Fig. 15.20 Relapsing polychondritis

Further reading

Abedini R, Kamyab Hesari K, Daneshpazhooh M, et al. Validity of trichoscopy in the diagnosis of primary cicatricial alopecias. Int J Dermatol 2016;55(10):1106–14.

Childs JM, Sperling LC. Histopathology of scarring and nonscarring hair loss. Dermatol Clin 2013;31(1):43–56.

Elston DM. Vertical vs. transverse sections: both are valuable in the evaluation of alopecia. Am J Dermatopathol 2005; 27(4):353–6.

Elston DM. What's new in the histologic evaluation of alopecia and hair-related disorders? Dermatol Clin 2012; 30(4):685–94.

Elston DM, Ferringer T, Dalton S, et al. A comparison of vertical versus transverse sections in the evaluation of alopecia biopsy specimens. J Am Acad Dermatol 2005; 53(2):267–72.

Elston DM, McCollough ML, Bergfeld WF, et al. Eosinophils in fibrous tracts and near hair bulbs: a helpful diagnostic feature of alopecia areata. J Am Acad Dermatol 1997; 37(1):101–6.

Elston DM, McCollough ML, Warschaw KE, et al. Elastic tissue in scars and alopecia. J Cutan Pathol 2000;27(3): 147–52.

Jackson AJ, Price VH. How to diagnose hair loss. Dermatol Clin 2013;31(1):21–8.

LaSenna C, Miteva M. Special stains and immunohistochemical stains in hair pathology. Am J Dermatopathol 2016;38(5):327–37.

Peckham SJ, Sloan SB, Elston DM. Histologic features of alopecia areata other than peribulbar lymphocytic infiltrates. J Am Acad Dermatol 2011;65(3):615–20.

Templeton SF, Santa Cruz DJ, Solomon AR. Alopecia: histologic diagnosis by transverse sections. Semin Diagn Pathol 1996;13(1):2–18.

Trachsler S, Trueb RM. Value of direct immunofluorescence for differential diagnosis of cicatricial alopecia. Dermatology 2005;211(2):98–102.

Wohltmann WE, Sperling L. Histopathologic diagnosis of multifactorial alopecia. J Cutan Pathol 2016;43(6):483–91.

CHAPTER 6

Panniculitis

Dirk M. Elston

The inflammatory infiltrate in septal panniculitis spills over into the lobule. The inflammation in lobular panniculitis often involves the septum; therefore septal and lobular panniculitis are best differentiated by the architecture of the lobule. In septal panniculitis, the lobule is intact; lipocytes are similar in size and shape, and the scan appearance resembles a bowl of toasted oat cereal. In lobular panniculitis, the lobule is necrotic; lipophages are common, and in most instances free lipid accumulates in pools that vary in size and shape. The scan appearance resembles the surface of a bowl of chicken soup. Important exceptions to this rule include conditions that result in solidification of fat (sclerema, subcutaneous fat necrosis of the newborn, and steroid-induced fat necrosis). In each of these conditions, the solidified fat cannot coalesce. Pancreatic panniculitis results in calcification of the necrotic membranes, and also prevents coalescence of lipid.

Septal panniculitis

Erythema nodosum is the major form of septal panniculitis. Infections can occasionally produce necrosis and inflammation within the septum, without necrosis of the fat lobule. Alpha$_1$-antitrypsin deficiency can occasionally result in liquefactive necrosis of the septum without necrosis of the lobule.

Erythema nodosum

Key Features

- Septal panniculitis (little to no necrosis of lobule)
- Neutrophils in septum in acute phase
- Mononuclear cells and granulomatous inflammation in chronic phase
- Miescher granuloma: central cleft within granuloma

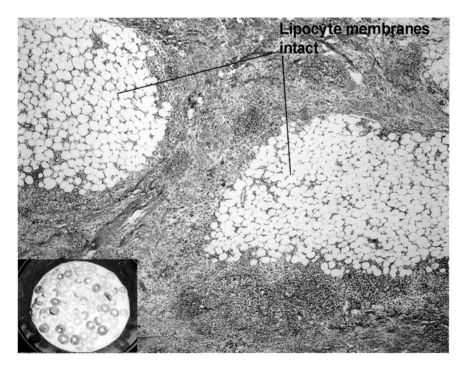

Fig. 16.1 Septal panniculitis

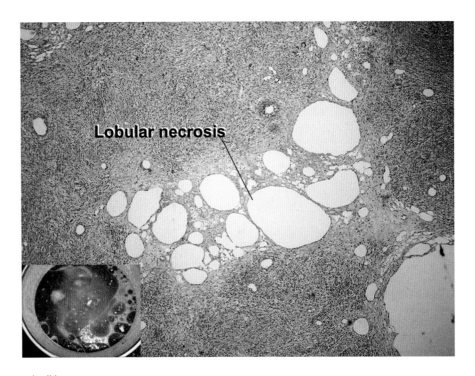

Fig. 16.2 Lobular panniculitis

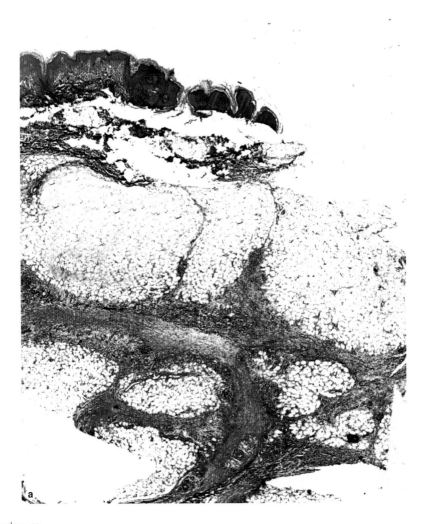

Fig. 16.3 Erythema nodosum

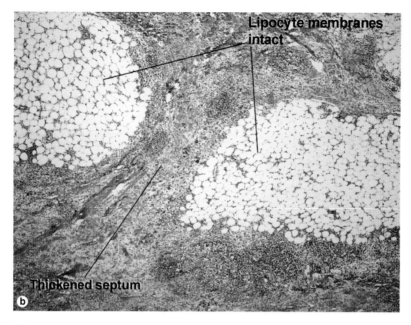

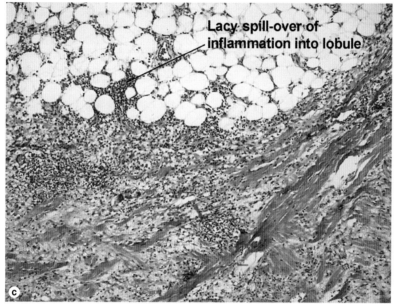

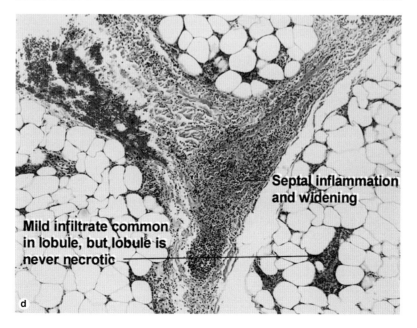

Fig. 16.3, cont'd

Lobular panniculitis

Lupus panniculitis (lupus profundus)

Key Features

- Necrosis of fat lobule ("chicken soup")
- Fibrin and hyaline rings around fat
- Nodular lymphoid infiltrates

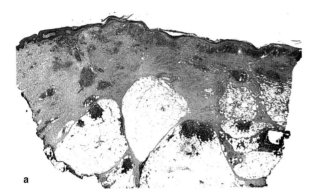

a

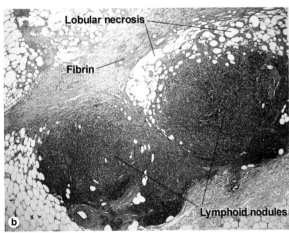

Lobular necrosis

Fibrin

Lymphoid nodules

b

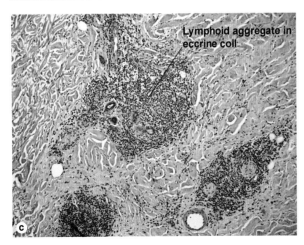

Lymphoid aggregate in eccrine coil

c

Fig. 16.4 Lupus panniculitis

Although connective tissue disease can produce less specific patterns of granulomatous panniculitis, the features noted earlier are highly characteristic of lupus panniculitis. Plasma cells are common in the nodular lymphoid foci. Overlying features of lupus erythematosus may be present. The overlying dermis may be sclerotic. Lipomembranous changes may be present (eosinophilic "frost on the windowpane" or "ferning" pattern at the edge of the lipid vacuole).

> **PEARL**
>
> Subcutaneous panniculitis-like lymphoma may have an identical histologic appearance. Features that favor lupus include interface dermatitis, lymphoid follicles with reactive germinal centers, mixed cellular infiltrate with plasma cells, and lack of T-cell receptor-gamma gene rearrangement. It should, however, be noted that interface change and dermal mucin have been noted in some patients with lymphoma.

Pancreatic panniculitis

Key Features

- Necrosis of the fat lobule with calcium soap outlining necrotic lipocytes

Pancreatic panniculitis may occur in the setting of pancreatitis or pancreatic neoplasm.

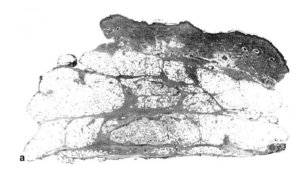

a

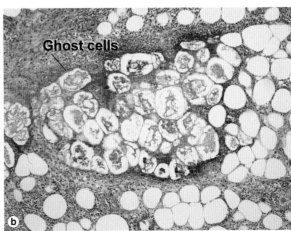

Ghost cells

b

Fig. 16.5 Pancreatic panniculitis

Subcutaneous fat necrosis of the newborn

Key Features

- Necrosis of the fat lobule with crystallization of fat (solid fat cannot coalesce like "chicken soup")
- Radial crystals in lipocytes
- Granulomatous inflammation

Differential Diagnosis

- Steroid-induced fat necrosis (aka poststeroid panniculitis) looks identical
- Sclerema neonatorum has identical crystals, but no inflammation

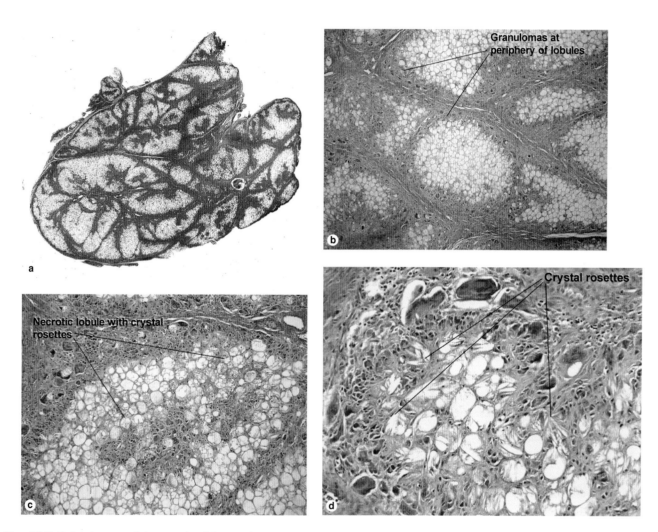

Fig. 16.6 Subcutaneous fat necrosis of the newborn

Eosinophilic panniculitis

Key Features

- Eosinophils in septum and lobule
- Necrosis variable

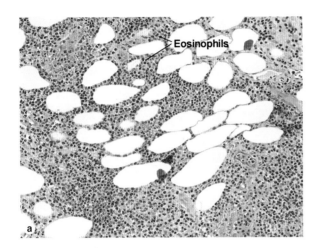

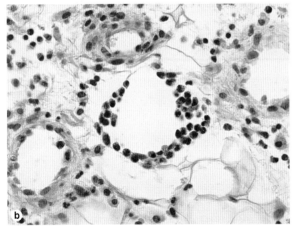

Fig. 16.7 Eosinophilic panniculitis

Causes

- Churg–Strauss syndrome
- Helminthic parasite
- Arthropod
- Hypereosinophilic syndrome

Suppurative and granulomatous panniculitis

Key Features

- Lobular panniculitis
- Suppurative and granulomatous infiltrate
- Usually infectious etiology
- May be factitial

Predominantly granulomatous lesions may be associated with lipodystrophy or connective tissue disease.

Nodular vasculitis/erythema induratum (EI) of Bazin

Key Features

- Necrosis of the fat lobule ("chicken soup")
- Multinucleated giant cells
- Nodular neutrophilic vasculitis often present in septum
- Caseation necrosis common

EI commonly involves the calves. Liquefied fat may drain from the lesions. Some authorities use the term *nodular vasculitis* when patients are purified protein derivative (PPD) negative, and EI when they are PPD positive. Polymerase chain reaction has been used to identify mycobacterial antigens within lesional tissue.

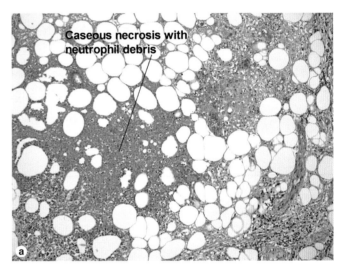

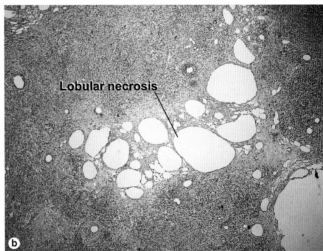

Fig. 16.8 Erythema induratum

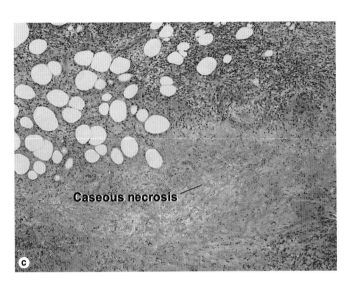

Fig. 16.8, cont'd

Alpha₁-antitrypsin deficiency

Key Features

- Neutrophilic infiltrate
- Fat necrosis and granulomatous infiltrate variable
- Liquefactive necrosis of the septum may be seen

Differential Diagnosis

Infectious etiologies should be excluded. Neutrophilic panniculitis may also occur in myelodysplastic syndromes.

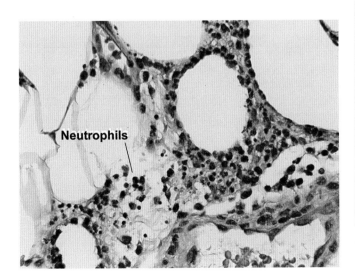

Fig. 16.9 Alpha₁-antitrypsin deficiency

Lipodermatosclerosis (stasis panniculitis)

Key Features

- Necrosis of the fat lobule ("chicken soup")
- Lipomembranous change ("frost on the windowpane")
- Overlying stasis change

PEARL

Lipomembranous change may be noted in many forms of lobular panniculitis, including lupus panniculitis.

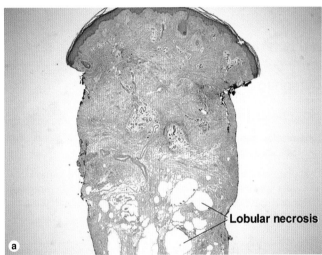

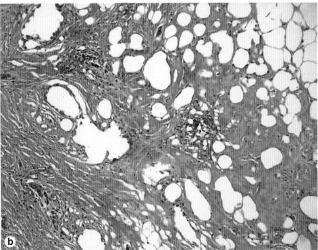

Fig. 16.10 Lipodermatosclerosis

continued

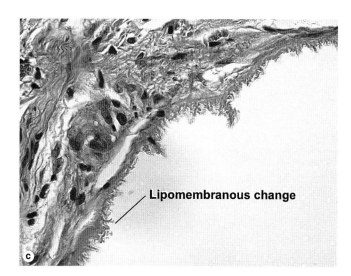

Lipomembranous change

Fig. 16.10, cont'd

Cytophagic histiocytic panniculitis

Key Features

- Lobular panniculitis
- "Beanbag cells"

Cytophagic histiocytic panniculitis may follow infection or may be induced by lymphoma. The patient often dies of a hemorrhagic diathesis. Beanbag cells are histiocytes that have engulfed inflammatory cells and erythrocytes.

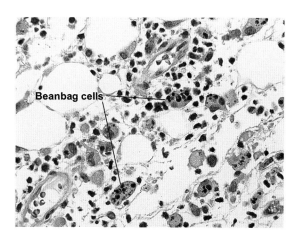

Beanbag cells

Fig. 16.11 Cytophagic histiocytic panniculitis

Traumatic fat necrosis ("mobile encapsulated lipoma")

Key Features

- Resembles lobular panniculitis
- Fibrous capsule

Subcutaneous panniculitis-like lymphoma

Key Features

- Resembles lobular panniculitis
- May closely resemble lupus panniculitis
- Atypical lymphocytes rimming lipocytes
- Natural killer and gamma–delta phenotypes may be seen

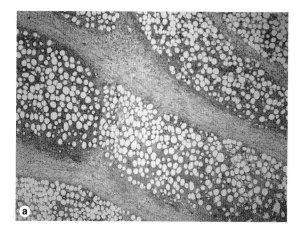

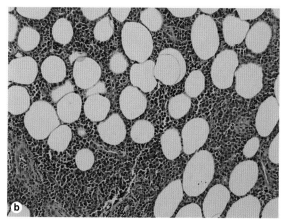

Fig. 16.12 Subcutaneous panniculitis-like lymphoma

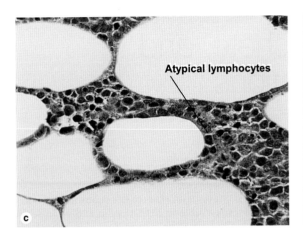

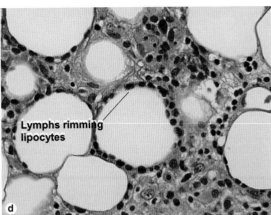

Fig. 16.12, cont'd

Further reading

Geraminejad P, DeBloom JR 2nd, Walling HW, et al. Alpha-1-antitrypsin associated panniculitis: the MS variant. J Am Acad Dermatol 2004;51(4):645–55.

Gonzalez EG, Selvi E, Lorenzini S, et al. Subcutaneous panniculitis-like T-cell lymphoma misdiagnosed as lupus erythematosus panniculitis. Clin Rheumatol 2006;26(2):244–6.

Heymann WR. Panniculitis. J Am Acad Dermatol 2005;52(4):683–5.

Ma L, Bandarchi B, Glusac EJ. Fatal subcutaneous panniculitis-like T-cell lymphoma with interface change and dermal mucin, a dead ringer for lupus erythematosus. J Cutan Pathol 2005;32(5):360–5.

Massone C, Kodama K, Salmhofer W, et al. Lupus erythematosus panniculitis (lupus profundus): clinical, histopathological, and molecular analysis of nine cases. J Cutan Pathol 2005;32(6):396–404.

McBean J, Sable A, Maude J, et al. Alpha1-antitrypsin deficiency panniculitis. Cutis 2003;71(3):205–9.

Phelps RG, Shoji T. Update on panniculitis. Mt Sinai J Med 2001;68(4–5):262–7.

Requena L, Sánchez Yus E. Panniculitis. Part II. Mostly lobular panniculitis. J Am Acad Dermatol 2001;45(3):325–61.

Schneider JW, Jordaan HF. The histopathologic spectrum of erythema induratum of Bazin. Am J Dermatopathol 1997;19(4):323–33.

Sutra-Loubet C, Carlotti A, Guillemette J, et al. Neutrophilic panniculitis. J Am Acad Dermatol 2004;50(2):280–5.

Bacterial, spirochete, and protozoan infections

Dirk M. Elston

🌐 An infectious disease atlas can be found in the online content for this book.

Bacterial diseases

Impetigo

Key Features

- Neutrophilic crust
- Chains or clusters of cocci

Impetigo recruits neutrophils to the stratum corneum. Organisms are commonly visible in hematoxylin and eosin sections. Gram stain and culture may be required.

Differential Diagnosis

Collections of neutrophils within the stratum corneum: psoriasis, tinea, impetigo, *Candida,* seborrheic dermatitis, syphilis (PTICSS)

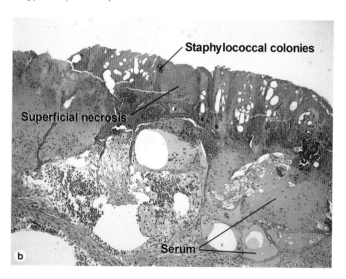

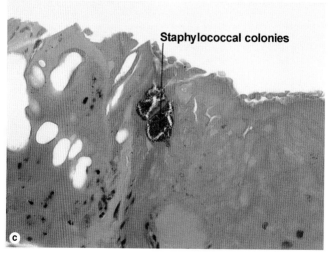

Fig. 17.1 Impetigo

Bullous impetigo

Key Features

- Subcorneal bulla
- Acantholysis in granular layer

Differential Diagnosis

Staphylococcal scalded-skin syndrome and pemphigus foliaceus demonstrate acantholysis at the same level.

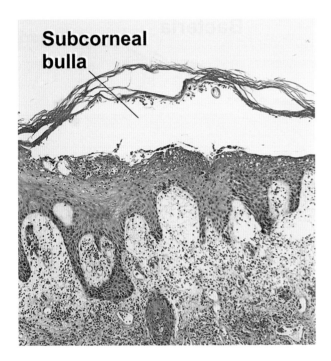

Fig. 17.2 Bullous impetigo

Suppurative folliculitis

Key Features

- Suppurative inflammation in or around a follicle
- Focal crusts in the stratum corneum
- Vertical column of suppurative inflammation in the dermis

The follicle may not be visible in every plane of section. In some sections, only a focus of inflammatory cells may be noted in the dermis. The microscopic differential diagnosis includes bacterial infection (including furunculosis and hot-tub folliculitis), fungal infection, chemical folliculitis, acne, rosacea, and pustular drug eruption.

Botryomycosis

Key Features

- Large staphylococcal grains in tissue
- Abscesses and sinus tracts

Clinically, botryomycosis may resemble a mycetoma. The grains represent huge staphylococcal colonies.

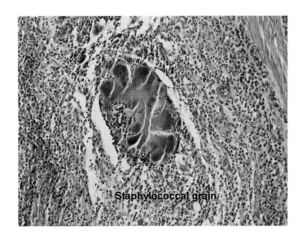

Fig. 17.3 Botryomycosis

Pitted keratolysis

Key Features

- Acral skin
- Dell or pit in stratum corneum
- Rods and cocci at base of dell

Pitted keratolysis is rarely biopsied because it is readily distinguished by its appearance and smell (so-called *toxic sock syndrome*). Both micrococci and diphtheroids are generally present (*Kytococcus sedentarius* and *Corynebacterium*).

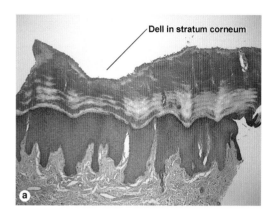

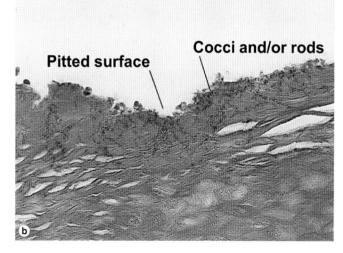

Fig. 17.4 Pitted keratolysis

Erythrasma

Key Features

- Rods forming vertical filaments in stratum corneum
- Inflammation variable

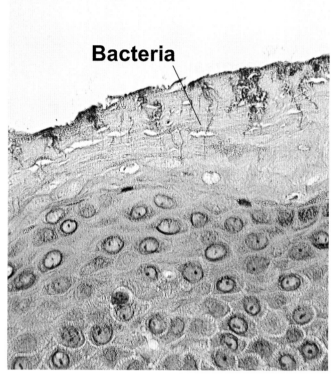

Fig. 17.5 Erythrasma

Ecthyma gangrenosum

Key Features

- Necrosis of deep dermal vessels
- Amphophilic bacilli surrounding vessels (light blue haze)
- Lack of inflammatory infiltrate around vessels
- Variable hemorrhage and cutaneous necrosis

Ecthyma gangrenosum is usually a manifestation of *Pseudomonas* sepsis.

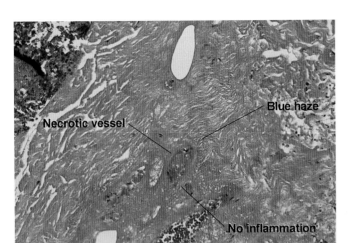

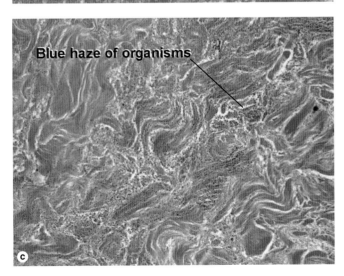

Fig. 17.6 Ecthyma gangrenosum

Rhinoscleroma

Key Features

- Sheets of plasma cells
- Russell bodies
- Mikulicz cells (resemble globi of leprosy)

Rhinoscleroma is caused by *Klebsiella rhinoscleromatis*. The inflammatory infiltrate is mixed and contains many plasma cells. Russell bodies are plasma cells filled with bright pink immunoglobulin ("pregnant plasma cells"). The nucleus may no longer be visible. Mikulicz cells are histiocytes containing large, round collections of bacilli.

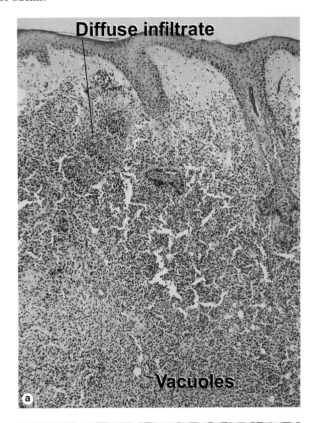

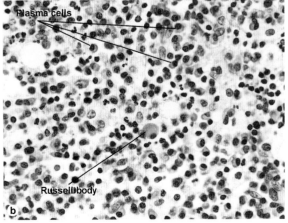

Fig. 17.7 Rhinoscleroma

Chancroid

Key Features

- Ulcer
- Zone of necrosis, fibrin, and neutrophils at surface
- Granulation tissue
- Many plasma cells below granulation tissue
- Gram stain and culture may demonstrate bacteria

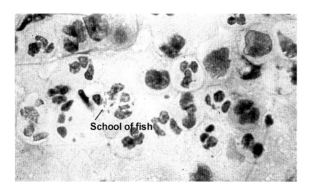

Fig. 17.8 Chancroid

Granuloma inguinale

Key Features

- Pseudoepitheliomatous hyperplasia with neutrophilic abscesses
- Organisms within histiocytes (Donovan bodies)

The organism may be seen best in very thin, plastic-embedded sections, processed as for electron microscopy.

Differential Diagnosis

Pseudoepitheliomatous hyperplasia with intraepidermal pustules (PEH and pus): "Here come big green leafy veggies":

- Here – **h**alogenoderma
- Come – **c**hromomycosis
- Big – **b**lastomycosis
- Green – **g**ranuloma inguinale
- Leafy – **l**eishmaniasis
- Veggies – pemphigus **v**egetans

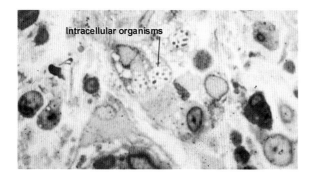

Fig. 17.9 Granuloma inguinale

Malakoplakia

Key Features

- Chronic gram-negative bacterial infection
- Globilike bacterial colonies within histiocytes (von Hansenman cells)
- Concentric calcifications (Michaelis–Gutmann bodies)

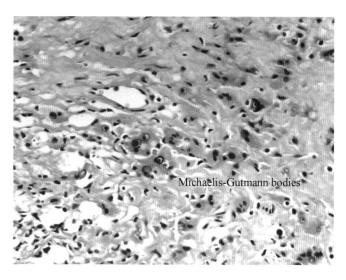

Fig. 17.10 Malakoplakia

Leprosy

Indeterminate leprosy may only demonstrate mild inflammation and onion-skin fibrosis around nerves. Borderline leprosy shows features intermediate between lepromatous and tuberculoid disease. New classification systems often divide disease into multibacillary (lepromatous end of spectrum) and paucibacillary (tuberculoid end) forms.

Lepromatous leprosy

Key Features

- Perivascular lymphohistiocytic infiltrate
- Ample amphophilic cytoplasm
- May form sheets of histiocytes with grenz zone
- Globi

Globi are amphophilic collections of mycobacteria. The organisms stain strongly with a Fite stain.

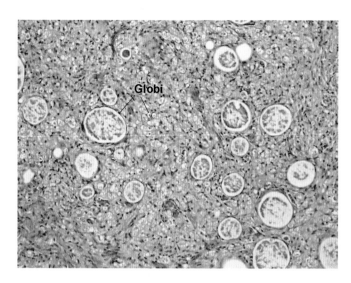

Fig. 17.11 Lepromatous leprosy

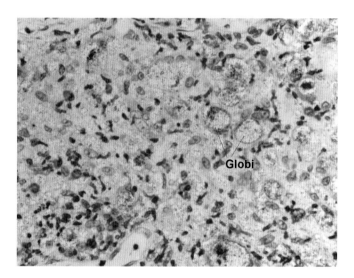

Fig. 17.12 Lepromatous leprosy (Fite stain)

Tuberculoid leprosy

Key Features

- Epithelioid granulomas running east–west in the dermis ("lavender sausages")
- Unlikely to find organisms with Fite stain

Tuberculoid leprosy is characterized by a high degree of cell-mediated immunity. Organisms are rare. The granulomatous infiltrate follows deep neurovascular bundles. Lesions are commonly anesthetic.

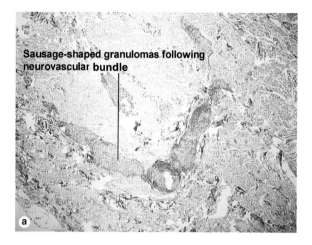

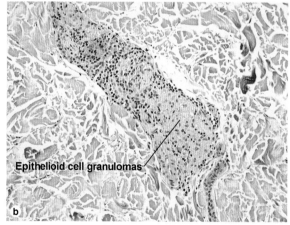

Fig. 17.13 Tuberculoid leprosy

Histoid leprosy

Key Features

- Usually the result of long-acting dapsone
- Fibrous nodules
- Globi present

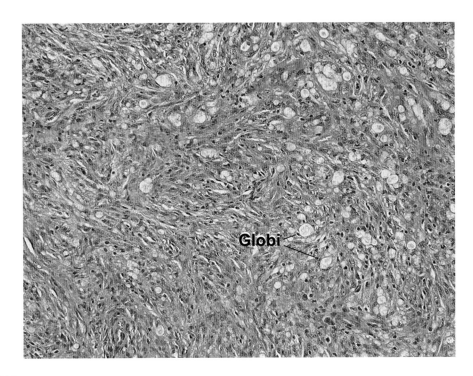

Fig. 17.14 Histoid leprosy

Leprosy reactions

Type 1: Reversal or downgrading reaction

Key Features

- Lymphoid and granulomatous inflammation
- Centered about neurovascular bundle

Reversal reactions commonly occur after antibiotic therapy is initiated. In response to antibiotic treatment, the patient regains a greater degree of cellular immunity. The increased type IV immune response inflicts damage on the neurovascular bundle.

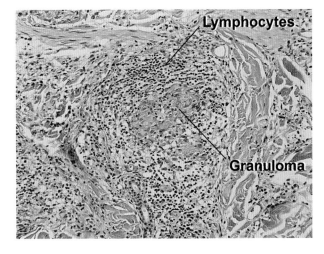

Fig. 17.15 Reversal reaction

Type 2: Erythema nodosum leprosum

Key Features

- Leukocytoclastic vasculitis superimposed upon preexisting lesions of leprosy
- Onion-skin fibrosis around nerves
- Globi

Erythema nodosum leprosum represents a type III immune response. There are no circulating immune complexes. Instead, the antigen–antibody complexes form locally within lesions.

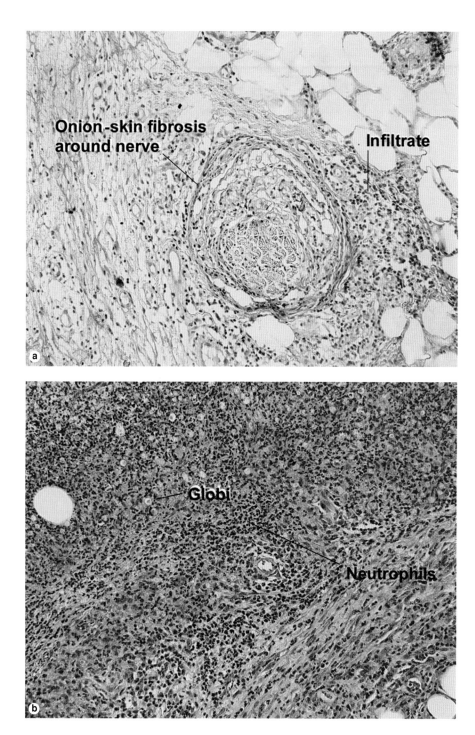

Fig. 17.16 Erythema nodosum leprosum

Type 3: Lucio phenomenon

Key Features

- Usual setting is diffuse lepromatous leprosy (lepra bonita) where the skin is taut without wrinkles, but nodules are absent

- Massive load of organisms, inflammation, and thrombosis in arterioles
- Stellate infarcts

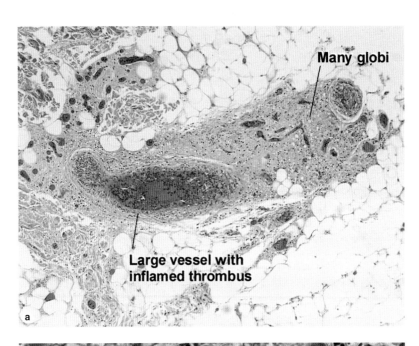

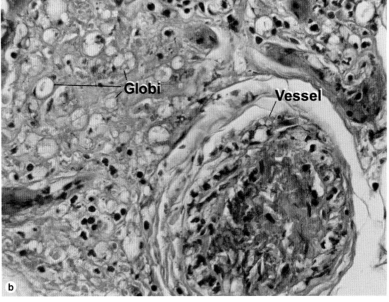

Fig. 17.17 Lucio phenomenon (courtesy of David M. Scollard, MD, PhD)

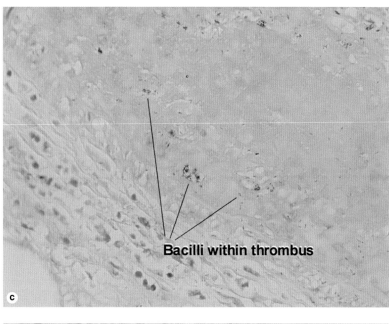

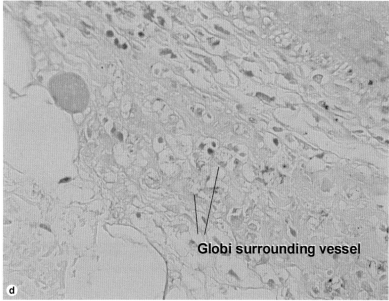

Fig. 17.17, cont'd

Tuberculosis

Key Features

- Early reactions suppurative
- Become granulomatous with central caseous necrosis

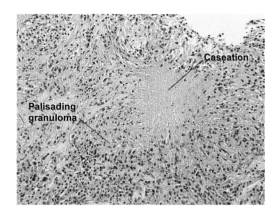

Fig. 17.18 Primary inoculation tuberculosis

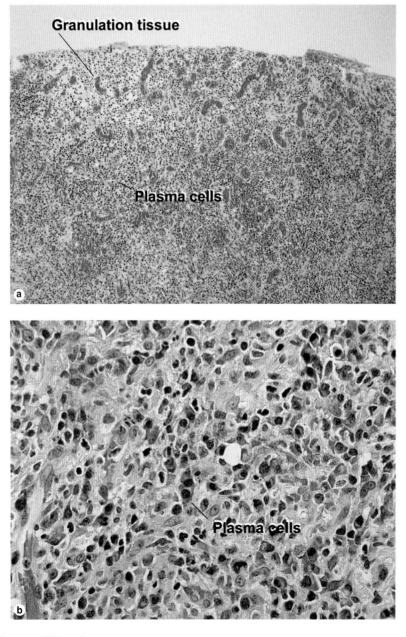

Fig. 17.19 (A and B) Chancre H&E stain

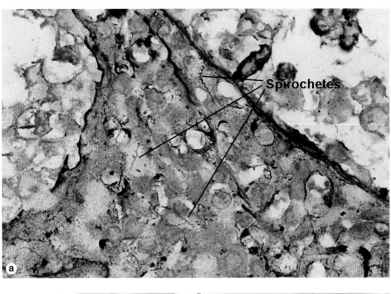

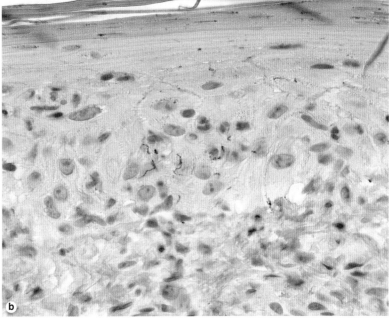

Fig. 17.20 *Treponema pallidum.* **(A)** Steiner stain. **(B)** Immunostain

Spirochete-mediated diseases

Syphilitic chancre

Key Features

- Ulcer
- Zone of necrosis, fibrin, and neutrophils at surface
- Granulation tissue
- Many plasma cells below granulation tissue
- Immunostain or silver stains may demonstrate spirochetes

Syphilitic chancres and chancroid have a similar histology. Chancroid typically produces a deeper, softer, more painful ulcer, as well as suppurative lymphadenitis. Stains, culture, and serology are typically required.

Secondary syphilis

Key Features

- Vacuolar interface dermatitis with either slender psoriasiform acanthosis or effacement
- Neutrophils in the stratum corneum
- Plasma cells present in about two thirds of cases
- Endothelial swelling obliterates the lumen of small vessels
- Perivascular lymphocytes and histiocytes with visible cytoplasm
- Interstitial "busy" dermis

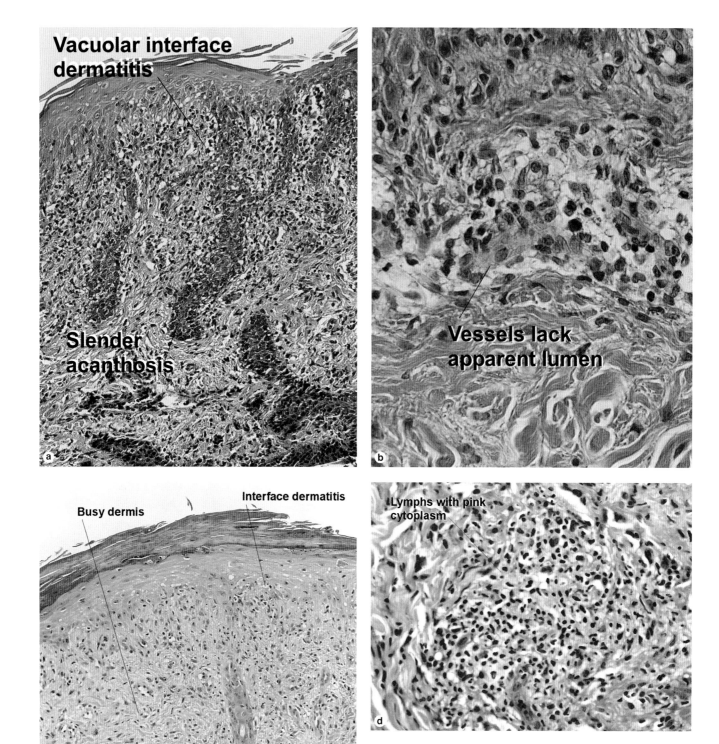

Fig. 17.21 Secondary syphilis

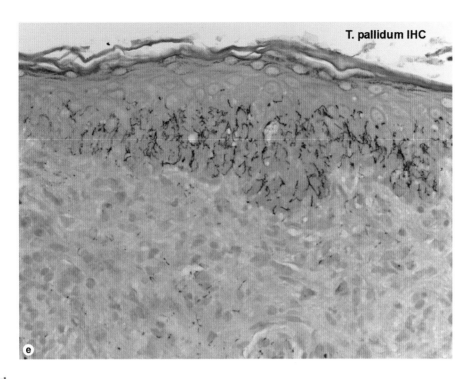

T. pallidum IHC

Fig. 17.21, cont'd

Secondary syphilis is highly variable in its clinical presentation, and almost as variable in its histologic appearance. Any suspicious feature should prompt an immunostain or silver stain, clinical evaluation, and serologic studies. False-negative prozone reactions are the result of massive antibody excess. Antigen–antibody complexes form most efficiently with mild antigen excess and can be inhibited by massive antibody excess. The serum may need to be diluted manyfold in order to test positive.

A biopsy frequently suggests the diagnosis. Whereas most other forms of vacuolar interface dermatitis are associated with effacement of the rete, secondary syphilis characteristically demonstrates a combination of vacuolar interface dermatitis and acanthosis with long, slender rete. This pattern has been referred to as an "icicle" or "icepick" pattern of acanthosis. Some students have found it helpful to remember that syphilis (a sexually transmitted disease) produces long, slender, "sexy" rete ridges with associated vacuolar interface dermatitis. Neutrophils are commonly present in the stratum corneum. Plasma cells are present in about two thirds of cases. Small dermal blood vessels appear to have no

lumen because of endothelial swelling. Another helpful feature is the presence of perivascular lymphocytes and histiocytes with visible cytoplasm. It may be difficult to decide at scanning power whether the infiltrate is granulomatous or lymphoid. A subtle interstitial infiltrate is often present as well, giving the impression of a hypercellular "busy dermis." It should be noted that although many cases of secondary syphilis conform to the description given earlier, those with five or fewer diagnostic features are more likely to show interface dermatitis with effacement of the rete pattern together with a busy dermis, endothelial swelling, and/or lymphocytes with too much cytoplasm.

Tertiary syphilis

Key Features

- Granulomatous
- Organisms not generally visible

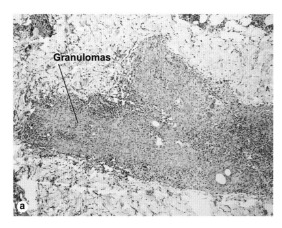

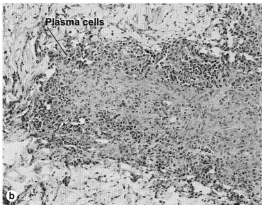

Fig. 17.22 Tertiary syphilis

Lyme disease

Erythema migrans

Key Features

- Highly variable perivascular infiltrate (often superficial and deep lymphoid, but many variations occur)
- May contain plasma cells
- May contain eosinophils
- Spirochetes may be present around superficial dermal vessels in silver-stained sections

The histologic features are nonspecific. The diagnosis is usually made clinically or by culture.

Acrodermatitis chronica atrophicans

Key Features

- Dermal atrophy with thin, attenuated collagen bundles
- Fat and large subcutaneous vessels appear close to surface
- Sparse lymphohistiocytic band throughout the dermis

In the evolving stage, lesions with a morphea-like appearance may show an interstitial granulomatous infiltrate, resembling granuloma annulare.

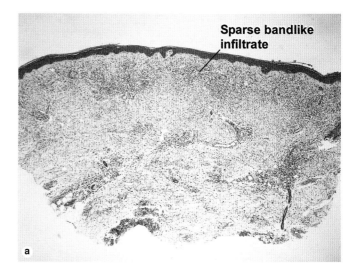

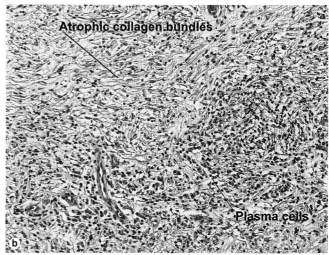

Fig. 17.23 Acrodermatitis chronica atrophicans

Protozoan diseases

Leishmaniasis

Key Features

- Granulomatous dermatitis
- Plasma cells common
- Intracellular organisms
- Organisms often line up at periphery of vacuole

The organisms are similar in size and shape to histoplasmosis. A kinetoplast is present, but may be difficult to see. The distribution of the organisms within the histiocyte is helpful. *Histoplasma* organisms are evenly spaced and surrounded by a pseudocapsule. In contrast, *Leishmania* organisms lack a pseudocapsule. They may be randomly spaced or lined up at the periphery of a vacuole, like light bulbs on a make-up mirror or movie marquee. Culture, polymerase chain reaction, and quantitative nucleic acid sequence–based amplification are sensitive techniques used to detect, type, and quantify *Leishmania* in tissue.

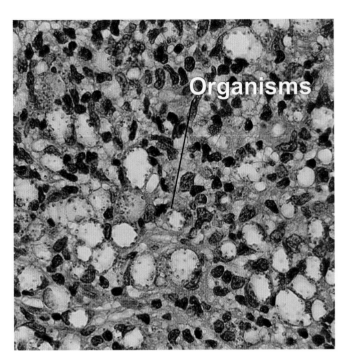

Fig. 17.24 Leishmaniasis

Acanthamoeba

Key Features

- Necrosis of deep vessels
- Organisms in vessel wall

At first glance, amoeba trophozoites may look like large histiocytes with somewhat refractile nuclei. Glance again. They have a characteristic appearance, as noted in Fig. 17.23. Vascular invasion and necrosis are typical. Lobular fat necrosis has been reported. Disseminated disease is frequently associated with human immunodeficiency virus (HIV) infection or immunosuppressive drugs. Cultures on an agar plate seeded with a lawn of *Escherichia coli* will demonstrate characteristic tracks.

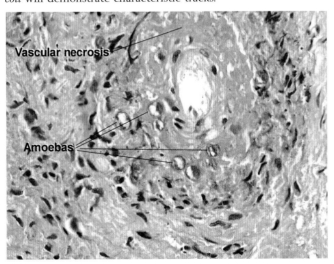

Fig. 17.25 *Acanthamoeba* infection

Further reading

Crotty MP, Krekel T, Burnham CA, et al. New gram-positive agents: the next generation of oxazolidinones and lipoglycopeptides. J Clin Microbiol 2016;54(9):2225–32.

Engelkens HJ, ten Kate FJ, Vuzevski VD, et al. Primary and secondary syphilis: a histopathological study. Int J STD AIDS 1991;2(4):280–4.

Flamm A, Parikh K, Xie Q, et al. Histologic features of secondary syphilis: A multicenter retrospective review. J Am Acad Dermatol 2015;73(6):1025–30.

Kaur C, Thami GP, Mohan H. Lucio phenomenon and Lucio leprosy. Clin Exp Dermatol 2005;30(5):525–7.

Lockwood DN, Nicholls P, Smith WC, et al. Comparing the clinical and histological diagnosis of leprosy and leprosy reactions in the INFIR cohort of Indian patients with multibacillary leprosy. PLoS Negl Trop Dis 2012;6(6):e1702.

Mathur MC, Ghimire RB, Shrestha P, et al. Clinicohistopathological correlation in leprosy. Kathmandu Univ Med J (KUMJ) 2011;9(36):248–51.

McBroom RL, Styles AR, Chiu MJ, et al. Secondary syphilis in persons infected with and not infected with HIV-1: a comparative immunohistologic study. Am J Dermatopathol 1999;21(5):432–41.

Moreno C, Kutzner H, Palmedo G, et al. Interstitial granulomatous dermatitis with histiocytic pseudorosettes: a new histopathologic pattern in cutaneous borreliosis. Detection of Borrelia burgdorferi DNA sequences by a highly sensitive PCR-ELISA. J Am Acad Dermatol 2003;48(3):376–84.

Pandhi RK, Singh N, Ramam M. Secondary syphilis: a clinicopathologic study. Int J Dermatol 1995;34(4):240–3.

Raval RC. Various faces of Hansen's disease. Indian J Lepr 2012;84(2):155–60.

Vargas-Ocampo F. Analysis of 6000 skin biopsies of the national leprosy control program in Mexico. Int J Lepr Other Mycobact Dis 2004;72(4):427–36.

Wilson TC, Legler A, Madison KC, et al. Erythema migrans: a spectrum of histopathologic changes. Am J Dermatopathol 2012;34(8):834–7.

Wohlrab J, Rohrbach D, Marsch WC. Keratolysis sulcata (pitted keratolysis): clinical symptoms with different histological correlates. Br J Dermatol 2000;143(6):1348–9.

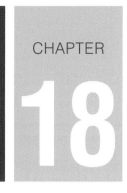
Fungal infections

Dirk M. Elston

Tinea

Key Feature

- Nonpigmented hyphae in stratum corneum

The stratum corneum may be basket-weave or compact and eosinophilic. It may contain parakeratosis or clusters of neutrophils.

Differential Diagnosis

Collections of neutrophils within the stratum corneum: psoriasis, tinea, impetigo, *Candida,* seborrheic dermatitis, syphilis (PTICSS).

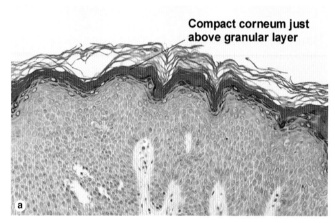

Compact corneum just above granular layer

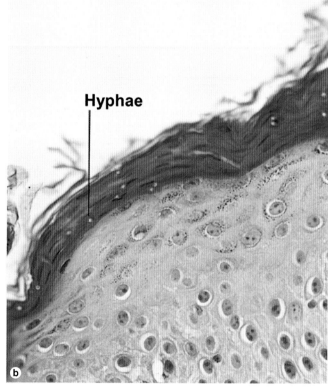

Hyphae

PAS stain

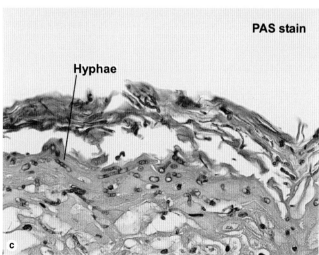

Hyphae

Fig. 18.1 Tinea

The stratum corneum in tinea is commonly basket-weave, but a narrow zone of compact eosinophilic stratum corneum is present just above the granular layer. Round hyphae cut on end are often visible in this compact layer.

If it scales, scrape it. If it scales and you don't know what it is, PAS it.

Bullous tinea

Key Features

- Massive papillary dermal edema
- Nonpigmented hyphae in stratum corneum

Reticular (netlike) degeneration of the epidermis is typically present. The infiltrate is typically polymorphous (predominantly lymphoid, with some neutrophils and eosinophils).

Differential Diagnosis

The massive papillary dermal edema resembles that of polymorphous light eruption, perniosis, or Sweet syndrome. Bullous tinea lacks the nodular and diffuse neutrophilic infiltrate and karyorrhexis of Sweet syndrome. Polymorphous light eruption and perniosis typically have a purely lymphoid infiltrate, and perniosis demonstrates edema surrounding lymphocytes in vessels.

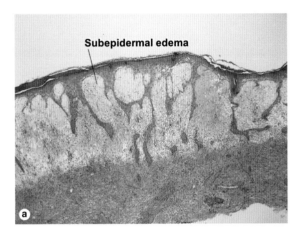

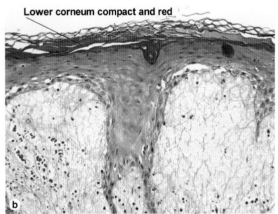

Fig. 18.2 Bullous tinea

Onychomycosis

Key Features

- Periodic acid–Schiff (PAS)-positive hyphae in subungual debris

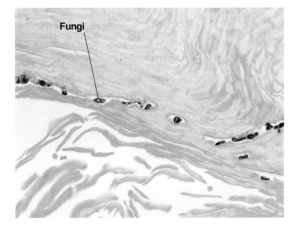

Fig. 18.3 Onychomycosis (periodic acid–Schiff)

Tinea versicolor

Key Features

- Loose lamellar or basket-weave hyperkeratosis
- Groups of round spores and short curved hyphae in the stratum corneum ("ziti and meatballs")

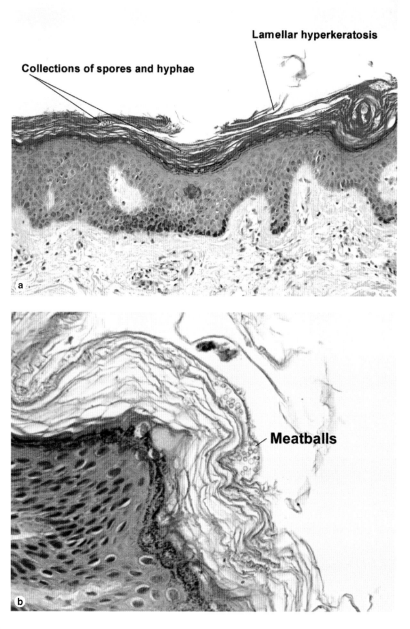

Fig. 18.4 Tinea versicolor

Candidiasis

Key Features

- Pseudohyphae in stratum corneum
- Often vertically oriented
- Neutrophils common in stratum corneum
- Hyperkeratosis and crusting common

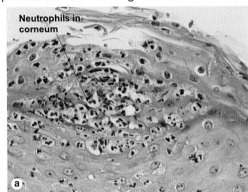

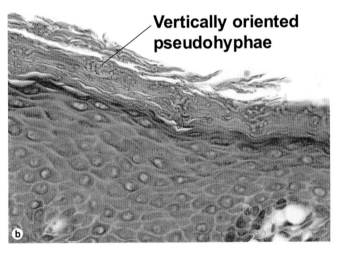

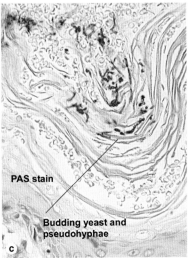

Fig. 18.5 Candidiasis

Differential Diagnosis

Collections of neutrophils within the stratum corneum: PTICSS (see earlier)

Budding yeast may sometimes be seen, or the pseudohyphae may resemble dermatophyte hyphae. Dermatophyte hyphae tend to be oriented east–west within the stratum corneum, whereas *Candida* pseudohyphae are often oriented north–south.

Coccidioidomycosis

Key Features

- Large spherules with gray, lacy, and granular cytoplasm
- Uniform in size and shape
- Refractile wall
- Endospores sometimes present

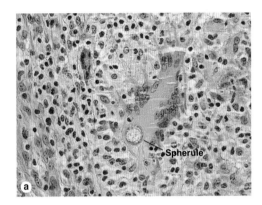

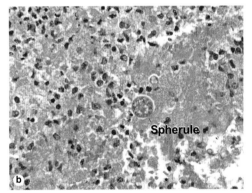

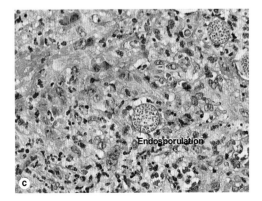

Fig. 18.6 Coccidioidomycosis

Coccidioidomycosis is endemic to southwestern United States and California. The organism grows easily on agar at room temperature. As such, cultures are highly infectious; deep fungal infections should never be cultured in the office setting.

Cryptococcosis

Key Features

- Pleomorphic yeast, varies markedly in size and shape
- Clear gelatinous capsules containing small groups of organisms ("gelatinous condominiums")
- Amount of capsular material is inversely proportional to granulomatous infiltrate

Whereas most other deep fungal organisms have a characteristic size and shape, *Cryptococcus* varies markedly in size and shape. The organisms are "gregarious" and cluster within clear spaces that correspond to the mucinous capsule. The capsule stains red with mucicarmine. Although they never appear brown in tissue, the organisms stain with a Fontana–Masson melanin stain.

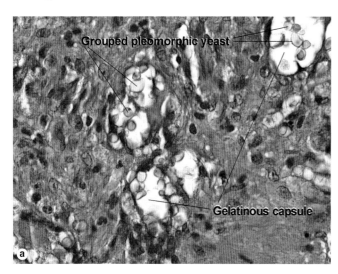

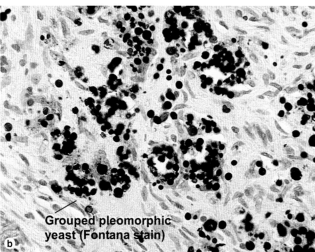

Fig. 18.7 Cryptococcosis

Umbilicated, molluscum-like lesions are often associated with human immunodeficiency virus (HIV).

Blastomycosis

Key Features

- Pseudoepitheliomatous hyperplasia with intraepidermal pustules
- Organisms are few in number, usually within giant cells, uniform in size and shape
- Thick, refractile, asymmetrical wall
- Dark nucleus
- If budding is seen, it is broad based

Blastomycosis is caused by *Blastomyces dermatitidis*. Skin lesions are typically slowly advancing verrucous plaques, with central scarring and a heaped edge.

Differential Diagnosis

Pseudoepitheliomatous hyperplasia with intraepidermal pustules (PEH and pus): "Here come big green leafy veggies":

- Here – *h*alogenoderma
- Come – *c*hromomycosis
- Big – *b*lastomycosis
- Green – *g*ranuloma inguinale
- Leafy – *l*eishmaniasis
- Veggies – pemphigus *v*egetans

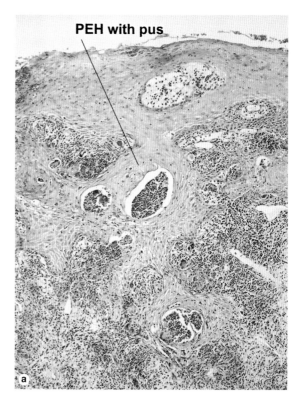

Fig. 18.8 Blastomycosis pseudoepitheliomatous hyperplasia (PEH)

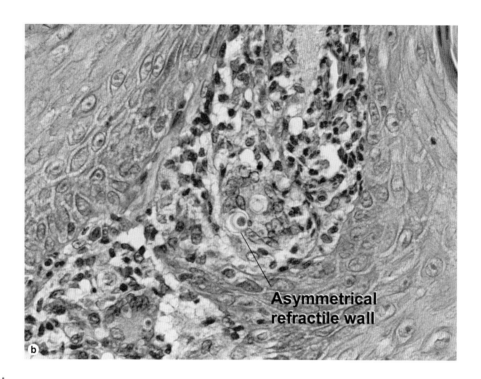

Fig. 18.8, cont'd

Paracoccidioides infection (South American "blastomycosis")

Key Features

- Small yeast (*Paracoccidioides braziliensis*)
- Lacks the thick refractile wall and eccentric nucleus of *Blastomyces* dermatitidis
- Narrow-based budding
- Mariner's wheel pattern of budding occasionally

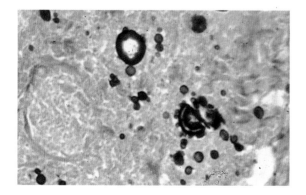

Fig. 18.9 *Paracoccidioides* infection (Grocott methenamine silver)

Histoplasmosis

Key Features

- Small uniform dots within histiocytes
- Each surrounded by a pseudocapsule
- Evenly spaced within histiocyte

Despite the name, *Histoplasma capsulatum* lacks a true capsule. The organisms are similar in size and shape to *Leishmania*, but lack a kinetoplast. The distribution of the organisms within the histiocyte is helpful. *Histoplasma* organisms are evenly spaced and surrounded by a pseudocapsule. In contrast, *Leishmania* organisms lack a pseudocapsule. They may be randomly spaced or lined up at the periphery of a vacuole like light bulbs on a make-up mirror or movie marquee. In cavitary lesions or within vascular spaces, histoplasmosis may grow in a mycelial (hyphal) phase.

Differential Diagnosis

"pH girl"
Differential of parasitized histiocytes

- *Penicillium marneffei* (looks strikingly similar to histoplasmosis)
- *Histoplasmosis
- *Granuloma inguinale
- *Rhinoscleroma
- *Leishmaniasis

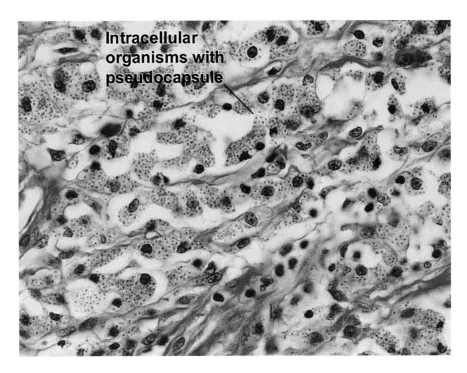

Fig. 18.10 Histoplasmosis

African histoplasmosis

Key Features

- Numerous large intracellular organisms in histiocytes and multinucleated giant cells
- Evenly spaced distribution of organisms in giant cells

Histoplasma duboisii infection differs from the usual *H. capsulatum* infection by the size of the organism and the presence of multinucleated giant cells. The organism is similar in size and shape to the lobomycosis organism, but lacks the characteristic "pop-bead" chains of lobomycosis.

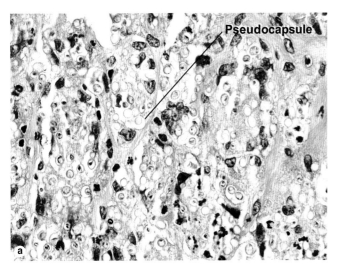

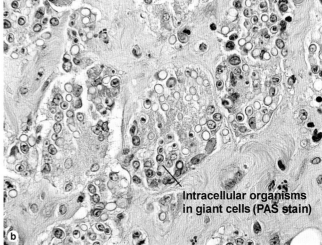

Fig. 18.11 African histoplasmosis

Lobomycosis (keloidal blastomycosis)

Key Features

- Large organisms (similar in size to African histoplasmosis)
- Often within histiocytes and multinucleated giant cells
- Characteristic pop-bead chains

Lobomycosis is caused by *Lacazia loboi*. The organism is similar in size and shape to African histoplasmosis, but chains are present, resembling a child's pop-beads. In biopsies from dolphins, the organism is significantly smaller than in human tissue.

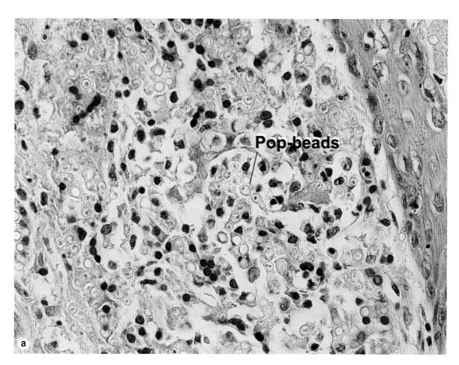

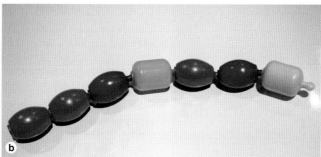

Fig. 18.12 (A) Lobomycosis. **(B)** Pop-beads for comparison

Sporotrichosis

Key Features

- Stellate abscess, surrounded by granuloma
- Rare cigar-shaped yeasts

Sporotrichosis forms characteristic stellate abscesses. Pseudoepitheliomatous hyperplasia is sometimes present. Some cases from Japan have numerous organisms, but generally, the organisms are few in number and culture is more sensitive than special stains. Among the organisms that form stellate abscesses, some demonstrate lymphangitic spread (nodules along lymph vessels), whereas others demonstrate ulceroglandular spread (ulcer with suppurative lymph node). Clinicopathologic correlation can narrow the differential diagnosis.

Differential Diagnosis

Stellate abscesses in skin: "CLATS"

- *C*at scratch
- *L*ymphogranuloma venereum
- *A*typical mycobacteria (usually *Mycobacterium marinum*)
- *T*ularemia
- *S*porotrichosis

PEARL

Lymphangitic syndromes	Ulceroglandular syndromes
Sporotrichosis	Tularemia
Leishmaniasis	Lymphogranuloma venereum
Atypical mycobacteria	Cat scratch
Nocardia	Glanders
Blastomyces	Melioidosis
	Chancroid
	Plague
	Tuberculosis

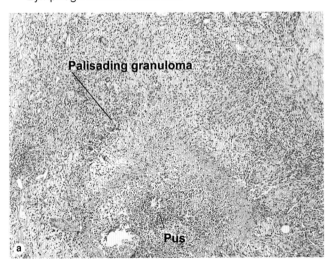

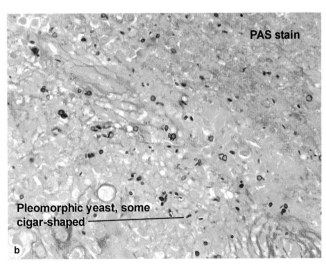

Fig. 18.13 Sporotrichosis

Mycetomas

Eumycetoma

Key Features

- Sinus tracts filled with neutrophils (resemble stellate abscesses)
- Grains within suppurative foci
- Grains made up of fungal hyphae
- Club-shaped Splendore–Hoeppli phenomenon at periphery of grain

Eumycetomas are true fungal mycetomas. The grains are composed of fungal hyphae, which may be pigmented. At the periphery of the grain, red, club-shaped accumulations of immunoglobulin appear as the Splendore–Hoeppli phenomenon.

PEARL

Dark-grain eumycetoma organisms are sometimes remembered by the mnemonic: "My lousy greasy jeans are black":

- My – *Madurella mycetomatis*
- Lousy – *Leptosphaeria* spp.
- Greasy – *M. grisea*
- Jeans – *Exophiala jeanselmei*
- Are black – pigmented

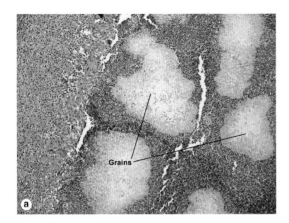

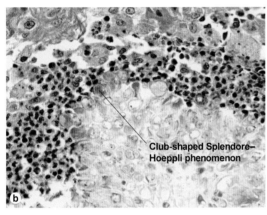

Fig. 18.14 Eumycetoma

Actinomycetomas

Key Features

- Sinus tracts filled with neutrophils (resemble stellate abscesses)
- Grains within suppurative foci
- Grains made up of filamentous bacteria
- Smooth Splendore–Hoeppli phenomenon at periphery of grain

Actinomycetomas are caused by filamentous bacteria but are discussed in this chapter because of their resemblance to fungal mycetomas. The grains are typically light in color. *Actinomadura* species commonly cause pink- to red-grain mycetomas, although some *A. madurae* grains are white or yellow.

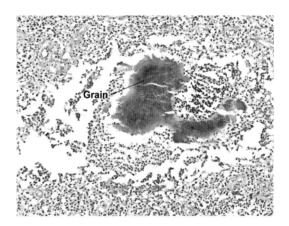

Fig. 18.15 Actinomycetoma

Dark-grain eumycetoma	Nonpigmented eumycetoma	Actinomycetoma
Madurella mycetomatis	Pseudoallescheria boydii	Nocardia brasiliensis
Leptosphaeria sp.	Acremonium sp.	N. asteroides
M. grisea	Fusarium sp.	N. transvalensis
Exophiala jeanselmei	Cylindrocarpon destructans	Actinomyces israelii
	Neotestudina sp.	Streptomyces somaliensis
	Dermatophytes	Actinomadura pelletieri
		A. madurae

Tinea nigra

Key Features

- Acral skin
- Gold to brown hyphae in stratum corneum

Tinea nigra is usually caused by *Hortaea werneckii*. It is more common in hot, humid climates, and typically occurs on a palm or sole.

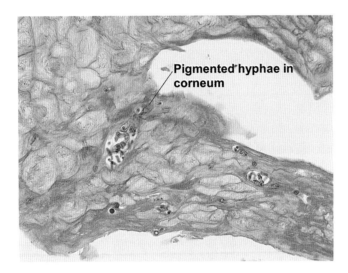

Fig. 18.16 Tinea nigra

Phaeohyphomycosis

Key Features

- Pigmented hyphae in tissue
- Commonly thick walled with vesicular swellings and visible bubbly cytoplasm

Phaeohyphomycosis is caused by a wide variety of black molds (dematiaceous fungi, mildew organisms). A cavity surrounded by histiocytes and giant cells may be seen. This pattern is referred to as a *phaeomycotic "cyst."* Most patients with phaeomycotic cysts are immunocompetent, and the most common organism is *Exophiala jeanselmei*. Most patients with invasive phaeohyphomycosis are immunocompromised, and the most common organism is *Bipolaris spicifera*.

PEARL

Pigment can sometimes be inconspicuous in the hyphal wall. Clues that the organism is a black mold include the combination of a thick refractile wall and bubbly cytoplasm. Some black mold hyphae form characteristic round swellings. Using a Fontana–Masson melanin stain to identify lightly pigmented dematiaceous fungi is problematic, as some nonpigmented molds (including zygomycetes and dermatophytes) will stain.

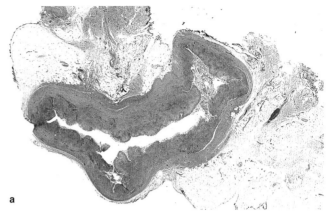

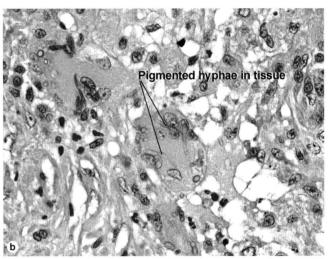

Fig. 18.17 Phaeohyphomycosis

Chromomycosis (chromoblastomycosis)

Key Features

- Pseudoepitheliomatous hyperplasia with intraepidermal pustules
- Medlar bodies: "copper pennies," "sclerotic bodies"

Round, copper-colored Medlar bodies are often seen in groups within giant cells or suppurative foci. Sometimes, they are noted within a wood splinter. Internal septation may be noted.

PEARL

Chromomycosis is caused by:

- Compact – *Fonsecaea compacta*
- Dead – *Cladosporium carrionii*
- Wet – *Rhinocladiella aquaspersa*
- Warty – *Phialophora verrucosa*
- Feet – *Fonsecaea pedrosoi*

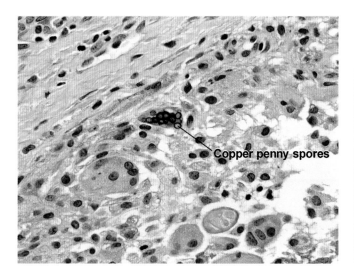

Fig. 18.18 Chromomycosis

Zygomycosis

Mucorales infection (mucormycosis)

Key Features

- Broad, hollow-appearing, lumpy, bumpy, refractile hyphae
- Blood vessel invasion
- Tissue necrosis

Although 90-degree branching is typical, some hyphae will appear to branch at more acute angles. The hyphae are nonseptate, but twists and bends in the wall commonly mimic a septum. An excellent clue to the nonseptate nature of the organism is that the hyphae appear hollow, as there are no septa to retain cytoplasm. Tissue sent for culture must be diced carefully, as homogenization easily renders the nonseptate hyphae nonviable. Causative organisms include *Rhizopus, Absidia, Mucor, Cunninghamella, Apophysomyces, Rhizomucor, Saksenaea, Mortierella,* and *Cokeromyces* species. They stain poorly with fungal stains such as PAS and Gomori methenamine silver (GMS: Grocott), but may stain well with a Gram stain.

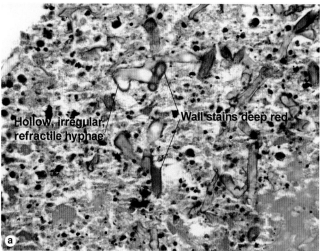

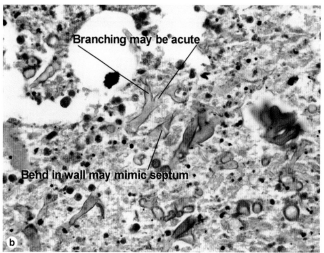

Fig. 18.19 *Rhizopus* infection

Entomophthorales infection (entomophthoromycosis)

Key Features

- Indolent infections
- Resemble zygomycetes in tissue

Conidiobolus coronatus causes perinasal disease. *Basidiobolus ranarum* causes broader subcutaneous lesions in nonfacial skin. The Splendore–Hoeppli phenomenon is commonly seen as an eosinophilic sleeve around the hyphae. *Pythiosis,* an aquatic hyphal organism, has a similar appearance.

Hyalohyphomycosis (including aspergillosis and fusariosis)

Key Features

- Narrow, nonpigmented hyphae in tissue
- Prominent, blue, bubbly cytoplasm

- Inconspicuous, delicate wall
- Septate
- Forty-five-degree-angle branching
- Invade vessels, causing tissue necrosis
- *Fusarium* may demonstrate vesicular swellings like a black mold, but lacks the thick refractile wall characteristic of *Bipolaris* (the most common invasive black mold)

The term *hyalohyphomycosis* is used for invasive infections by any nonpigmented mold, excluding zygomycetes. As a group, they tend to be vasculotropic and cause tissue necrosis. They are septate organisms, and the septa typically retain bubbly, blue cytoplasm within the delicate hyphal walls. The blue cytoplasm is always more conspicuous than the nearly invisible wall. The only exception is when a Splendore–Hoeppli phenomenon (eosinophilic immunoglobulin) coats the fungal wall. The immunoglobulin is never refractile like chitin. Dead hyphae will swell to the diameter of a zygomycete, but the dead wall will be pale-staining and will never be thick and refractile like a zygomycete.

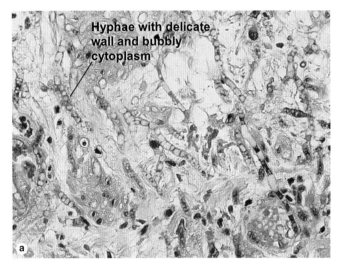 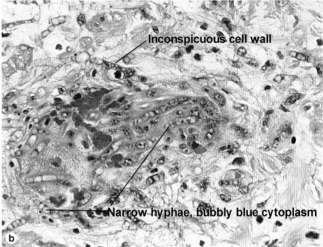

Fig. 18.20 Aspergillosis

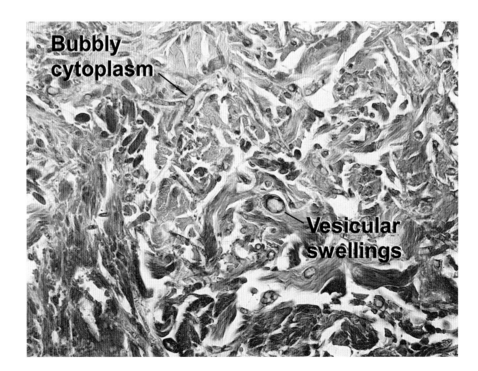

Fig. 18.21 Fusariosis

Protothecosis

Key Features

- Morula (like a soccer ball)
- Nonmorulating forms have characteristic "eyeball" appearance

The organism (genus *Prototheca*) is found in tree slime and generally classified as an achloric (nonpigmented) algae.

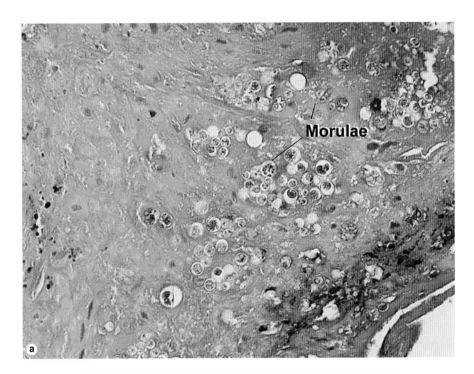

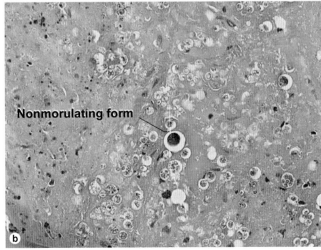

Fig. 18.22 Protothecosis

Rhinosporidiosis

Key Features

- Huge sporangia with many endospores
- Nonsporulating trophocyte form resembles *Coccidioides*, but with a central small nucleus

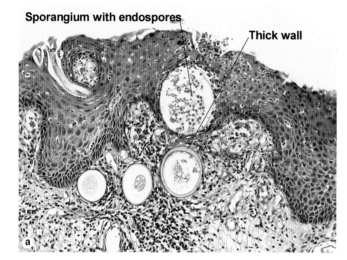

Sporangium with endospores

Thick wall

a

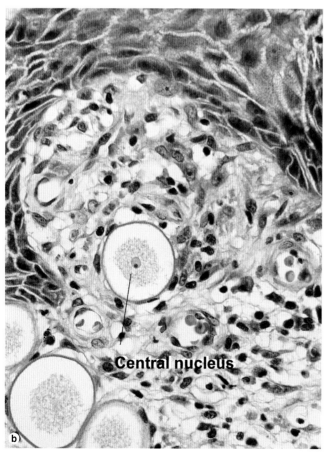

Central nucleus

b

Fig. 18.23 Rhinosporidiosis

Rhinosporidium has been classified as a fungus or protist. Granulomas are present in about 50% of cases. A suppurative response may be present when sporangia rupture. Transepithelial elimination of sporangia may be seen. The organism requires synergistic bacteria for growth. Culture of the organism has been accomplished when it is grown with the cyanobacterium *Microcystis aeruginosa*. The organisms are naturally found together in pond water.

Further reading

Arseculeratne SN, Panabokke RG, Atapattu DN. Lymphadenitis, trans-epidermal elimination and unusual histopathology in human rhinosporidiosis. Mycopathologia 2002;153(2):57–69.

Bracca A, Tosello ME, Girardini JE, et al. Molecular detection of Histoplasma capsulatum var. capsulatum in human clinical samples. J Clin Microbiol 2003;41(4):1753–5.

Haubold EM, Cooper CR Jr, Wen JW, et al. Comparative morphology of Lacazia loboi (syn. Loboa loboi) in dolphins and humans. Med Mycol 2000;38(1):9–14.

Hu S, Chung WH, Hung SI, et al. Detection of Sporothrix schenckii in clinical samples by a nested PCR assay. J Clin Microbiol 2003;41(4):1414–18.

Husain S, Alexander BD, Munoz P, et al. Opportunistic mycelial fungal infections in organ transplant recipients: emerging importance of non-Aspergillus mycelial fungi. Clin Infect Dis 2003;37(2):221–9.

Kantrow SM, Boyd AS. Protothecosis. Dermatol Clin 2003;21(2):249–55.

Makannavar JH, Chavan SS. Rhinosporidiosis – a clinicopathological study of 34 cases. Indian J Pathol Microbiol 2001;44(1):17–21.

Minotto R, Bernardi CD, Mallmann LF, et al. Chromoblastomycosis: a review of 100 cases in the state of Rio Grande do Sul, Brazil. J Am Acad Dermatol 2001;44(4):585–92.

Perfect JR. The triple threat of cryptococcosis: it's the body site, the strain, and/or the host. MBio 2012;3(4):pii: e00165-12.

Ramesh A, Deka RC, Vijayaraghavan M, et al. Entomophthoromycosis of the nose and paranasal sinus. Indian J Pediatr 2000;67(4):307–10.

Revankar SG, Patterson JE, Sutton DA, et al. Disseminated phaeohyphomycosis: review of an emerging mycosis. Clin Infect Dis 2002;34(4):467–76.

Shinozaki M, Okubo Y, Sasai D, et al. Development and evaluation of nucleic acid-based techniques for an auxiliary diagnosis of invasive fungal infections in formalin-fixed and paraffin-embedded (FFPE) tissues. Med Mycol J 2012;53(4):241–5.

Talhari S, Talhari C. Lobomycosis. Clin Dermatol 2012;30(4):420–4.

Viral infections, helminths, and arthropods

Dirk M. Elston

Viral infections

Warts

Verruca vulgaris

Key Features

- Exophytic
- Papillomatosis

- Compact eosinophilic hyperkeratosis
- Coarse hypergranulosis in dells
- Vertical tiers of round parakeratosis common above peaks
- Blood and serum common above peaks
- Koilocytes variable

The biopsy will demonstrate a compact stratum corneum, coarse hypergranulosis, and papillomatosis. The papillomatosis often curves inward. Vascular ectasia is common. Koilocytes (vacuolated cells with hyperchromatic shriveled nuclei) may be present. Red cytoplasmic inclusions may sometimes be present.

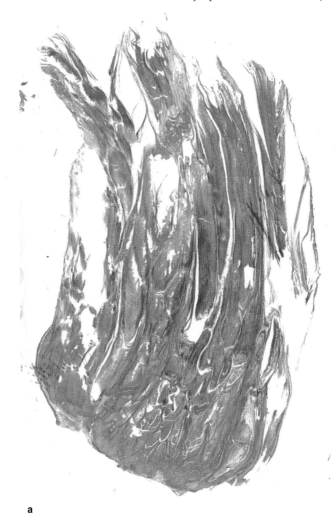

a

Fig. 19.1 Verruca vulgaris

continued

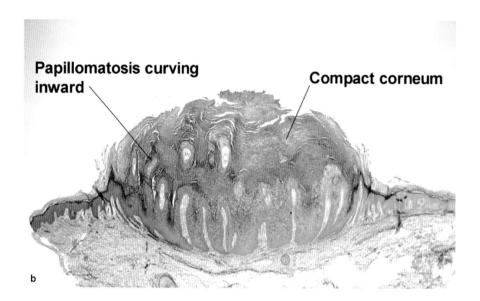

Fig. 19.1, cont'd

Myrmecia

Key Features

- Deep palmoplantar wart with anthill-like appearance clinically
- Endophytic
- Coarse red cytoplasmic inclusions

Myrmecia are associated with human papillomavirus 1 (HPV-1).

Verruca plana (flat wart)

Key Features

- Coarse basket-weave hyperkeratosis
- Hypergranulosis common
- "Bird's eye" cells (like koilocytes but lack shriveled nuclei)

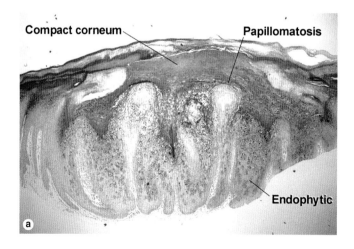

Fig. 19.2 Myrmecia

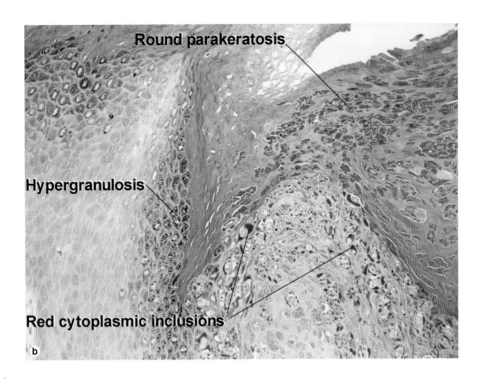

Fig. 19.2, cont'd

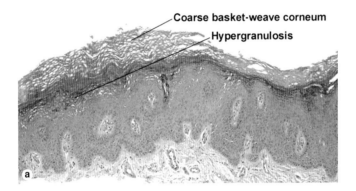

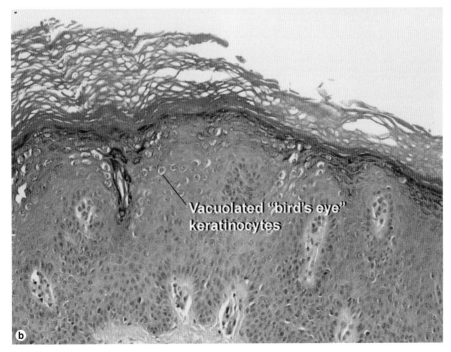

Fig. 19.3 **(A and B)** Verruca plana.

continued

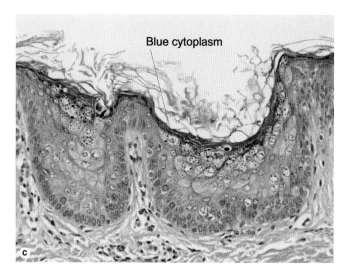

Fig. 19.3, cont'd (C) Verruca plana with changes characteristic of epidermodysplasia verruciformis

Epidermodysplasia verruciformis (EDV)

Key Feature

- Widespread, flat warts with foamy blue cytoplasm

Condyloma acuminatum

Key Features

- Benign acanthoma on genital skin
- Areas of compact stratum corneum, round parakeratosis, and coarse hypergranulosis generally present
- Vacuolated keratinocytes, typically with large gray nuclei
- True koilocytes rare

Condylomata acuminata commonly have horn cysts and resemble seborrheic keratoses. The two are differentiated by areas of compact stratum corneum, round parakeratosis, coarse hypergranulosis, and vacuolated keratinocytes with large gray nuclei. In situ hybridization can identify the HPV type.

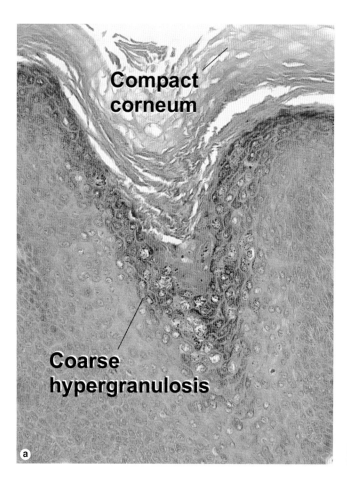

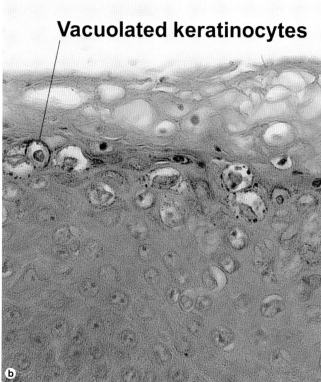

Fig. 19.4 (A and B) Condyloma accuminatum.

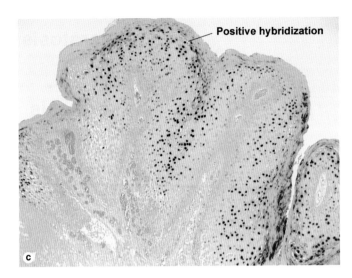

Fig. 19.4, cont'd (C) Condyloma accuminatum in situ hybridization for low-risk HPV (types 6 and 11)

Bowenoid papulosis

Key Features

- HPV-16 most commonly
- Atypia

Bowenoid papulosis presents as discrete pink, brown, or gray lesions in the genitalia. They are typically sessile rather than papillomatous or cauliflower-like. The histologic spectrum ranges from that of a condyloma with buckshot scatter of atypical cells to full-thickness atypia, indistinguishable from Bowen disease.

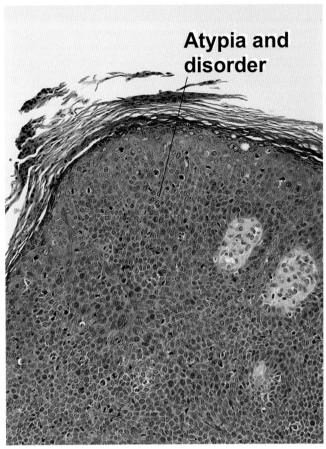

Fig. 19.5 Bowenoid papulosis

Heck disease

Key Features

- Focal oral hyperplasia
- Hyperkeratosis with round parakeratosis
- Epithelial pallor
- HPV-13 and -32

Type of wart	HPV type
Common	1, 2, 4
Flat (verruca plana)	3, 5
Plantar	1 (myrmecia), 2, 4 (mosaic)
Epidermodysplasia verruciformis	5, 8, and many others
Buschke–Löwenstein tumor	6, 11
Butcher's	7 and others
Laryngeal papillomas	6, 11
Genital dysplasia	16, 18, 31, 33, 35, and others
Heck focal oral hyperplasia	13, 32
Subungual squamous cell carcinoma	16

Verrucous cyst (cystic papilloma)

Key Features

- Cyst with wartlike lining

Verrucous cysts may arise as a result of papillomavirus infection of a hair follicle. On plantar surfaces, they may arise from eccrine ducts, and the lining is more likely to resemble myrmecia.

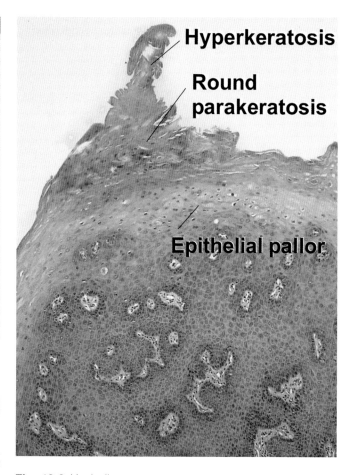

Fig. 19.6 Heck disease

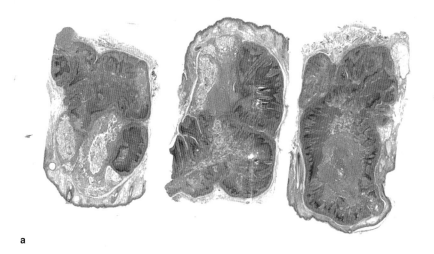

a

Fig. 19.7 Verrucous cyst

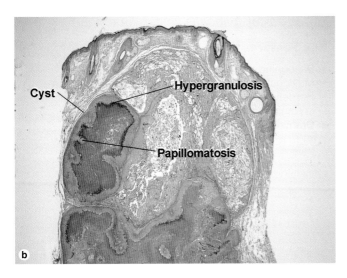

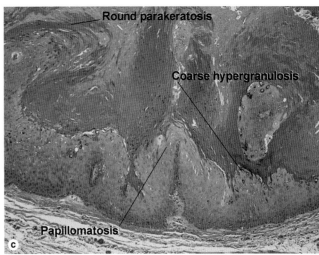

Fig. 19.7, cont'd

Herpetic infections

Herpes simplex

Key Features

- Ballooning degeneration of keratinocytes
- Multinucleated keratinocytes with nuclear molding

- Herpetic cytopathic effect (basophilic eggshell of chromatin at the periphery of the nucleus)
- Mild features of leukocytoclastic vasculitis may be present

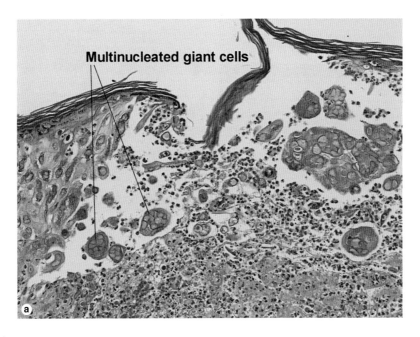

Fig. 19.8 Herpes simplex

continued

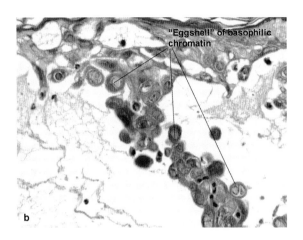

"Eggshell" of basophilic chromatin

Fig. 19.8, cont'd

Herpes zoster (varicella-zoster virus: VZV)

Key Features

- Ballooning degeneration of keratinocytes
- Multinucleated keratinocytes with nuclear molding
- Herpetic cytopathic effect (basophilic eggshell of chromatin at the periphery of the nucleus)
- Dramatic leukocytoclastic vasculitis typical

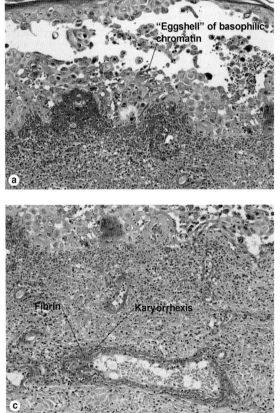

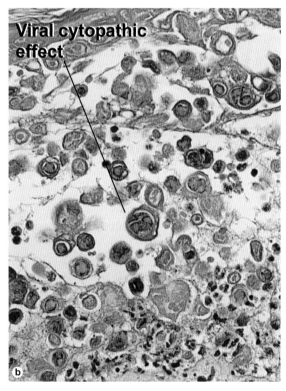

Fig. 19.9 Herpes zoster (shingles)

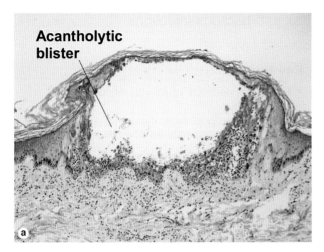

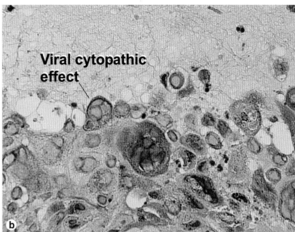

Fig. 19.10 Varicella (chicken pox)

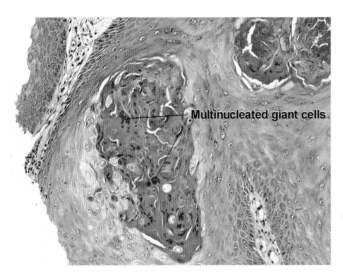

Fig. 19.11 Verrucous zoster

Chicken pox (VZV)

Key Features

- Ballooning degeneration of keratinocytes
- Multinucleated keratinocytes with nuclear molding
- Herpetic cytopathic effect (basophilic eggshell of chromatin at the periphery of the nucleus)
- Mild features of leukocytoclastic vasculitis may be present

Verrucous VZV infection

Key Features

- Compact hyperkeratosis
- Variable papillomatosis
- Follicular herpetic cytopathic effect

Multinucleated giant cells with basophilic nuclear rims and nuclear molding are noted within follicular epithelium. This pattern is typically seen in immunosuppressed patients, especially in the setting of human immunodeficiency virus (HIV) infection.

Cytomegalovirus

Key Features

- Large endothelial cells with owl's-eye nuclei
- Cytoplasm may be ample or scant

In HIV patients, cytomegalovirus probably does not cause ulcers, but reactivates within ulcers. Viral cytopathic changes may be found in ulcers of various causes. This alerts the clinician to look for evidence of cytomegalovirus retinal involvement.

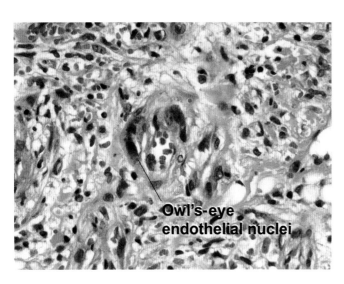

Fig. 19.12 Cytomegalovirus infection

Pox and parapox infections

Smallpox (variola)

Key Features

- Epidermal necrosis, often with reticular degeneration
- Eosinophilic cytoplasmic inclusions
- Nuclear inclusions may also be seen

In scrapings, Guarnieri bodies appear black with Gispen's modified silver stain. Guarnieri bodies are aggregations of the smaller Paschen bodies.

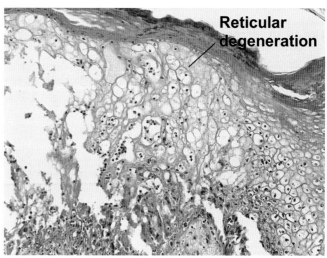

Fig. 19.13 Smallpox

Monkey pox

Key Features

- Ballooning degeneration of basal keratinocytes
- Epidermal necrosis
- Spongiosis
- Bandlike polymorphous infiltrate
- Superficial and deep perivascular and periadnexal infiltrate
- Multinucleated syncytial keratinocytes
- Animal contact

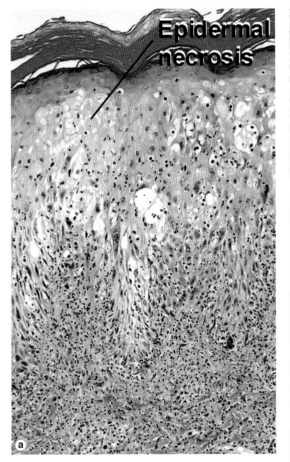

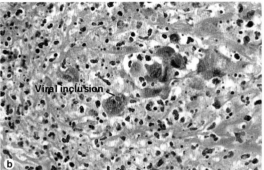

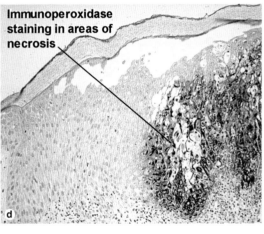

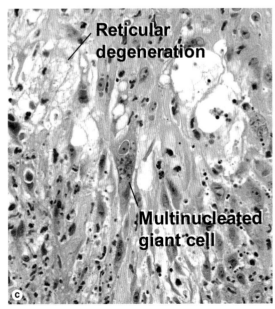

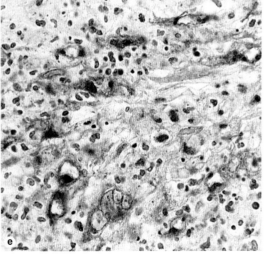

Fig. 19.14 Monkey pox (courtesy of Erik Stratman, MD.)

Molluscum contagiosum

Key Features

- Cup-shaped lesion with scalloped border
- Henderson–Paterson bodies (molluscum bodies)

Molluscum contagiosum is readily recognized by the characteristic cytoplasmic inclusions. These vary from eosinophilic to basophilic as the inclusion bodies mature.

Orf and milker's nodules

Key Features

- Epidermal necrosis
- Viral inclusion bodies (may be both cytoplasmic and intranuclear)
- Animal contact

Orf and milker's nodules are caused by distinct viruses, but have a similar histologic appearance. Each lesion evolves through a series of clinical stages, and the histologic appearance varies by stage. During the verrucous phase, the epidermis demonstrates endophytic strandlike proliferations. The dermal papillae are edematous with dilated vessels. A dense, predominantly lymphoid infiltrate is present. Plasma cells and histiocytes are often present. Viral inclusion bodies, clumping of keratohyalin, and cytoplasmic vacuolation may still be seen.

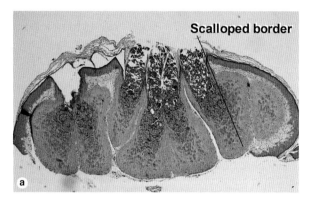

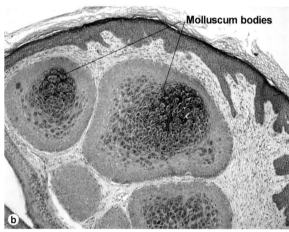

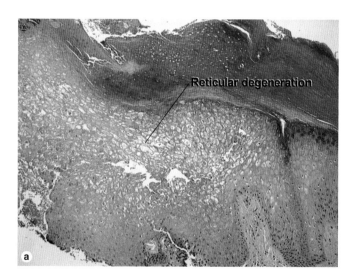

Fig. 19.16 Orf nodules

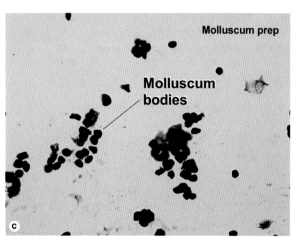

Fig. 19.15 Molluscum contagiosum

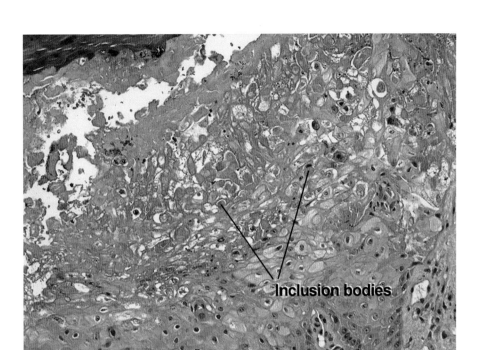

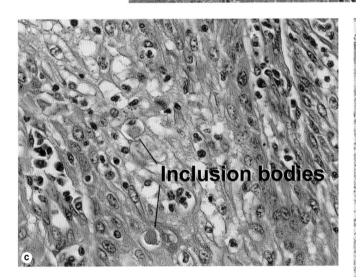

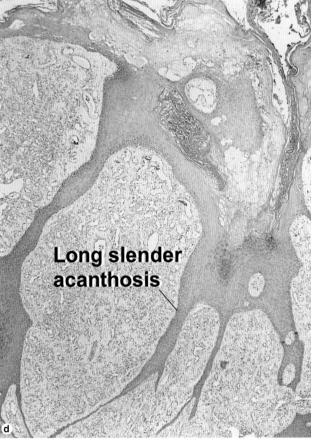

Fig. 19.16, cont'd

Gianotti–Crosti syndrome

Key Features

- Papular acrolocated syndrome
- Associated with various viruses, notably hepatitis B virus (HBV) in Italy
- In the United States, papulovesicular acrolocated syndrome is rarely associated with HBV
- Minor crusting
- Spongiosis
- Papillary dermal edema
- Superficial perivascular lymphoid infiltrate

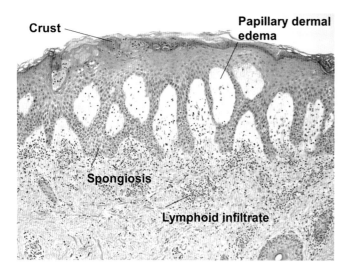

Fig. 19.17 Gianotti–Crosti syndrome

Hand, foot, and mouth syndrome

Key Features

- Oval vesicles or ulcers on the sides of the digits, palms, soles, mouth, and buttocks
- Coxsackie A16 and others
- Reticular and ballooning degeneration of keratinocytes

Oral hairy leukoplakia

Key Features

- HIV-associated Epstein–Barr virus (EBV) infection
- Nuclear stippling characteristic
- In situ hybridization (Epstein–Barr encoding region [EBER]) is helpful for confirmation

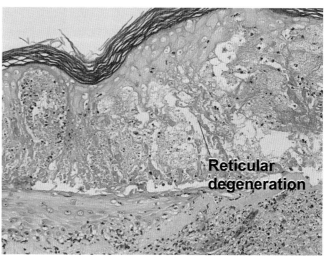

Fig. 19.18 Hand, foot, and mouth syndrome

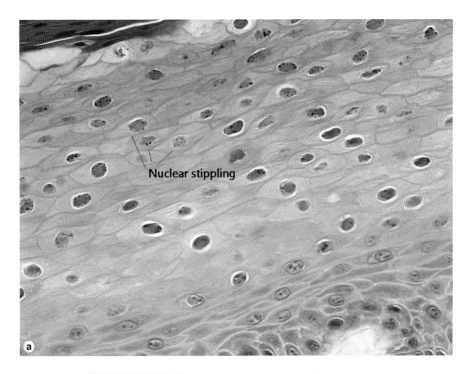

Nuclear stippling

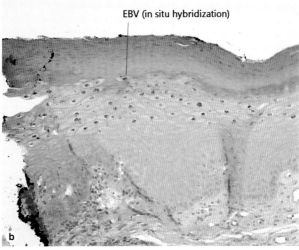

EBV (in situ hybridization)

Fig. 19.19 Oral hairy leukoplakia

Oral white sponge nevus (for comparison)

Key Features

- Not virally induced
- Lacks nuclear stippling
- Red band of dyskeratosis surrounds nucleus

Viral-associated trichodysplasia (trichodysplasia spinulosa)

Key Features

- HIV-associated polyomavirus infection of the hair follicle
- Characteristic eosinophilic inclusion bodies

Flukes, tapeworms, and roundworms

Flukes

Schistosomiasis

Key Features

- Ova with stippled contents
- Mixed inflammatory response, commonly granulomatous

Schistosomes are trematodes (flukes). When cutaneous involvement occurs, it usually involves genital skin. *Schistosoma haematobium* is typically implicated.

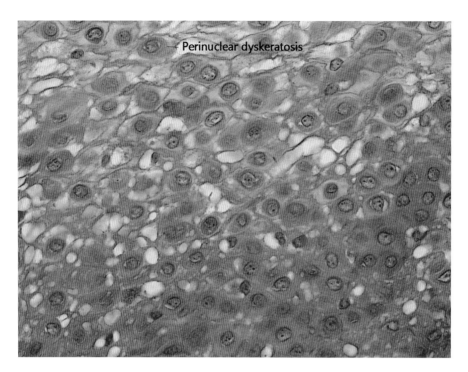

Fig. 19.20 Oral white sponge nevus for comparison

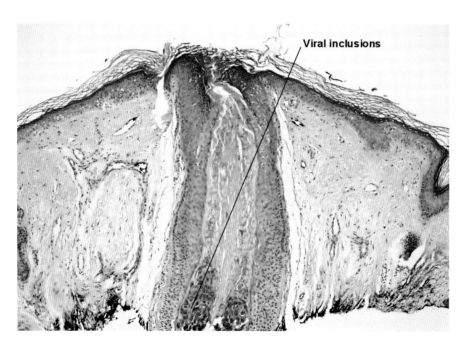

Fig. 19.21 Viral-associated trichodysplasia

Identification of schistosome ova:

- *S. haematobium* – thin wall with thin vertical spine (Fig. 19.23)
- *S. mansoni* – thick refractile wall with thick angular spine (Fig. 19.24)
- *S. japonicum* – round with refractile wall and no visible spine (Fig. 19.25)

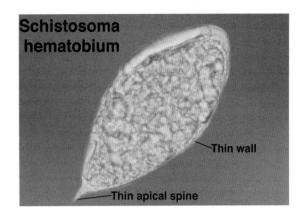

Fig. 19.23 Schistosoma hematobium

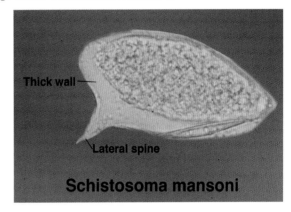

Fig. 19.24 Schistosoma mansoni

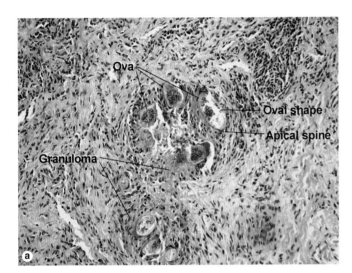

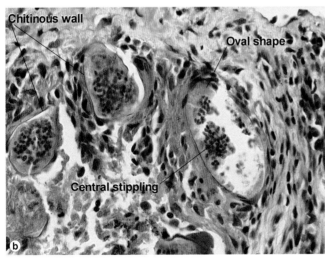

Fig. 19.22 Cutaneous schistosomiasis

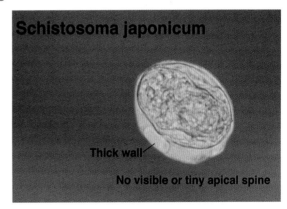

Fig. 19.25 Schistosoma japonicum

Flatworms

- Secretory tegument, rows of subtegumental cells
- Calcareous bodies
- Smooth muscle
- No gut

Spirometra worms, the cause of sparganosis, are typical cestodes. They lack a gut and must absorb nutrients through the tegumental cells. They cannot excrete waste and so calcify it internally as calcareous bodies.

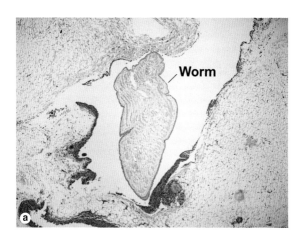

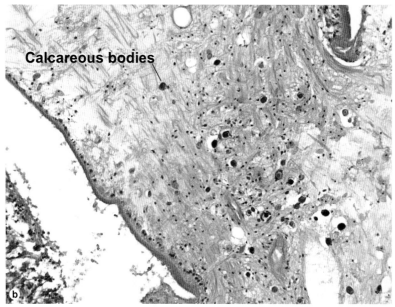

Fig. 19.26 Sparganosis

Sparganum proliferum

Key Features

- Multilocular cyst
- High-power views show features of a flatworm

Differential Diagnosis

The features of other tapeworm cysts are similar. Some tapeworms demonstrate scolices (rings of hooks). The cysts can degenerate to little more than a rim of epithelium.

Roundworms

Elephantiasis

Key Features

- Filarial roundworm within lymphatic vessel
- Inflammatory response leads to lymphedema

Table 19.1 Ridge patterns of *Dirofilaria* species

Species	Ridge pattern
D. tenuis	Wide/broken
D. repens	Narrow/sharp
D. ursi	Spaced far apart/round
D. immitis	None

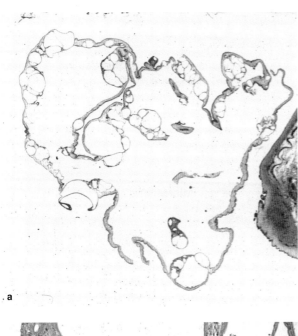

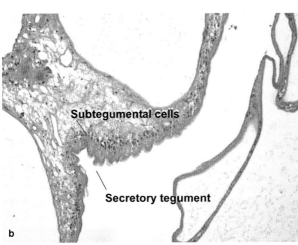

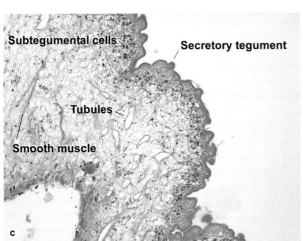

Fig. 19.27 Sparganum proliferum (courtesy of Richard Bernert, MD.)

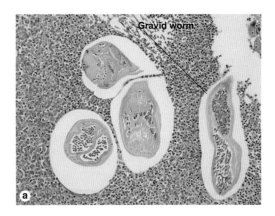

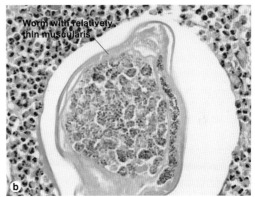

Fig. 19.28 Elephantiasis (courtesy of Brooke Army Medical Center teaching file.)

Onchocerciasis

Onchocerciasis is caused by *Onchocerca volvulus,* an obligate human pathogen spread by *Simulium* blackflies.

Onchocercoma

Key Features

- Well-defined ball of convoluted worms
- Male and female
- Females gravid
- Thin layer of striated muscle
- Corrugated cuticle

An onchocercoma represents a "mating ball" of convoluted worms. The females demonstrate microfilaria within the paired uteri. Because of their thin musculature they have been likened to married adults who no longer go to the gym and have "gone to flab." This is in stark contrast to zoonotic dirofilarial worms that possess a thick muscular layer. In human dirofilarial infestations, a solitary "bachelor" worm is typically identified. Like other bachelors (with little to do besides work out at the gym), the musculature is well developed.

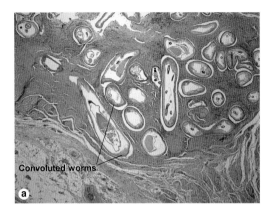

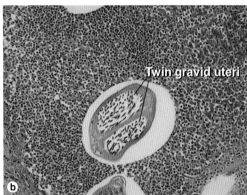

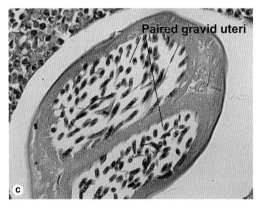

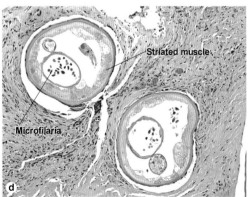

Fig. 19.29 Onchocercoma

Onchocerca *microfilaria*

Key Features

- Large microfilaria in lymphatics and free in the dermis
- Large cephalic and caudal spaces
- Paired oval terminal nuclei

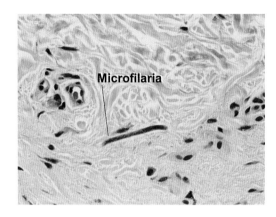

Fig. 19.30 *Onchocerca* microfilaria

Dirofilariasis

Key Features

- Thick muscular layer interrupted by lateral cords
- Internal chitinous ridge

Early lesions may demonstrate abscesses with a mix of neutrophils and eosinophils. Later biopsies show a 1- to 3-cm granulomatous nodule surrounded by dense eosinophilic fibrin. Because humans are accidental hosts, there is only a single adult worm, and reproduction cannot occur. Microfilaria are not seen. Most human cases are associated with *Dirofilaria tenuis*. *Aedes*, *Anopheles*, and *Culex* mosquitoes act as vectors for most *Dirofilaria*. *D. ursi* is transmitted by *Simulium* blackflies.

All *Dirofilaria* demonstrate an internal lateral thickening of the cuticle in the area of the lateral cords. In *D. tenuis*, it appears as a prominent 10-μm pointed ridge. The cuticle is multilayered with criss-cross fibers at right angles. A gut is present, and twin nongravid uteri are noted in females. At the ends of the worm, longitudinal ridges are absent. In this area, the uteri form loops, with four or more seen in cross-section.

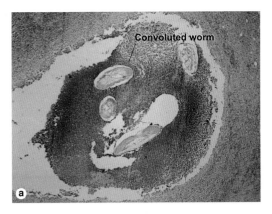

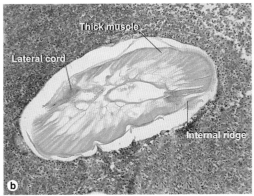

Fig. 19.31 Subcutaneous *Dirofilaria tenuis*

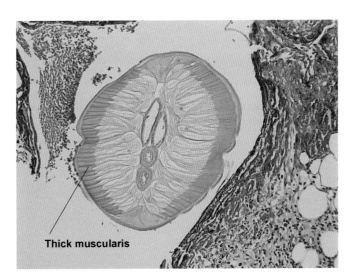

Fig. 19.32 Dirofilaria ursi

Hookworm

- Ridged cuticle
- Characteristic twists gives the organism its name

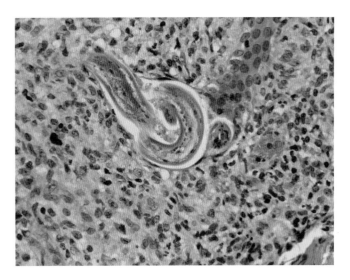

Fig. 19.33 Hookworm

Pinworm

- Enterobiasis (pinworm infestation) typically affects the anus, but perianal and vulvar abscesses may occur
- Bilateral external ridges appear like dark lateral thorns

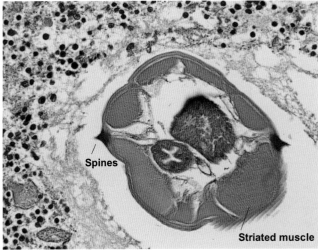

Fig. 19.34 Pinworm

Gnathostomiasis

- Eosinophilia, migratory lesions, and exposure risk
- Cuticle, intestinal cells and characteristic large lateral chords

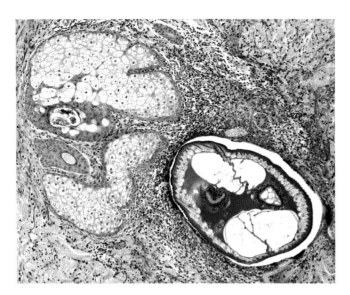

Fig. 19.35 Gnathostomiasis. Movat stain (courtesy of Javier Banquera.)

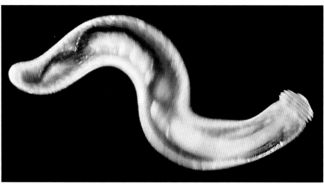

Fig. 19.37 Gnathostomiasis. PTAH stain (courtesy of Javier Banquera.)

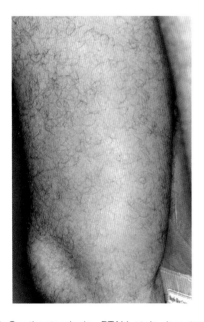

Fig. 19.36 Gnathostomiasis. PTAH stain (courtesy of Javier Banquera.)

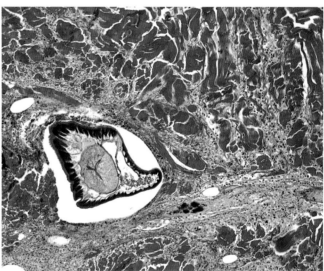

Fig. 19.38 Gnathostomiasis. PTAH stain (courtesy of Javier Banquera.)

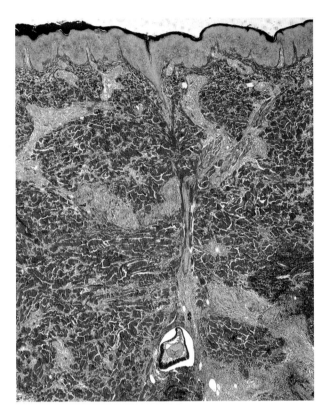

Fig. 19.39 Gnathostomiasis. PTAH stain (courtesy of Javier Banquera.)

Arthropods

Scabies

Key Features

- Mite, ova, or scybala in stratum corneum
- Chitin scrolls and pigtails
- Dermal infiltrate may resemble an insect bite
- Subepidermal bulla with eosinophils occasionally present

The dermal host response to scabies mites often resembles an insect bite reaction. There may be a wedge-shaped perivascular lymphoid infiltrate with eosinophils. The diagnosis rests on demonstration of the mite, eggs, or feces. Oval spaces in the stratum corneum should prompt deeper sections looking for an intact mite. Fragmented mites and ova curl inward, forming scrolls in the stratum corneum. Intact mites have internal striated muscle and dorsal spines. In crusted scabies, many mites are seen within a thick and crusted stratum corneum.

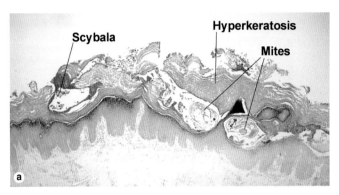

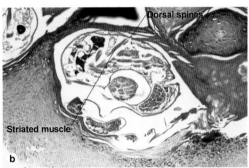

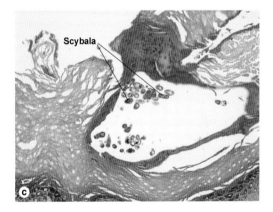

Fig. 19.40 Scabies

PEARL

Scabies can mimic bullous pemphigoid with eosinophil-filled bullae and positive immunofluorescence. In children, scabies can induce a Langerhans cell infiltrate and mimic Langerhans cell histiocytosis. Cases with CD30+ cells can mimic lymphomatoid papulosis.

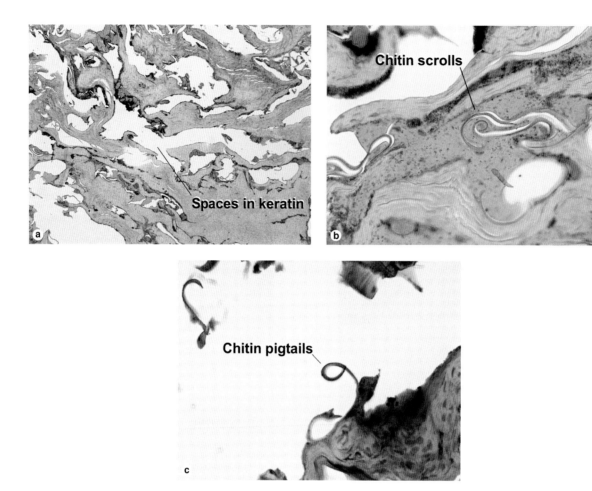

Fig. 19.41 Crusted ("Norwegian") scabies

Bites and stings

Insect bite

Key Features

- Dense, wedge-shaped, perivascular lymphoid infiltrate
- Eosinophils
- Variable vascular damage
- Variable atypical lymphocytes

Insect sting

Key Features

- Findings are highly variable
- Fire ant stings produce an urticarial reaction, followed by a late-phase reaction with fibrin and eosinophils or a neutrophil-filled pustule

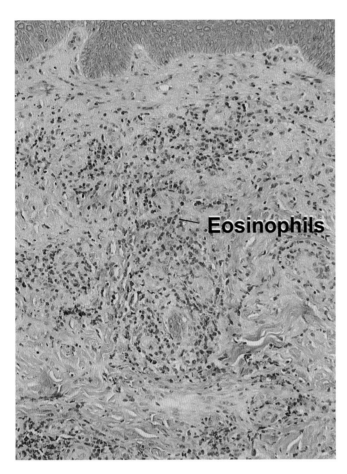

Fig. 19.42 Insect bite

Tick

Key Features

- Pigmented mouthparts embedded in skin
- Neutrophilic inflammation and necrosis of the dermis
- Thick chitinous wall
- Striated muscle
- Blood-filled gut

Tick bite

Key Features

- Wedge-shaped area of necrosis
- Early-stage neutrophilic
- Late-stage polymorphous with variable eosinophils and atypical lymphocytes
- CD30+ cells may be numerous
- Variable vascular damage

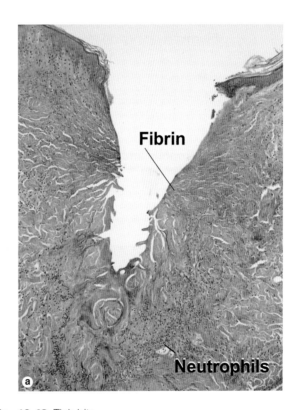

Fig. 19.43 Tick bite

Continued

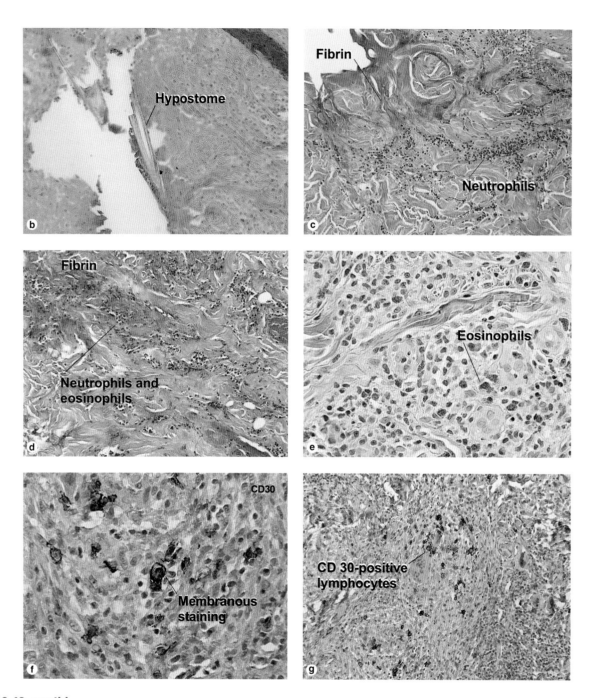

Fig. 19.43, cont'd

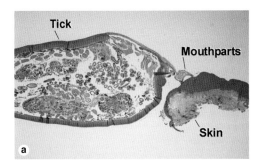

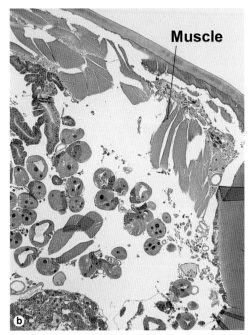

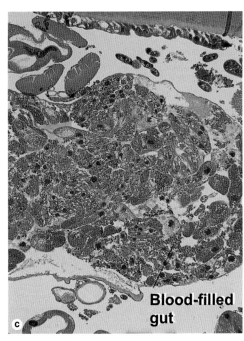

Fig. 19.44 Tick

Spider bite

Key Features

- Findings are highly variable
- Brown recluse bites demonstrate cutaneous necrosis with an underlying neutrophilic band and variable small- and large-vessel vasculitis

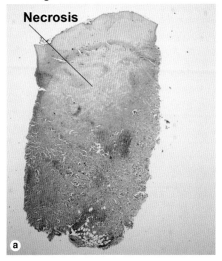

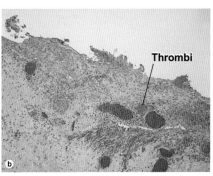

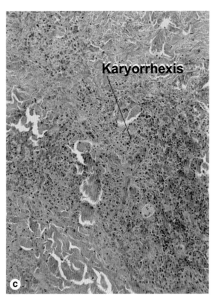

Fig. 19.45 Brown recluse bite

Myiasis

Key Features

- Fly larva with thick, corrugated, chitinous wall
- Pigmented setae
- Striated muscle
- Gut

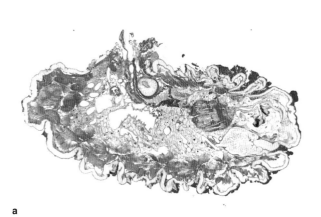

a

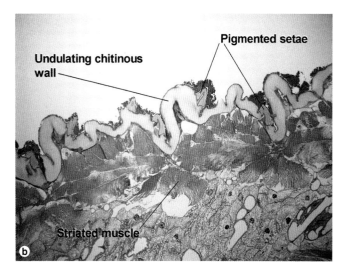

b

Fig. 19.46 Myiasis

Tungiasis

Key Features

- Acral skin
- Embedded organism near surface
- Gravid female flea
- Red, hollow tubules
- Blood in gut
- Striated muscle

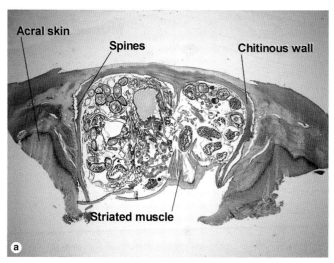

a

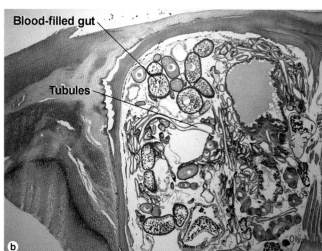

b

Fig. 19.47 Tungiasis

Further reading

Bayer-Garner IB. Monkeypox virus: histologic, immunohistochemical and electron-microscopic findings. J Cutan Pathol 2005;32(1):28–34.

Brar BK, Pall A, Gupta RR. Bullous scabies mimicking bullous pemphigoid. J Dermatol 2003;30(9):694–6.

Burch JM, Krol A, Weston WL. Sarcoptes scabiei infestation misdiagnosed and treated as Langerhans cell histiocytosis. Pediatr Dermatol 2004;21(1):58–62.

Burroughs RF, Elston DM. What's eating you? Human Dirofilaria infections. Cutis 2003;72(4):269–72.

Crowson AN, Saab J, Magro CM. Folliculocentric herpes: a clinicopathological study of 28 patients. Am J Dermatopathol 2017;39(2):89–94.

Elston DM, Eggers JS, Schmidt WE, et al. Histological findings after brown recluse spider envenomation. Am J Dermatopathol 2000;22(3):242–6.

Fagan WA, Collins PC, Pulitzer DR. Verrucous herpes virus infection in human immunodeficiency virus patients. Arch Pathol Lab Med 1996;120(10):956–8.

Mukherjee A, Ahmed NH, Samantaray JC, et al. A rare case of cutaneous larva migrans due to Gnathostoma sp. Indian J Med Microbiol 2012;30(3):356–8.

Nikkels AF, Snoeck R, Rentier B, et al. Chronic verrucous varicella zoster virus skin lesions: clinical, histological, molecular and therapeutic aspects. Clin Exp Dermatol 1999;24(5):346–53.

Santesteban R, Feito M, Mayor A, et al. Trichodysplasia spinulosa in a 20-month-old girl with a good response to topical cidofovir 1. Pediatrics 2015;136(6):e1646–9.

Uthida-Tanaka AM, Sampaio MC, Velho PE, et al. Subcutaneous and cerebral cysticercosis. J Am Acad Dermatol 2004;50:S14.

Yang Y, Ellis MK, McManus DP. Immunogenetics of human echinococcosis. Trends Parasitol 2012;28(10):447–54.

Fibrous tumors

Dirk M. Elston, Christine J. Ko and Tammie Ferringer

 A soft tissue tumor atlas can be found in the online content for this book.

Dermatofibroma

Key Features

- Interstitial spindle cell proliferation
- Collagen trapping
- Overlying platelike acanthosis
- Follicular induction common
- Ringed lipidized siderophages or perivascular collagen donuts may be present
- Factor XIIIa+
- CD34–

All dermatofibromas demonstrate a proliferation of fibrohistiocytic cells. A curlicue pattern is typical. Another typical feature is that some areas of the tumor will be densely cellular, whereas others are sclerotic and hypocellular. The overlying epidermis is acanthotic and often demonstrates primitive follicular germs or sebaceous follicles. At the periphery of the tumor, collagen trapping (collagen balls) can be seen. The tumor may extend into the superficial fat in a lacy pattern.

When present, ringed lipidized siderophages are pathognomonic for dermatofibroma. These cells are like Touton giant cells with hemosiderin. They have central pink cytoplasm surrounded by a wreath of nuclei. There is both lipid and hemosiderin peripheral to the ring of nuclei.

Immunostaining can be helpful to separate cellular dermatofibromas from dermatofibrosarcoma protuberans. Large stellate cells within a dermatofibroma stain for factor XIIIa. The surrounding stroma will stain for CD34, but the central tumor is negative (except for endothelial cells).

Differential Diagnosis

- Densely cellular tumors are suspicious for dermatofibrosarcoma protuberans, even if overlying acanthosis and collagen trapping are present. CD34 and factor XIIIa staining should be performed.
- Long fascicles of parallel nuclei suggest a melanocytic tumor. Nodular lymphoid aggregates suggest desmoplastic malignant melanoma. S100 staining should be performed.
- Corkscrew nuclei running parallel to the epidermis suggest a dermatomyofibroma.

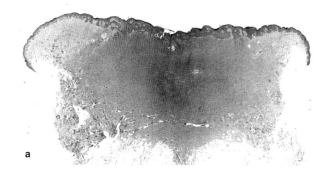

a

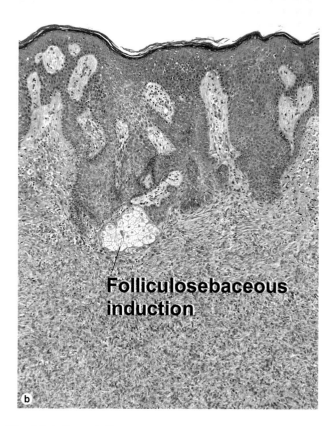

Folliculosebaceous induction

b

Fig. 20.1 Dermatofibroma

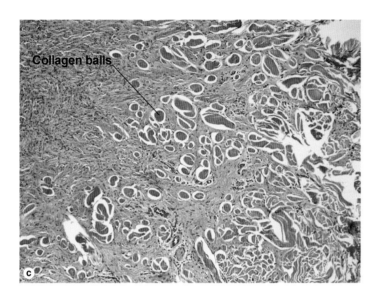

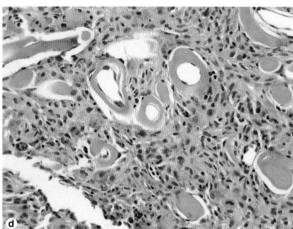

Fig. 20.1, cont'd (C and D) Demonstrate characteristic collagen balls and donuts

Aneurysmal dermatofibroma (sclerosing hemangioma)

Key Features

- Type of dermatofibroma
- Aneurysmal dilatation of vessels

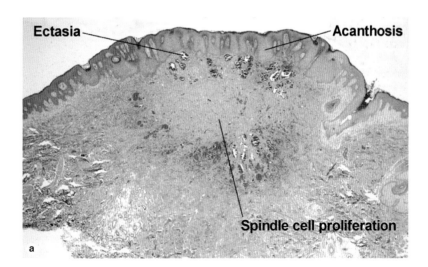

Fig. 20.2 Aneurysmal dermatofibroma

continued

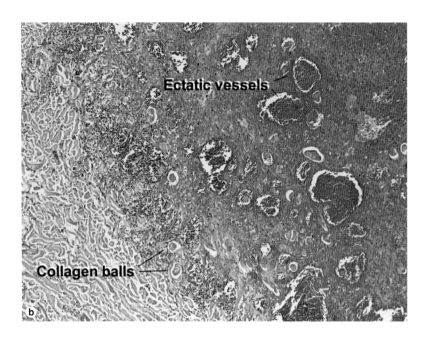

Fig. 20.2, cont'd

Fibrous histiocytoma

Key Features

- Type of dermatofibroma
- Large, histiocytoid, vesicular nuclei with prominent nucleoli

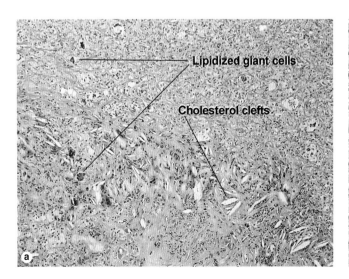

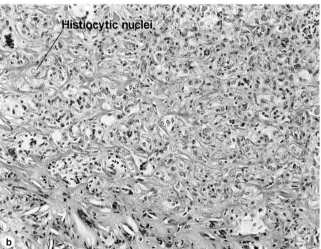

Fig. 20.3 Fibrous histiocytoma

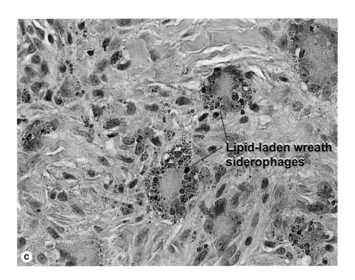

Fig. 20.3, cont'd

Dermatofibroma with monster cells

Key Features

- Very large cells with vesicular nuclei and prominent nucleoli
- Sometimes hyperchromatic
- Despite large alarming cells, these are completely benign lesions

Multinucleate cell angiohistiocytoma

Key Features

- Increased small capillaries and venules in the upper dermis
- Interstitial multinucleated cells
- Slightly thickened collagen bundles

This lesion is of uncertain histogenesis and may be reactive rather than neoplastic. Middle-aged to elderly women are most commonly affected with solitary or multiple grouped red-brown to violaceous asymptomatic papules to plaques on the dorsal hands, thighs, and legs.

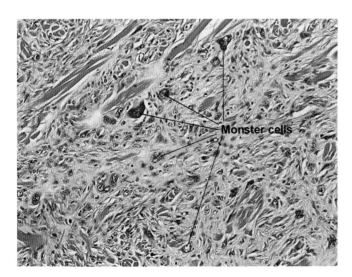

Fig. 20.4 Dermatofibroma with monster cells

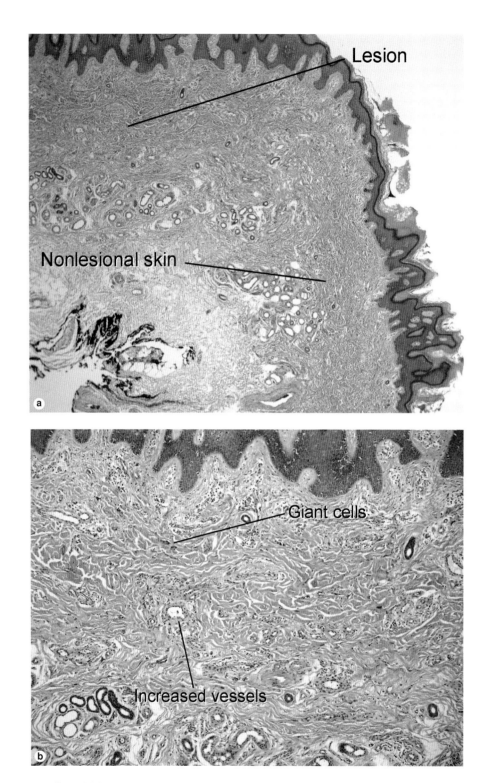

Fig. 20.5 Multinucleate cell angiohistiocytoma

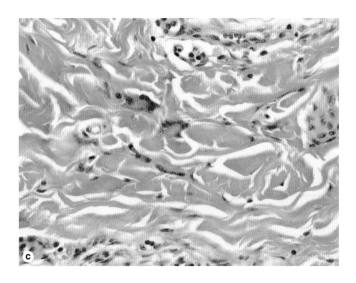

Fig. 20.5, cont'd

Adult myofibroma

Key Features

- Nodules with blue centers
- Myofibroblasts
- Peripheral fibrovascular proliferation

The shade of blue in the center of the nodule resembles that of cartilage. The peripheral vascular proliferation may have staghorn vessels and resemble hemangiopericytoma.

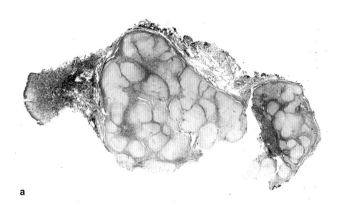

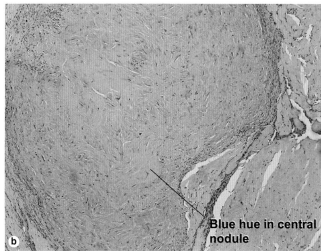

Blue hue in central nodule

Fig. 20.6 (A-C) Adult myofibroma.

Continued

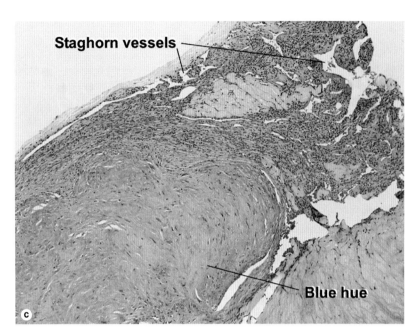

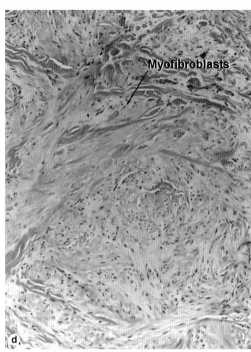

Fig. 20.6, cont'd (D) Juvenile myofibroma lacks the surrounding vascular proliferation

Juvenile myofibroma

Key Features

- Fascicles of corkscrew myofibroblasts
- Lacks blue hypocellular nodules and surrounding vascular proliferation

Dermatomyofibroma

Key Features

- Plaquelike tumor
- Spindle cells with east–west orientation

- Proliferation "respects" (doesn't displace) adnexal structures
- Corkscrew appearance of some myofibroblast nuclei
- Thick elastic fibers visible with Verhoeff–van Gieson stain

At scanning magnification, the most striking features of a dermatomyofibroma are the horizontal orientation of the spindle cell nuclei and the pattern of the proliferation with respect to the adnexal structures, especially hair follicles. The follicles are normal in appearance, and the proliferation extends up to each follicle, then continues on the other side without any displacement of the follicle.

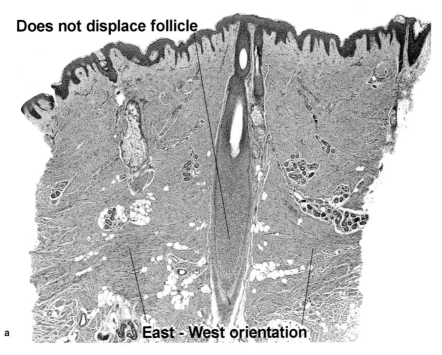

Does not displace follicle

East - West orientation

a

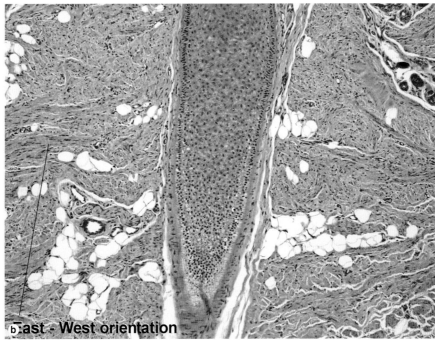

East - West orientation

b

Fig. 20.7 Dermatomyofibroma.

Continued

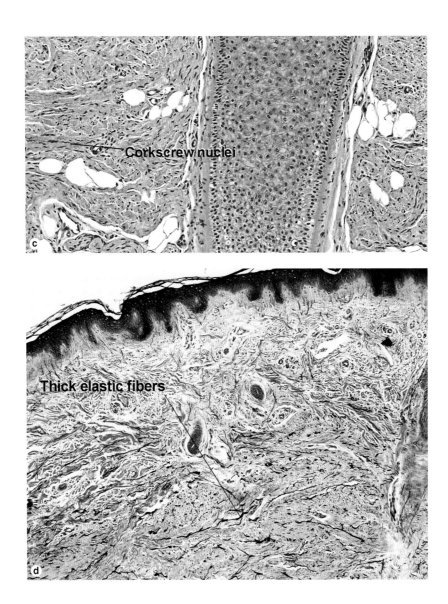

Fig. 20.7, cont'd (D) Verhoeff-Van Gieson elastic stain

Fibromatosis

Key Features

- Myofibroblastic proliferation
- Locally infiltrative, but does not metastasize
- Corkscrew-shaped myofibroblasts

The fibromatoses include Dupuytren (hand) contracture, Peyronie (penis) disease, and Ledderhose (foot) plantar fibromatosis. All forms demonstrate corkscrew-shaped myofibroblasts and collagen. Ledderhose disease tends to form large, whorled nodules.

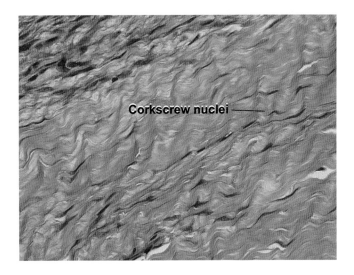

Fig. 20.8 Dupuytren contracture

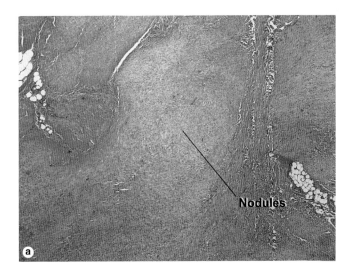

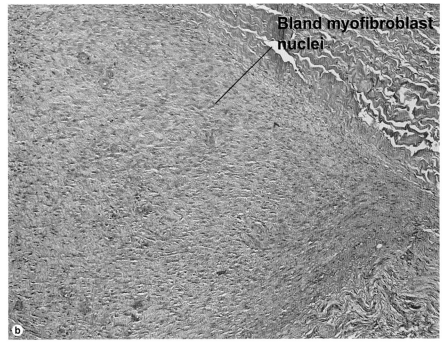

Fig. 20.9 Ledderhose disease

Infantile myofibromatosis

Key Features

- Myofibroblastic proliferation
- Locally infiltrative, but does not metastasize
- Corkscrew-shaped myofibroblasts

There is a tendency toward spontaneous regression. Superficial disease has an excellent prognosis. Visceral involvement may be fatal in some cases. In one series, more than half of the lesions were present at or soon after birth, approximately 80% were solitary, and 50% involved the head and neck. In the early stage, undifferentiated immature histiocytic cells may predominate. As the lesion matures, they develop characteristics of myofibroblasts. Regressing lesions become progressively less cellular and more fibrous.

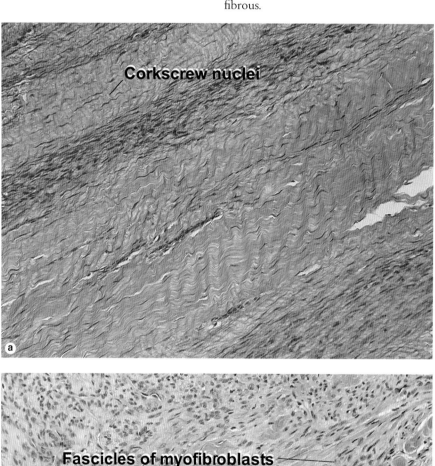

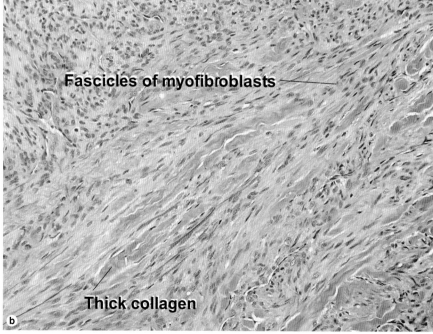

Fig. 20.10 Infantile myofibromatosis

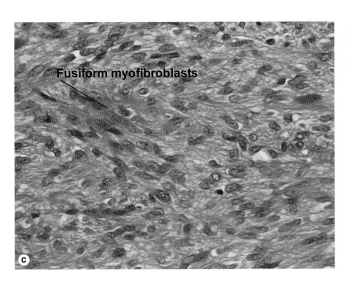

Fig. 20.10, cont'd

Juvenile hyaline fibromatosis

Key Features

- Autosomal recessive
- Nodular skin lesions of the hands, scalp, ears, and central face
- Gingival hypertrophy
- Joint contractures and osteopenia
- Nodular hyaline fibrosis in the dermis
- Linked to *CMG2* or *ANTXR2* mutations (gene encoding capillary morphogenesis protein-2 on chromosome 4q21)

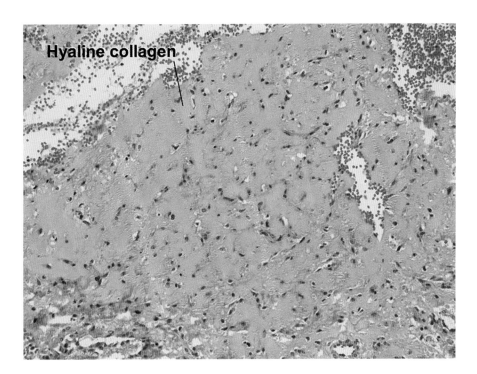

Fig. 20.11 Juvenile hyaline fibromatosis

Scar

Key Features

- Fibroblasts with east–west orientation
- Blood vessels with north–south orientation
- Loss of elastic tissue (see Chapter 13)

Hypertrophic scar

Key Features

- Whorled proliferation of fibroblasts and blood vessels

Keloid

Key Features

- Whorled proliferation of fibroblasts and blood vessels
- Central bundles of amorphous "bubble gum" collagen

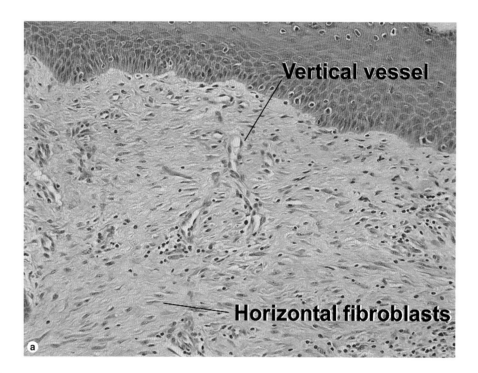

Fig. 20.12 (A) Scar.

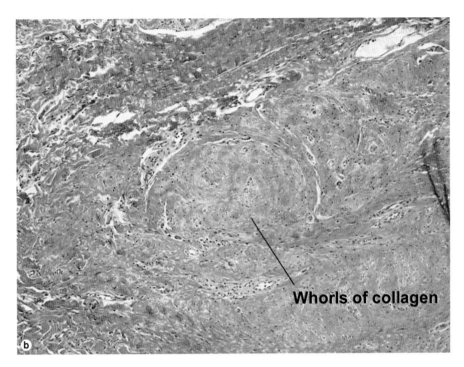

Whorls of collagen

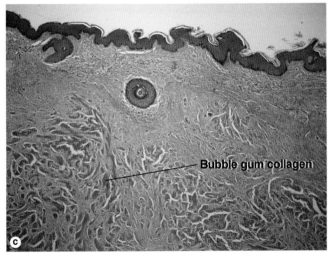

Bubble gum collagen

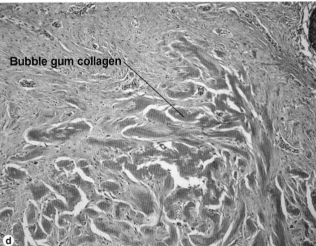

Bubble gum collagen

Fig. 20.12, cont'd **(B)** Hypertrophic scar. **(C and D)** Keloid forming within whorls of hypertrophic scar

Metaplastic synovial cyst

Key Features

- Cystic space lined by villous, synovium-like projections
- Some villous projections are fibrinous

This intradermal nodule usually occurs at the site of previous surgery or other trauma. This is a pseudocyst without true epithelial lining. Often inflamed granulation tissue or scar is present. Multinucleated giant cells and multiple normal mitotic figures may be noted.

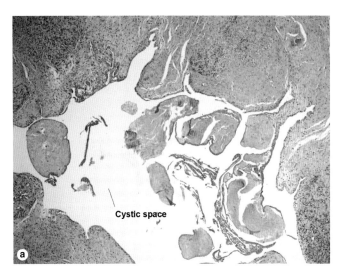

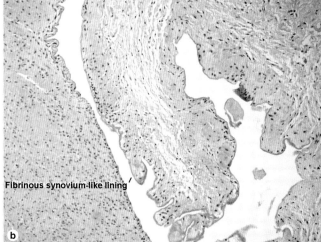

Fig. 20.13 Metaplastic synovial cyst

Fibrous hamartoma of infancy

Key Features

- Disorderly growth of benign tissues
- Myxoid areas, mature fibrous areas, and fat
- Organoid (compartmentalized) appearance
- Surrounding skin has features of "kid" skin

A young child's skin ("kid" skin) is characterized by delicate collagen bundles that stain deeply red. Many fibroblast nuclei are present. Lipocytes and adnexal structures tend to be small.

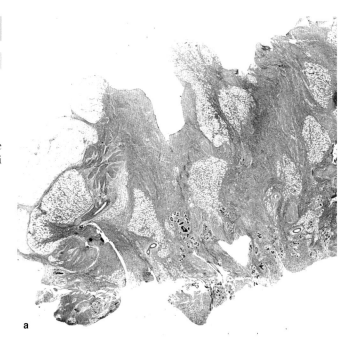

Fig. 20.14 Fibrous hamartoma of infancy

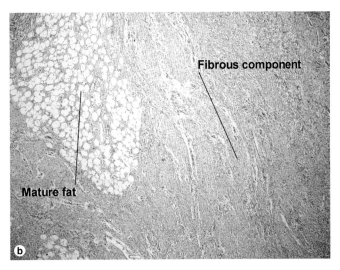

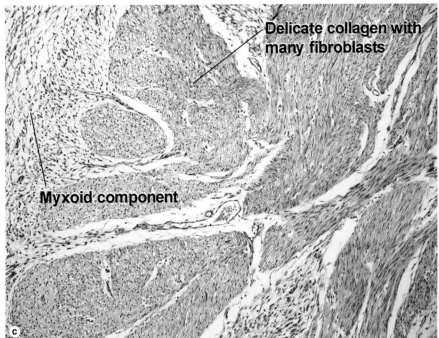

Fig. 20.14, cont'd

Infantile digital fibroma (inclusion body fibroma)

Key Features

- Acral skin
- Criss-cross fascicles
- Spindle cells with red inclusion bodies

Infantile digital fibroma is also called *recurrent infantile digital fibroma* or *aggressive digital fibromatosis*. It is benign, but often extends deeply and has a high recurrence rate after excision. The inclusions stain purple with phosphotungstic acid hematoxylin (PTAH) and red with both hematoxylin and eosin (H&E) and Masson's trichrome. They are actin positive.

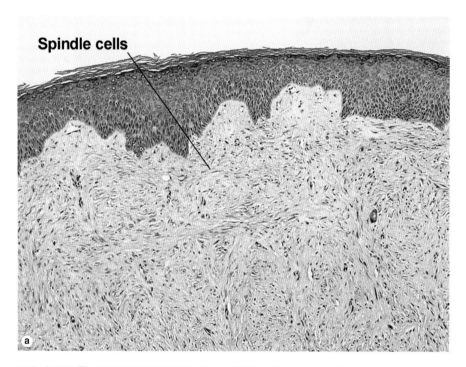

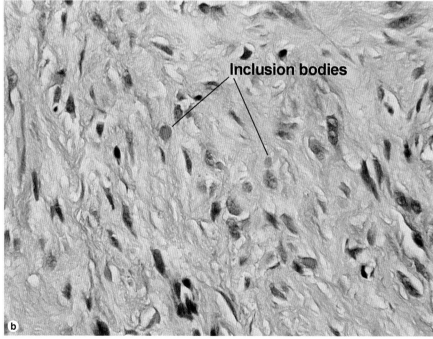

Fig. 20.15 Infantile digital fibroma

Giant cell tumor of the tendon sheath

Key Features

- Osteoclast-like giant cells
- Plump fibroblasts
- Focal, dense collagen
- Hemosiderin pigment common

Osteoclast-like giant cells have randomly distributed nuclei. The cytoplasm stains deeply pink to amphophilic and has scalloped edges where the cell exhibits molding against adjoining tissue.

Fibroma of tendon sheath

Key Features

- Giant cell tumor of tendon sheath without the giant cells
- Characteristic plump fibroblasts often present

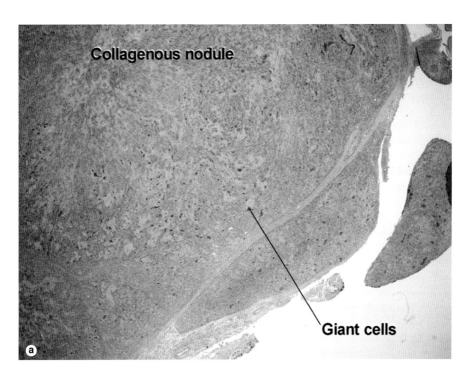

Fig. 20.16 Giant cell tumor of tendon sheath

continued

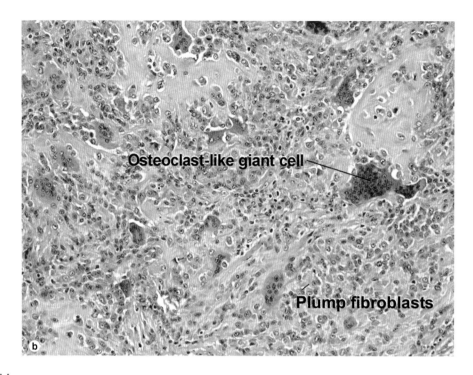

Fig. 20.16, cont'd

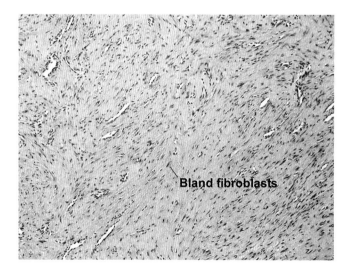

Fig. 20.17 Fibroma of tendon sheath

Giant cell tumor of the soft tissue

Key Features

- Well-circumscribed, multinodular soft tissue tumor
- Mononuclear and osteoclastic giant cells
- Peripheral rim of metaplastic bone in half of cases
- Hemorrhagic cystic spaces

These lesions, seen most on the limbs of adults, are the soft tissue counterpart of giant cell tumor of bone. They are also known as *giant cell tumor of low malignant potential*. Mitoses can be common but are typical figures. The mononuclear and osteoclastic giant cells are CD68 positive.

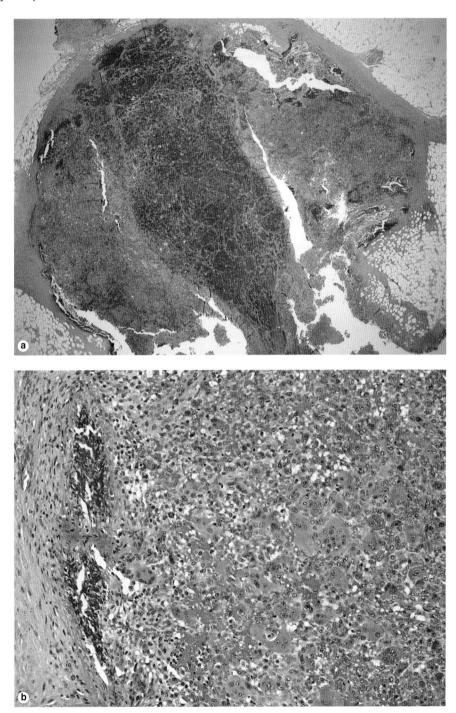

Fig. 20.18 Giant cell tumor of soft tissue

Elastofibroma dorsi

Key Features

- Large fibrous tumor
- Elastin deposits throughout tumor
- Beaded elastic fibers

As the name implies, elastofibroma dorsi is typically found on the back.

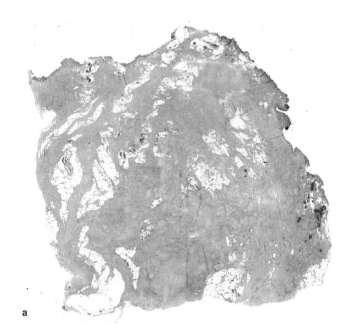

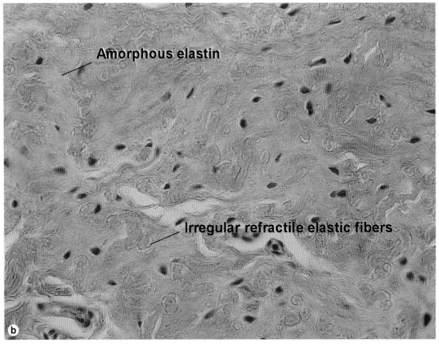

Fig. 20.19 Elastofibroma dorsi.

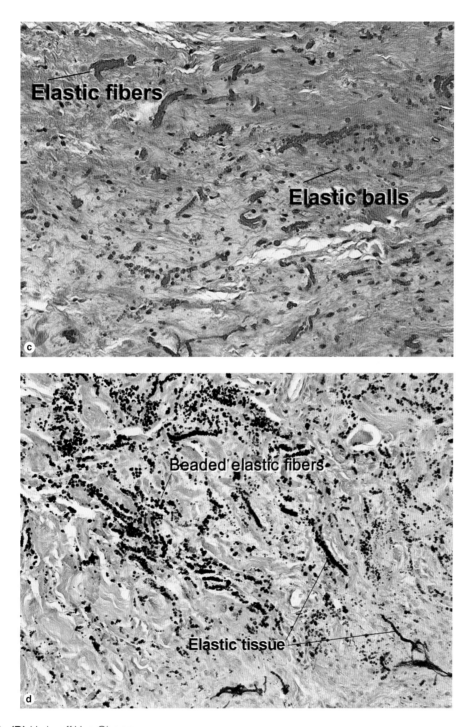

Fig. 20.19, cont'd **(D)** Verhoeff-Van Gieson

Sclerotic fibroma

Key Features

- Collagen pattern resembles van Gogh's *Starry Night*
- Hypocellular
- May be a marker for Cowden syndrome

Because of the association with Cowden syndrome, sclerotic fibromas should be considered a distinct entity. Similar hypocellular areas have been seen in other fibrous tumors, especially dermatofibromas.

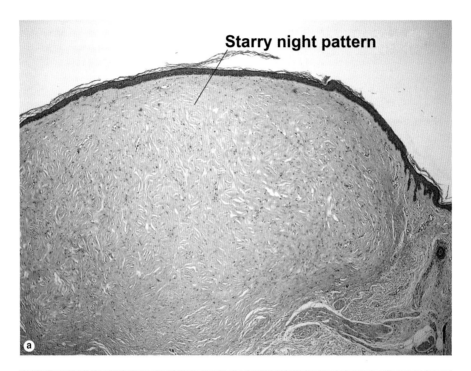

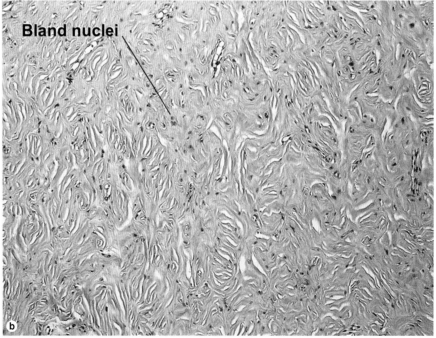

Fig. 20.20 Sclerotic fibroma

Pleomorphic fibroma

Key Features

- Scattered, large, hyperchromatic stellate nuclei
- Never hypercellular
- No mitoses

Despite the large hyperchromatic nuclei, pleomorphic fibromas are benign. They are peppered with hyperchromatic stellate nuclei that resemble the stellate nuclei in fibrous papules. Although the stellate cells resemble those of a fibrous papule, they are usually CD34 positive. Multinucleated cells may be present, but mitoses are absent. Tumors with overlapping features of sclerotic and pleomorphic fibroma have been described.

Collagenous fibroma (desmoplastic fibroblastoma)

Key Features

- Collagenous stroma with a blue hue
- Paucicellular with scattered spindled or stellate fibroblasts

These tumors most commonly involve the subcutis of adults in a variety of sites, including arms, legs, back, hands, and feet. Typically, they are well demarcated but can focally infiltrate surrounding tissue and vessels are inconspicuous, differentiating desmoplastic fibroblastoma from the more cellular fibromatosis. Mitoses are not a component. S100, CD34, and desmin are negative. Clonal abnormalities involving 11q12 have been reported.

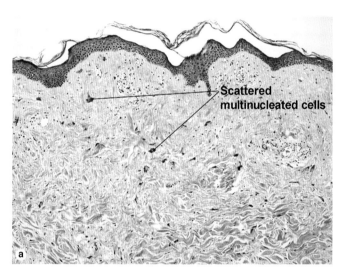

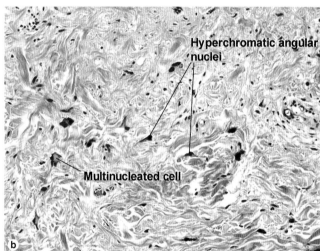

Fig. 20.21 Pleomorphic fibroma

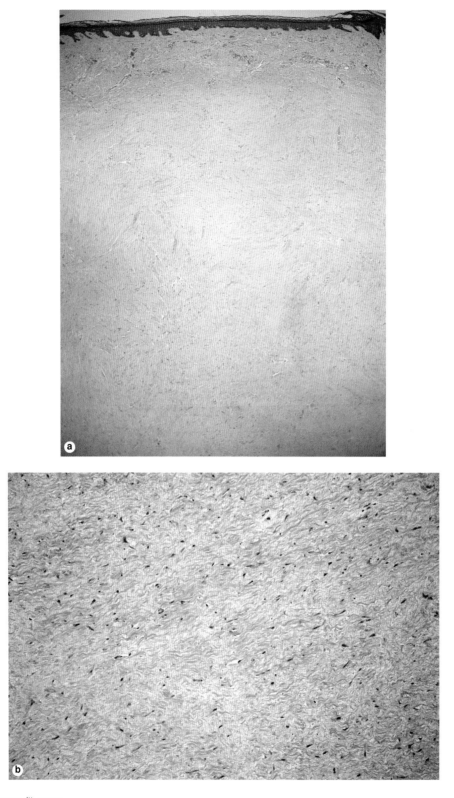

Fig. 20.22 Collagenous fibroma

Nuchal-type fibroma (collagenosis nuchae)

Key Features

- Poorly circumscribed tumor composed of thick collagen bundles with few fibroblasts

Nuchal fibromas tend to occur as diffuse induration and swelling of the posterior neck in young to middle-aged men, but can occur at other locations where they are referred to as *nuchal-type fibroma*. There is an association with scleredema and diabetes. Histologically, the lesions are indistinguishable from the fibromas in Gardner syndrome. Desmoid fibromatosis can be confused with nuchal fibroma, but desmoids are typically more cellular and prominently infiltrate the surrounding tissue.

Angiofibromas

Key Features

- Concentric perivascular fibrosis
- Stellate, factor XIIIa+ stromal cells

In tuberous sclerosis, we call them *adenoma sebaceum* or *Koenen periungual fibromas*. Multiple angiofibromas may also be seen in multiple endocrine neoplasia type I (MEN 1) and in type II neurofibromatosis.

On the face, we refer to the most common variant of solitary angiofibroma as *fibrous papule of the face*. On the penis, we call them *pearly penile papules*. Acquired digital fibrokeratoma is a closely related lesion.

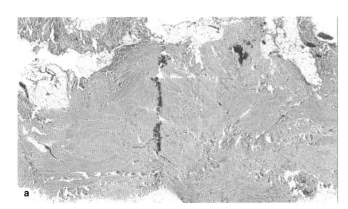

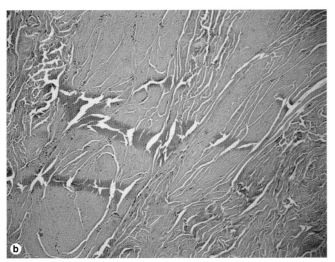

Fig. 20.23 Nuchal-type fibroma

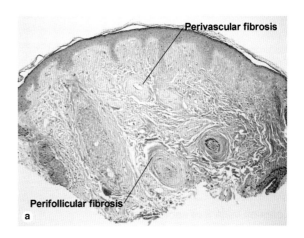

Fig. 20.24 Angiofibroma

Continued

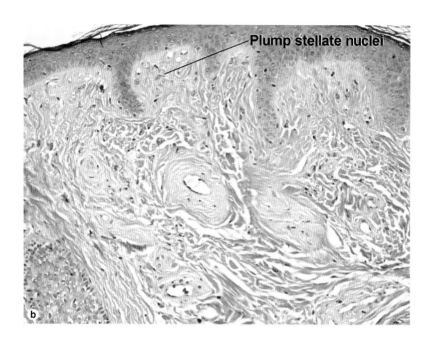

Fig. 20.24, cont'd

Fibrous papule of the face (benign fibrous papule, solitary angiofibroma)

A superficial shave biopsy of a fibrous papule may suggest a melanocytic lesion because of the large melanocytes at the dermal–epidermal junction. Before the advent of immunostains, the stellate dermal cells were thought to be degenerated melanocytes.

Key Features

- Common variant of angiofibroma
- Concentric perivascular fibrosis
- Stellate, factor XIIIa+ stromal cells
- Large pyramid-shaped melanocytes may be present at the dermal–epidermal junction

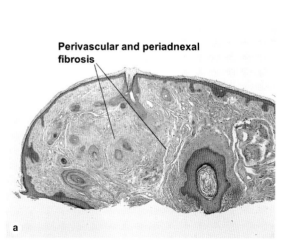
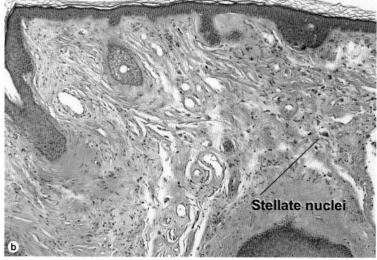

Fig. 20.25 Fibrous papule of the face

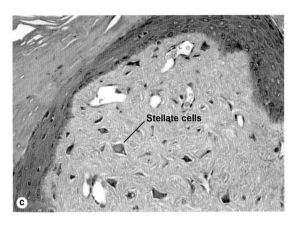

Fig. 20.25, cont'd

Acquired digital fibrokeratoma

Key Features

- Acral skin
- Hyperkeratosis, acanthosis, hypergranulosis
- Spindle cells and collagen often perpendicular to the surrounding skin surface
- Stellate, factor XIIIa+ stromal cells may be present

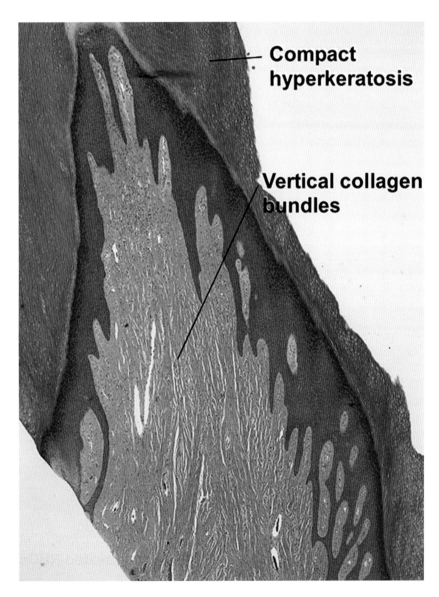

Fig. 20.26 Acquired digital fibrokeratoma

Nodular fasciitis

Key Features

- "Tissue culture" fibroblasts
- Erythrocyte extravasation
- Loose myxoid pattern
- Foci of inflammatory cells

With time, nodular fasciitis develops thick, red collagen bundles, but young lesions appear loose and myxoid, with erythrocyte extravasation and nodular aggregates of inflammatory cells. The stellate fibroblasts look like those in tissue culture.

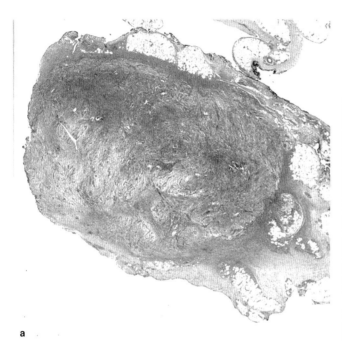

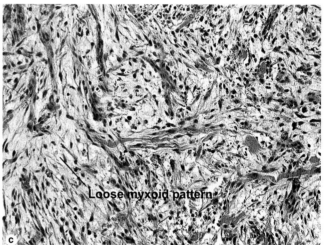

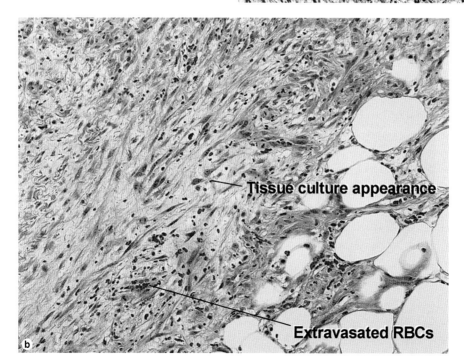

Fig. 20.27 Nodular fasciitis

Cranial fasciitis

Key Features

- Variant of nodular fasciitis that occurs on the head of a child

Proliferative fasciitis

Key Features

- Variant of nodular fasciitis
- Ganglion-like giant cells
- Collagen trapping at periphery

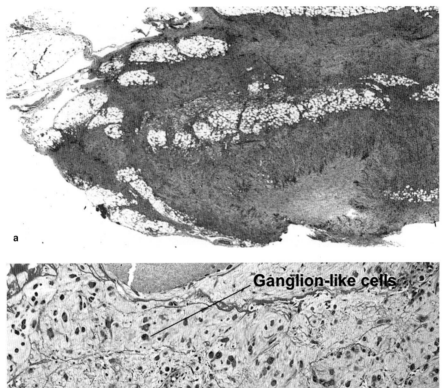

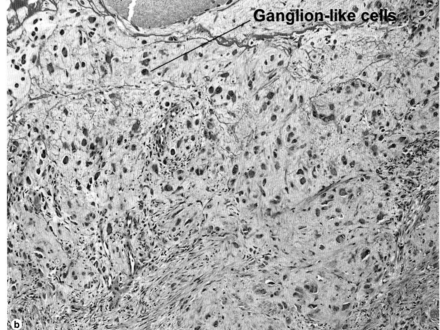

Fig. 20.28 Proliferative fasciitis

Intravascular fasciitis

Key Features

- Variant of nodular fasciitis that involves the lumen and wall of a peripheral vessel, usually a vein
- Clefts focally separate the proliferation from the vessel wall

Intravascular fasciitis typical presents as a small, sometimes elongate, mass on the upper extremity or head and neck of young adults. Although sometimes confused with vascular invasion of a malignancy, these lesions are benign and rarely recur. The histology is similar to nodular fasciitis consisting of fascicles of fibroblasts in a myxoid stroma with typical mitotic figures and red blood cell extravasation. There may be a greater number of multinucleate giant cells and less prominent mucoid matrix.

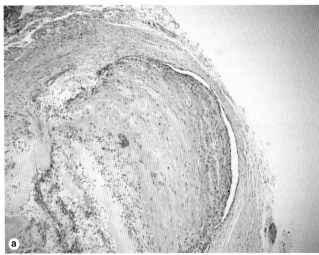

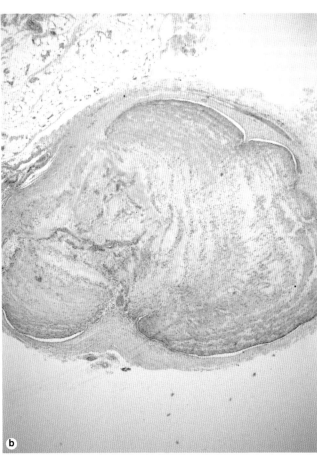

Fig. 20.29 Intravascular fasciitis

Ischemic fasciitis (atypical decubital fibroplasia)

Key Features

- Fibrinoid necrosis centrally surrounded by reactive, atypical-appearing, stellate or ganglion-like fibroblasts in a fibrotic to myxoid stroma
- Surrounded by a vascular proliferation (granulation tissue) in a zonal pattern
- Mitoses are frequent but not atypical, and there is no hypercellularity
- Thrombi may be present

Ischemic fasciitis presents as a subcutaneous mass, typically without overlying ulceration, in an elderly and/or immobilized person. It overlies a bony prominence, such as the hip or shoulder.

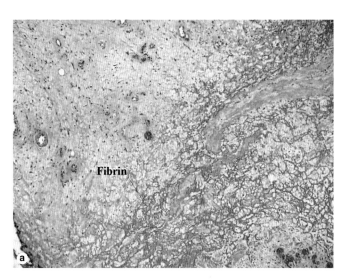

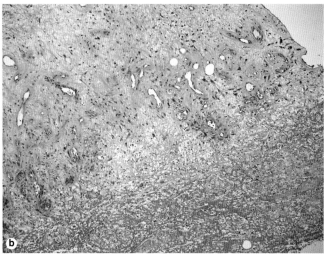

Fig. 20.30 Ischemic fasciitis

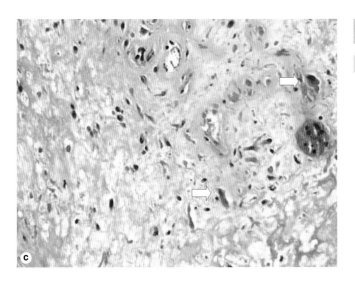

Fig. 20.30, cont'd Large stellate hyperchromatic nuclei

Key Features

- Plump, epithelioid fibroblasts palisading around chondroid foci with or without calcification, occasionally with osteoclast-like cells
- Distal extremities
- Commonly found in children and adolescents

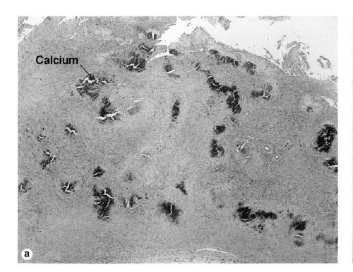

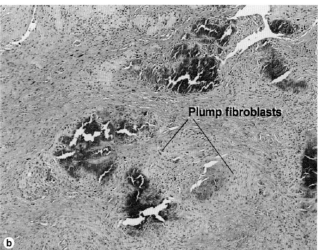

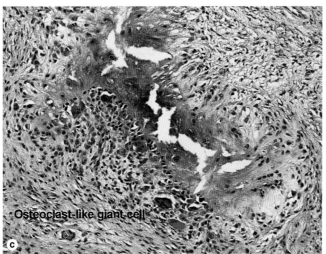

Fig. 20.31 Calcifying aponeurotic fibroma

Ossifying fibromyxoid tumor of soft parts

Key Features

- Well circumscribed and lobular
- Cords or nests of small, round to polygonal cells embedded in fibromyxoid matrix
- Often an incomplete shell of mature bone

This lesion usually presents as a subcutaneous mass involving the extremity of a middle-aged adult. Widespread immunoreactivity for S100 protein is noted. Malignant cases are distinguished by high nuclear grade, high cellularity, and mitotic rate of more than two mitoses in 50 high-powered fields (HPFs).

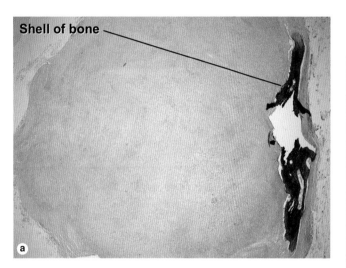

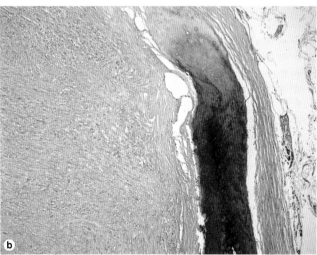

Fig. 20.32 Ossifying fibromyxoid tumor of soft parts

Borderline tumors

Desmoid tumor (aggressive fibromatosis)

Key Features

- Slender, elongated, bland, spindled myofibroblasts separated by collagen in long fascicles
- Bland nuclei
- Tendency for deep infiltration and recurrence
- Beta catenin expressed
- Most are sporadic but can be associated with Gardner syndrome

Extraabdominal desmoids originate from the fascia and connective tissue surrounding muscles, especially in the shoulder/pelvic girdle/thighs. Adolescents and young adults are most commonly affected.

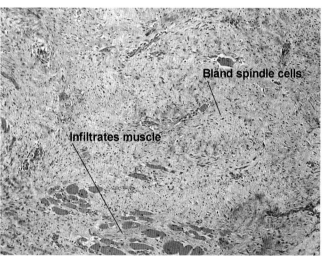

Fig. 20.33 Desmoid tumor

Plexiform fibrohistiocytic tumor

Key Features

- Plexiform fascicles of myofibroblast-like fusiform and spindle cells
- Nodules of histiocytic cells and osteoclast-like giant cells (biphasic tumor)
- Variable pleomorphism and mitotic rate

Plexiform fibrohistiocytic tumor is a tumor of intermediate malignant behavior that occurs in children and young adults. It commonly involves an arm.

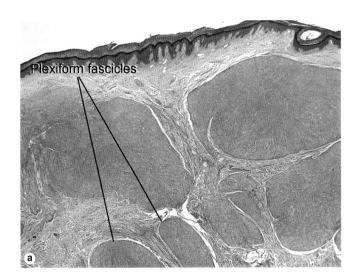

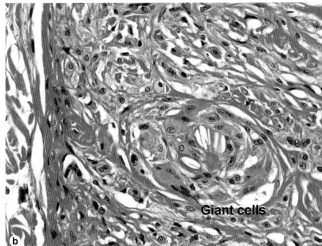

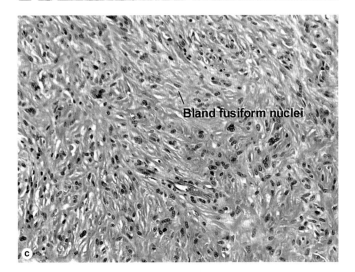

Fig. 20.34 Plexiform fibrohistiocytic tumor

Solitary fibrous tumor

Key Features

- Well-circumscribed tumor
- Patternless pattern of fascicles
- Hemangiopericytoma-like branching vascular network
- CD34+

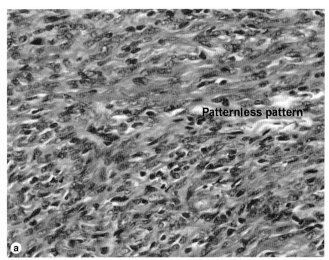

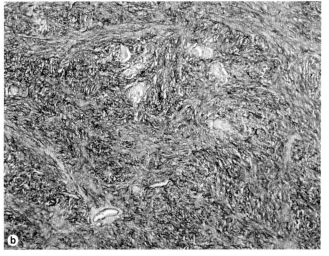

Fig. 20.35 Solitary fibrous tumor. **(B)** CD34

Malignant tumors

Dermatofibrosarcoma protuberans (DFSP)

Key Features

- Densely hypercellular
- Storiform (woven) pattern
- Infiltrates fat in a honeycomb pattern
- Forms fibrous layers in the fat, parallel to the surface epidermis
- Epidermal rete pattern usually effaced
- CD34+, factor XIIIa–

Dermatofibrosarcoma protuberans infiltrates the fat in a honeycomb pattern. As the tumor progresses, parallel layers of tumor form in the fat, like a layer cake with lipocytes (frosting) in between the layers. The nuclei appear as dark spindle cells when cut across, and as pale-gray oval nuclei when cut en face. Chromosomal translocations, especially t(17;22), are usually present. A pigmented dermatofibrosarcoma protuberans is referred to as a *Bednar tumor.*

PEARL

Occasionally, overlying acanthosis and collagen trapping may be present in a dermatofibrosarcoma protuberans. If the tumor is densely hypercellular and infiltrates fat, CD34 staining should be performed.

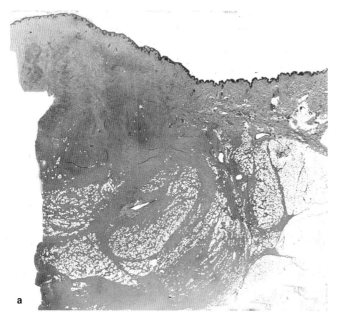

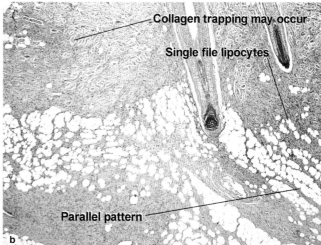

Fig. 20.36 Dermatofibrosarcoma protuberans

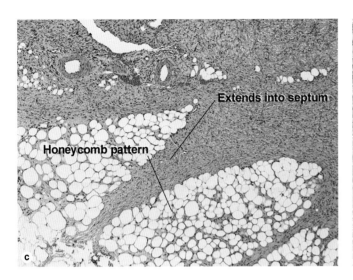

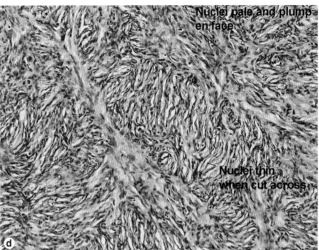

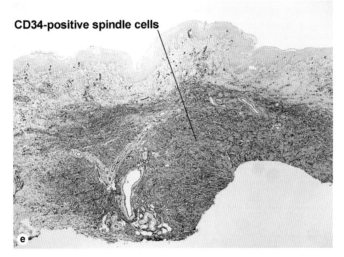

Fig. 20.36, cont'd

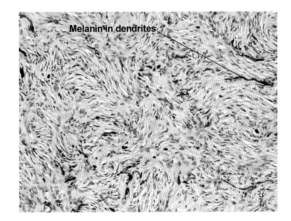

Fig. 20.37 Bednar tumor

Giant cell fibroblastoma

Key Features

- Juvenile variant of dermatofibrosarcoma protuberans
- Multinucleated giant cells lining vascular-like spaces

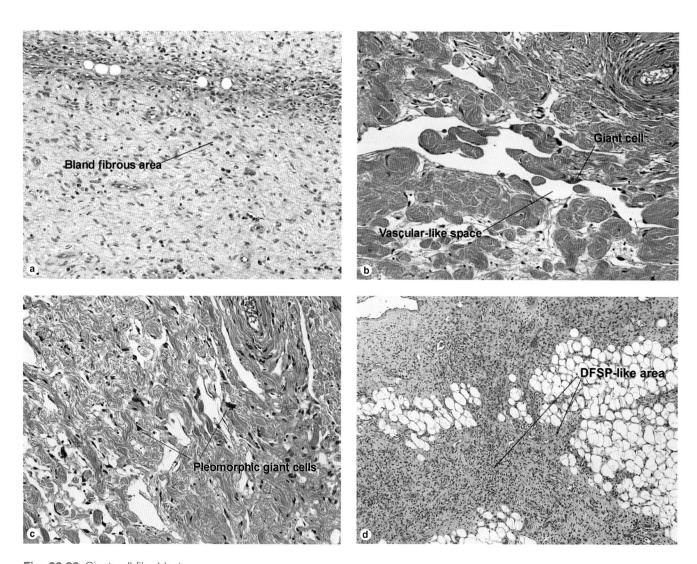

Fig. 20.38 Giant cell fibroblastoma

Fibrosarcoma

Key Features

- Densely hypercellular
- Herringbone or fir-tree pattern common
- Variable mitotic rate
- Nuclei may be large and hyperchromatic

Many fibrosarcomas tend to have a herringbone or fir-tree pattern. Dermatofibrosarcoma protuberans is a type of fibrosarcoma with a characteristic storiform and honeycomb pattern. In contrast, dermatofibromas and hemangiopericytomas have a curlicue pattern.

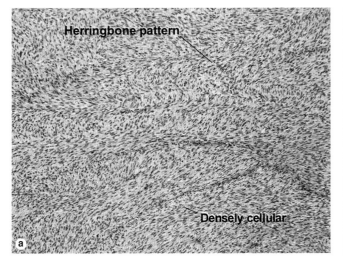

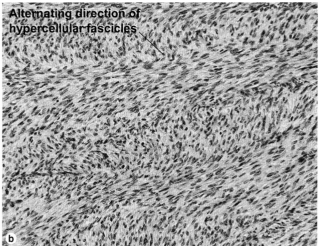

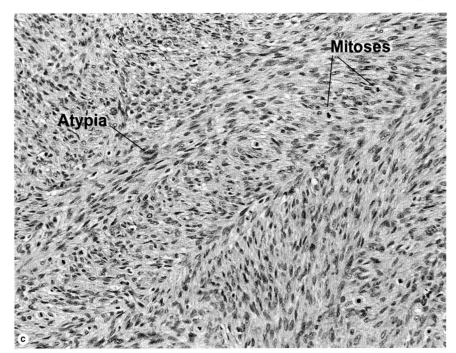

Fig. 20.39 Fibrosarcoma

Atypical fibroxanthoma (AFX)

Key Features

- CD10+, S100A6+, and procollagen+ but none of these stains is specific; it remains a diagnosis of exclusion
- Atypical pleomorphic or spindle cells

Some consider atypical fibroxanthoma to be a superficial variant of pleomorphic undifferentiated sarcoma.

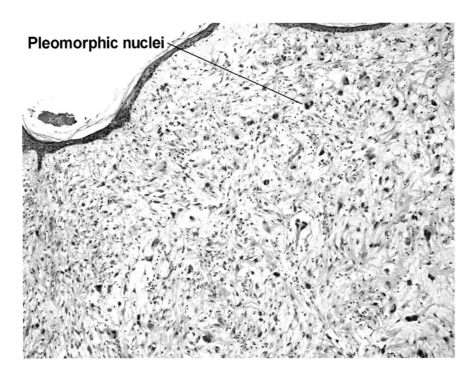

Fig. 20.40 Pleomorphic atypical fibroxanthoma (AFX)

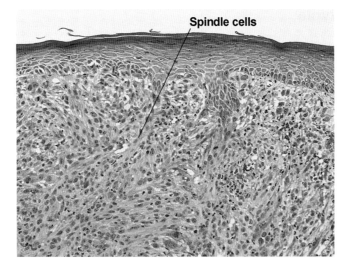

Fig. 20.41 Spindled atypical fibroxanthoma (AFX)

Pleomorphic undifferentiated sarcoma

Key Features

- Heterogeneous group of soft tissue sarcomas
- Pleomorphic, myxoid, inflammatory, and other variants

Newer classifications no longer include malignant fibrous histio-cytoma (MFH) as a distinct diagnosis, but rather as subtypes of pleomorphic undifferentiated sarcoma. Superficial dermal tumors, formerly called *superficial MFH*, mostly fall into the category of myxofibrosarcoma.

Epithelioid sarcoma

Key Features

- Mimics a palisaded granuloma
- Biphasic (transition between epithelioid and spindle cells)
- Central necrosis
- Stains for both keratin and vimentin

Epithelioid sarcomas tend to occur on the extremity in young people and may be misdiagnosed as pseudorheumatoid nodule, leading to a delay in treatment.

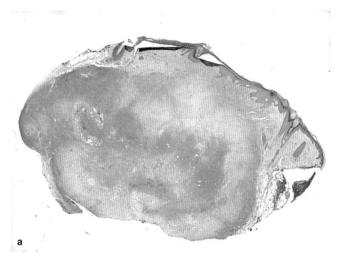

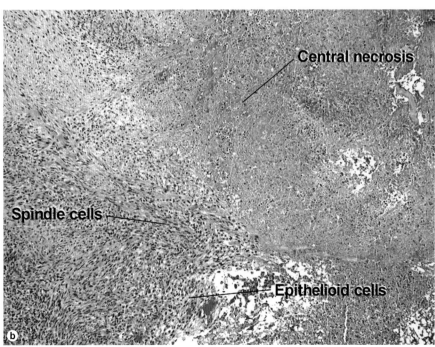

Fig. 20.42 Epithelioid sarcoma

continued

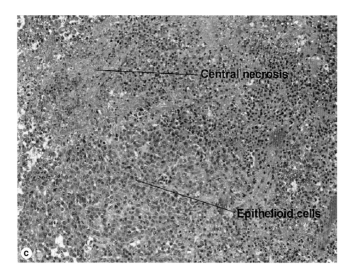

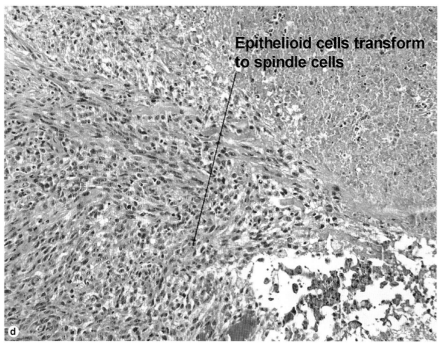

Fig. 20.42, cont'd

Synovial sarcoma

Key Features

- Can be biphasic tumor (mixed epithelial and spindle cells)
- Usually found in deep soft tissues
- Cytokeratin and epithelial membrane antigen positive
- t(X;18)(p11;q11)

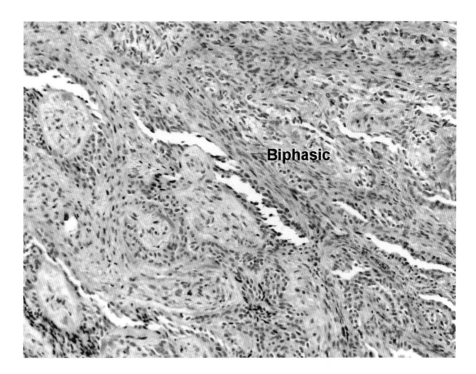

Fig. 20.43 Synovial sarcoma

Low-grade fibromyxoid sarcoma (LGFMS)

Key Features

- Abrupt transition from collagenous to myxoid areas
- Whorled or fascicular spindle cells
- Deceptively bland spindle cells and low mitotic rate
- Prominent vascularity with perivascular hypercellularity, especially in myxoid areas

LGFMS usually are deep-seated tumors of adults in their 30s and 40s that present on the proximal extremity or trunk. Hyalinizing spindle cell tumor with giant rosettes is a morphologic variant, where collagenous acellular central areas are cuffed by plump tumor cells. The majority of LGFMS are associated with t(7;16), fusing FUS and CREB3L2.

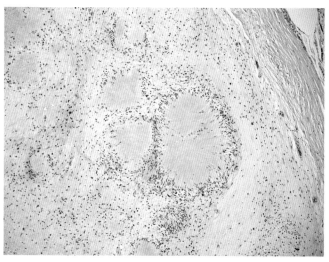

Fig. 20.45 Hyalinizing spindle cell tumor with giant rosettes

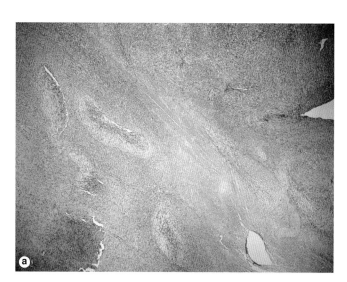

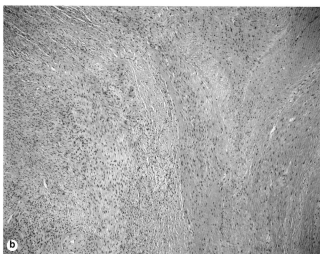

Fig. 20.44 Low-grade fibromyxoid sarcoma

Further reading

Argenta AE, Chen W, Davis A, et al. A review of eight unusual pediatric skin and soft-tissue lesions: diagnosis, workup, and treatment. J Plast Reconstr Aesthet Surg 2015;68(12):1637–46.

Billings SD, Folpe AL. Cutaneous and subcutaneous fibrohistiocytic tumors of intermediate malignancy: an update. Am J Dermatopathol 2004;26(2):141–55.

Clarke LE. Fibrous and fibrohistiocytic neoplasms: an update. Dermatol Clin 2012;30(4):643–56.

Costigan DC, Doyle LA. Advances in the clinicopathological and molecular classification of cutaneous mesenchymal neoplasms. Histopathology 2016;68(6):776–95.

Evans HL. Low-grade fibromyxoid sarcoma: a clinicopathologic study of 33 cases with long-term follow-up. Am J Surg Pathol 2011;35(10):1450–62.

Iijima S, Suzuki R, Otsuka F. Solitary form of infantile myofibromatosis: a histologic, immunohistochemical, and electron microscopic study of a regressing tumor over a 20-month period. Am J Dermatopathol 1999;21(4):375–80.

Koch M, Freundl AJ, Agaimy A, et al. Atypical fibroxanthoma - histological diagnosis, immunohistochemical markers and concepts of therapy. Anticancer Res 2015;35(11):5717–35.

Martín-López R, Feal-Cortizas C, Fraga J. Pleomorphic sclerotic fibroma. Dermatology 1999;198(1):69–72.

Parish LC, Yazdanian S, Lambert WC, et al. Dermatofibroma: a curious tumor. Skinmed 2012;10(5):268–70.

Stanford D, Rogers M. Dermatological presentations of infantile myofibromatosis: a review of 27 cases. Australas J Dermatol 2000;41(3):156–61.

Tani M, Komura A, Ichihashi M. Dermatomyofibroma (plaqueformige dermale fibromatose). J Dermatol 1997;24(12):793–7.

Terrier-Lacombe MJ, Guillou L, Maire G, et al. Dermatofibrosarcoma protuberans, giant cell fibroblastoma, and hybrid lesions in children: clinicopathologic comparative analysis of 28 cases with molecular data – a study from the French Federation of Cancer Centers Sarcoma Group. Am J Surg Pathol 2003;27(1):27–39.

Tumors of fat, muscle, cartilage, and bone

Tammie Ferringer

Fat

Lipoma

Key Features

- Well-circumscribed tumor with a thin capsule
- Mature lipocytes
- Inconspicuous septae

Lipomas typically present as asymptomatic, mobile, soft nodules in the deep soft tissue or subcutis. Histologically, they are thinly encapsulated tumors composed of sheets of mature adipocytes that are indistinguishable from the fat cells in the subcutaneous tissue. Each adipocyte has a single vacuole and an eccentric nucleus. The thin fibrous septa, which contain sparse blood vessels, are delicate and inconspicuous. Intramuscular lipomas, commonly of the forehead, consist of mature fat cells that displace muscle, splaying the fibers.

There are several rare syndromes in which multiple lipomas occur. Hundreds of slow-growing subcutaneous and deep or visceral lipomas develop in early adulthood in the autosomal-dominant condition familial multiple lipomatosis. Benign symmetric lipomatosis (Madelung disease) has a predilection for middle-aged men with a propensity to develop multiple lesions, especially in the region of the neck in a "horse-collar" distribution. Tender, circumscribed or diffuse fatty deposits of the lower legs, abdomen, and buttocks in obese patients exemplify adiposis dolorosa (Dercum disease), sometimes

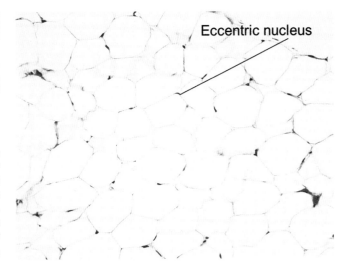

Fig. 21.2 Lipoma

associated with weakness and mental disturbances. Lipomas may also be a component of Gardner syndrome, Bannayan–Zonana syndrome, Cowden syndrome, and Proteus syndrome.

Angiolipoma

Key Features

- Lipoma with proliferation of capillary-sized blood vessels
- Erythrocytes and scattered fibrin microthrombi are commonly present in the lumens

Clinically, angiolipoma are often tender to palpation. They commonly occur in women, are multifocal, and have a predilection for the forearm.

Differential Diagnosis

The differential diagnosis of painful tumors can be remembered by the mnemonic "BANGLE":

- *B*lue rubber bleb nevus
- *A*ngiolipoma
- *N*euroma
- *G*lomus tumor
- *L*eiomyoma
- *E*ccrine spiradenoma

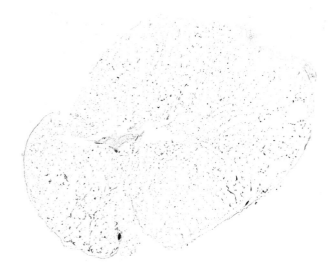

Fig. 21.1 Lipoma

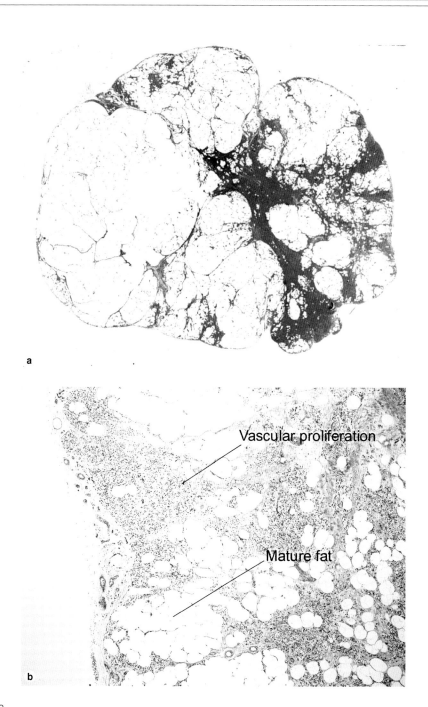

Fig. 21.3 Angiolipoma

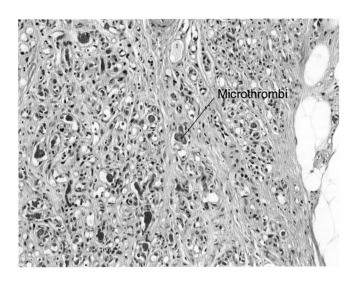

Fig. 21.4 Angiolipoma

Spindle cell lipoma

Key Features

- Well-circumscribed tumor of mature fat with interspersed zones of bland spindle cells and variable amounts of collagen
- In young lesions, the spindle cell areas are myxoid, with many mast cells
- No lipoblasts or mitotic figures
- CD34+ spindle cells
- Ropey collagen bundles

The most common presentation is a solitary lesion at the base of the neck, shoulder, or upper back in an older man. These lesions are generally firmer and more fixed to surrounding tissue than the usual lipoma.

Differential Diagnosis

When spindle cell and myxoid components predominate, there may be confusion with neural or fibroblastic proliferations, especially diffuse neurofibroma.

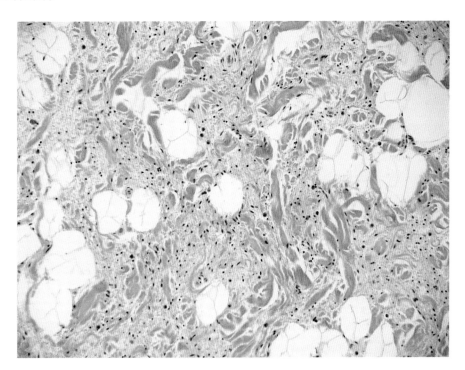

Fig. 21.5 Spindle cell lipoma

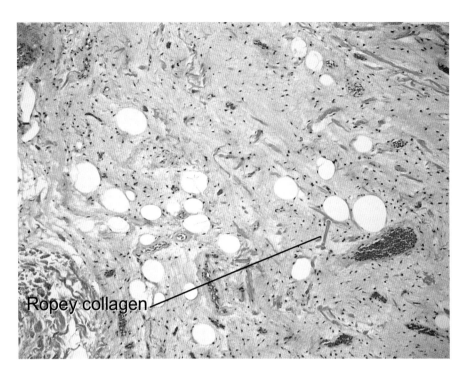

Fig. 21.6 Spindle cell lipoma

Fibrolipoma

- Well-circumscribed tumor of mature lipocytes containing large bundles of mature collagen

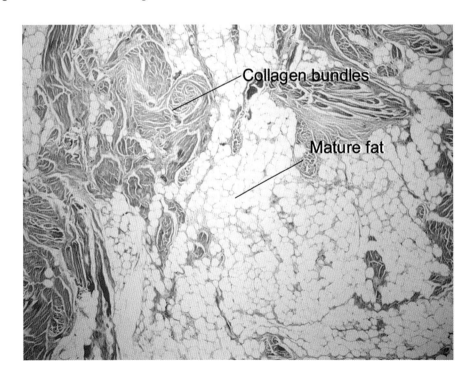

Fig. 21.7 Fibrolipoma

Pleomorphic lipoma

Key Features

- Well-circumscribed tumor of lipocytes with multinucleate floret cells containing overlapping nuclei arranged at the periphery like the petals of a flower
- Hyperchromatic nuclei may be present
- Myxoid areas and ropey collagen bundles may be present, as in spindle cell lipoma

Pleomorphic lipomas have a firm consistency and similar distribution to spindle cell lipomas on the neck and shoulder girdle of older men.

Differential Diagnosis

The sharp circumscription, superficial location, floret cells, paucity of mitotic activity, and absence of lipoblasts distinguish pleomorphic lipoma from pleomorphic liposarcoma. Lipoblasts are immature fat cells that may have an eccentric nucleus (signet-ring lipoblasts) or have a central scalloped nucleus indented by lipid vacuoles (mulberry lipoblasts). Liposarcoma typically arises in deep soft tissue, especially the retroperitoneum, but may involve the skin. Liposarcomas demonstrate an arborizing pattern of blood vessels that resembles "chicken wire."

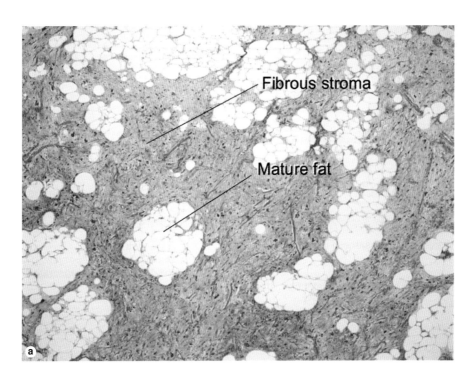

Fig. 21.8 Pleomorphic lipoma

continued

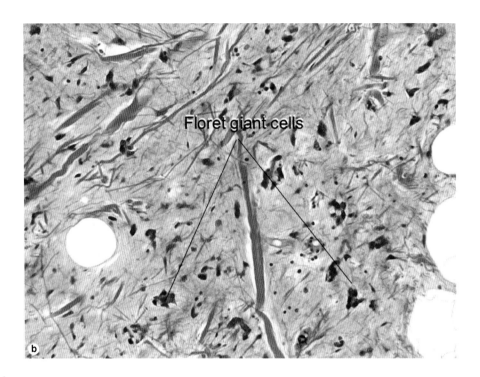

Fig. 21.8, cont'd

Atypical lipomatous tumor (ALT)

Key Features

- Represents well-differentiated liposarcoma
- Lipocytes vary in size
- Atypia noted near septae
- Positive for MDM2 and CDK4 by immunohistochemistry (IHC) or fluorescence in situ hybridization (FISH)

Pleomorphic and myxoid liposarcoma

Key Features

- Lipocytes vary in size
- Mulberry or signet-ring lipoblasts
- Arborizing (chicken-wire) vascular pattern

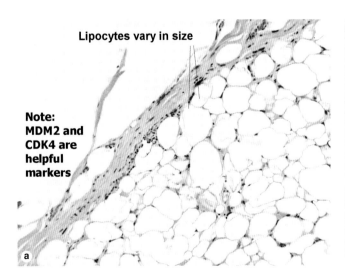

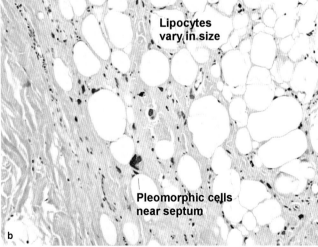

Fig. 21.9 Atypical lipomatous tumor (ALT)

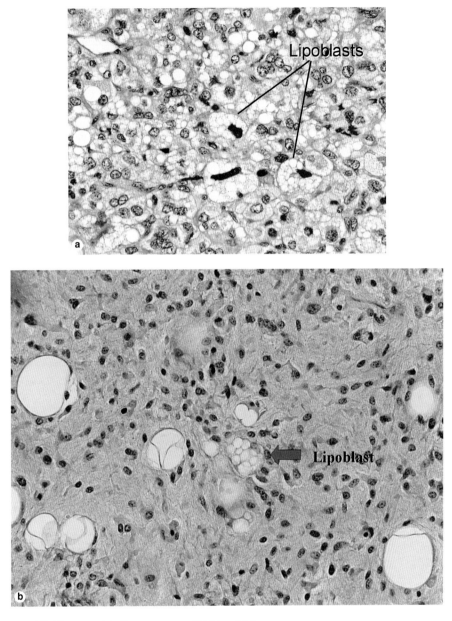

Fig. 21.10 Liposarcoma. **(A)** Pleomorphic liposarcoma. **(B)** Myxoid liposarcoma

Angiomyolipoma

Key Features

- Well-circumscribed tumor
- Smooth muscle radiating in a pinwheel fashion from the walls of muscular vessels
- Mature fat

Cutaneous angiomyolipomas are rare, solitary, painless subcutaneous nodules most commonly on the extremity of middle-aged men. Unlike renal angiomyolipomas, cutaneous lesions are not associated with tuberous sclerosis. Some consider these lesions to be angioleiomyomas with admixed mature fat.

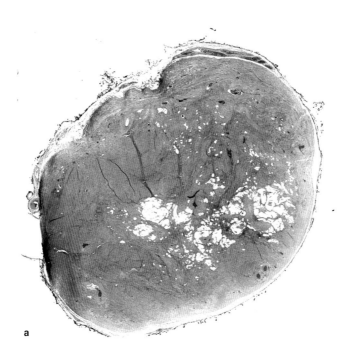

a

Fig. 21.11 (A–C) Angiomyolipoma

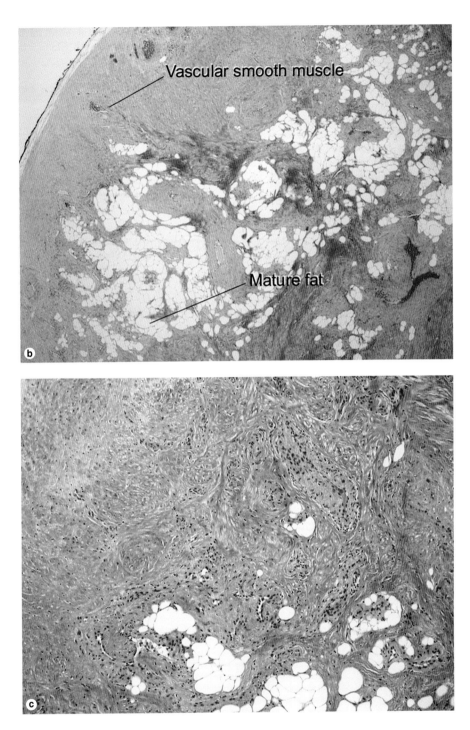

Fig. 21.11, cont'd

Hibernoma

Key Features

- Well-circumscribed tumor
- Multivacuolated "mulberry cells"

Hibernomas are rare tumors that demonstrate differentiation toward brown (fetal) fat. Whereas brown fat occurs anywhere in a fetus, hibernomas in adults most frequently arise in the subcutis of the shoulder girdle, posterior neck, and axilla. The gross brown color is a result of the prominent vascularity and many mitochondria within the tumor cells.

Mulberry cells with central round nuclei predominate in most hibernomas. Smaller cells with granular cytoplasm and univacuolated cells may sometimes be seen.

Differential Diagnosis

Lipoblasts of liposarcoma have hyperchromatic scalloped nuclei. The tumors are large, poorly circumscribed, and have an arborizing vascular pattern.

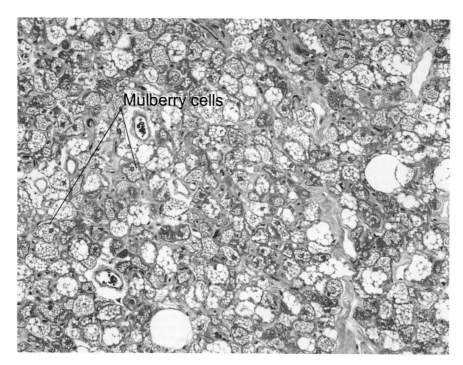

Fig. 21.12 Hibernoma

Nevus lipomatosis superficialis of Hoffmann and Zurhelle

Key Features

- Mature adipocytes replacing much of the dermis

Nevus lipomatosis superficialis presents as multiple soft yellow-tan papules or nodules on the hip or buttock that coalesce into plaques or form a linear arrangement. Rarely, there is disseminated body involvement with extensively folded skin ("Michelin tire baby syndrome").

Large acrochordons with a broad base may have a similar appearance.

Differential Diagnosis

The histologic differential diagnosis includes Goltz syndrome (focal dermal hypoplasia), an X-linked dominant syndrome with a blaschkoid distribution. Long-standing dermal nevi may also undergo extensive fatty degeneration but retain focal residual nevus.

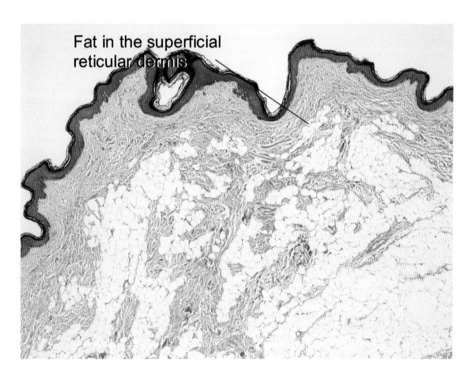

Fig. 21.13 Nevus lipomatosis superficialis

Mobile encapsulated lipoma (encapsulated fat necrosis, nodular–cystic fat necrosis)

Key Features

- Lobules of necrotic fat surrounded by fibrous capsule

These clinically mobile lesions are typically associated with prior trauma. The necrosing fat consists of nonnucleated adipocytes.

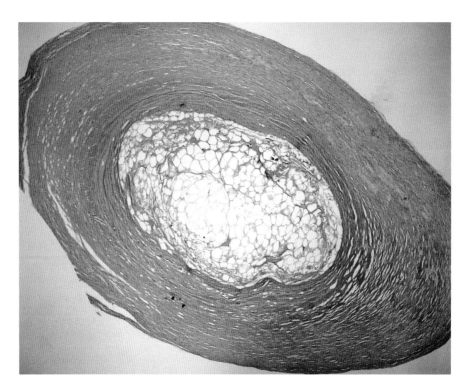

Fig. 21.14 Mobile encapsulated lipoma

Muscle

Smooth muscle hamartoma

Key Features

• Numerous haphazard bundles of smooth muscle in the dermis

Most are congenital plaques of the lumbosacral area or proximal extremity composed of perifollicular papules. Becker nevus and smooth muscle hamartoma are on the same developmental spectrum, but Becker nevus is hyperpigmented and hypertrichotic.

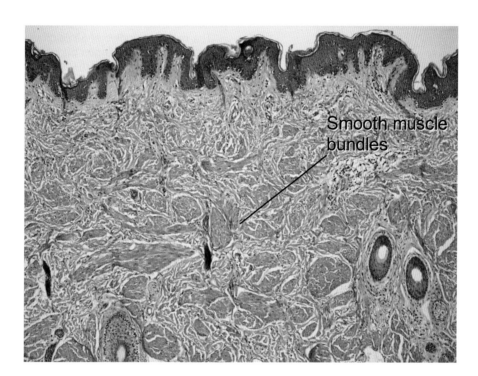

Fig. 21.15 Smooth muscle hamartoma

Leiomyoma

Leiomyomas are benign smooth muscle tumors. Smooth muscle is normally found in the skin as arrector pili muscles, in the walls of blood vessels, breast (periareolar muscle), and genital skin (dartos muscle). Smooth muscle tumors can arise from each of these sources and are known as *piloleiomyoma*, *angioleiomyoma*, and *leiomyoma of the genital skin*, respectively.

Smooth muscle cells are characterized by long, thin, cigar-shaped nuclei with blunt ends. A paranuclear vacuole, representing a glycogen "snack" for the muscle, is well demonstrated in cross-section.

Piloleiomyoma

Key Features

- Circumscribed but nonencapsulated dermal nodule
- Interlacing bundles of smooth muscle fibers resemble arrector pili muscle "on steroids"
- Mitotic activity is negligible
- Nuclear density matches that of normal smooth muscle

Piloleiomyomas, derived from the arrector pili muscle, typically present as multiple firm, red-brown lesions in the third decade.

They may be solitary, grouped, or in a linear pattern. Manipulation and exposure to cold result in pain.

Multiple lesions have been associated with papillary renal cell carcinoma and uterine leiomyomas (fibroids) in females. This constellation of findings, known as *Reed syndrome*, is inherited in an autosomal-dominant pattern and is due to a mutation in the fumarate hydratase gene.

Differential Diagnosis

Smooth muscle hamartomas consist of smaller bundles that are sparsely distributed in a broad patch or plaquelike lesion.

The muscle bundles of piloleiomyoma can be distinguished from collagen bundles by the blunt, cigar-shaped nuclei with adjacent vacuole rather than the short, tapered nuclei of the fibroblasts in collagen. The cytoplasm of smooth muscle cells is more conspicuous than in fibroblasts. A trichrome stain will stain muscle red and collagen green-blue. Immunoperoxidase markers for smooth muscle (smooth muscle actin and desmin) can also be used.

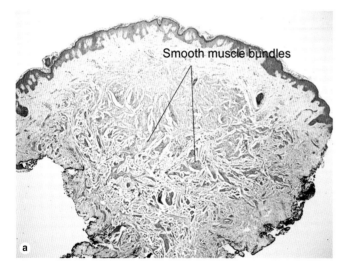
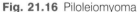
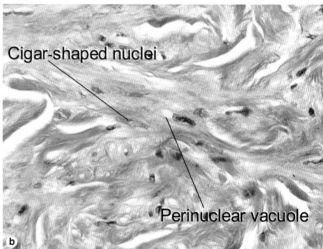

Fig. 21.16 Piloleiomyoma

Angioleiomyoma

Key Features

- Subcutaneous nodule of smooth muscle containing round and slitlike vascular spaces

Angioleiomyomas are usually tender subcutaneous nodules on the lower extremities of middle-aged adults. More than half of lesions are spontaneously painful. Each vessel has several layers of smooth muscle that merge with the intervascular smooth muscle fascicles.

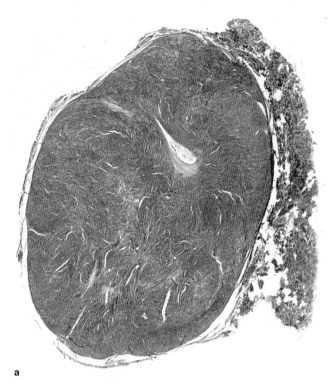

a

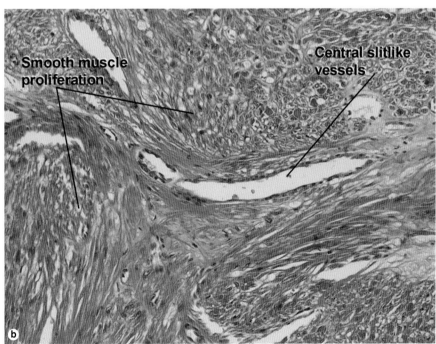

Fig. 21.17 Angioleiomyoma

Leiomyosarcoma

Key Features

- High cellularity
- Mitoses and nuclear atypia

Superficial or dermal leiomyosarcomas are neoplasms that arise from the pili or genital smooth muscle. They occur predominantly in middle-aged men on the extensor extremities. Lesions recur in 30% of cases but metastasis is extremely rare.

Subcutaneous leiomyosarcomas, presumably arising from vascular smooth muscle, are larger and have a greater tendency for metastasis to lung, other soft tissue sites, and the liver in one third of cases.

Similar to leiomyomas, leiomyosarcomas are composed of intertwined fascicles of fusiform cells with blunt-ended nuclei and eosinophilic cytoplasm. Leiomyosarcomas, however, are hypercellular with a high nuclear to cytoplasmic ratio. Mitotic figures are variable. Subcutaneous leiomyosarcomas have a greater degree of pleomorphism and nuclear atypia, have a higher mitotic rate, and may show focal necrosis.

Differential Diagnosis

Although a grenz zone is often present, dermal leiomyosarcomas may be *SLAM*med up against the epidermis and resemble other spindle cell neoplasms. IHC can aid in the microscopic differential diagnosis.

- *S*pindled squamous cell carcinoma (keratin+)
- *L*eiomyosarcoma (desmin+)
- *A*typical fibroxanthoma (diagnosis of exclusion)
- *M*elanoma (S100+)

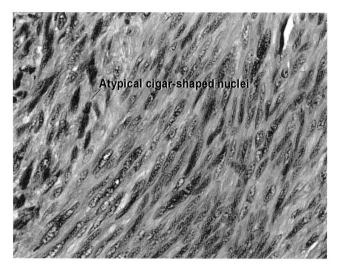

Fig. 21.18 Leiomyosarcoma

Cartilage and Bone

Osteoma cutis

Key Features

- Dermal or subcutaneous bone
- Haversian canals, osteocytes in lacunae, and osteoclasts similar to normal bone

Cutaneous bone formation may be primary or secondary. It is primary if no preceding cutaneous lesion is present. Primary cutaneous ossification can occur in Albright hereditary osteodystrophy and as osteoma cutis. Secondary bone formation occurs through metaplasia within a preexisting lesion such as a pilomatricoma, chondroid syringoma, intradermal nevus (nevus of Nanta), acne scar, scleroderma, or dermatomyositis.

The osteoblasts that form bone in cutaneous ossification originate in preexisting fibrous connective tissue and result in intramembranous rather than endochondral bone formation. An important exception would be chondroid syringoma in which endochondral bone formation may occur.

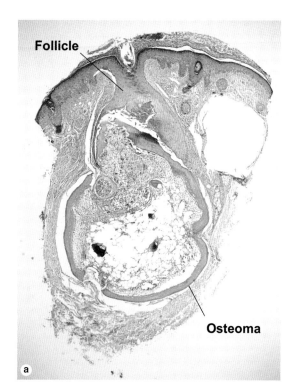

Fig. 21.19 Osteoma cutis

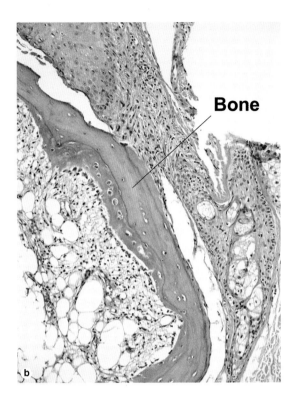

Fig. 21.19, cont'd

Accessory tragus (cartilaginous rest)

Key Features

- Fibrovascular polyp containing numerous vellus follicles
- Core of adipose tissue and cartilage may be seen

Accessory tragi are congenital lesions, typically in the preauricular area, but sometimes involving the neck. Rarely, they are associated with oculo-auriculo-vertebral syndrome (Goldenhar syndrome).

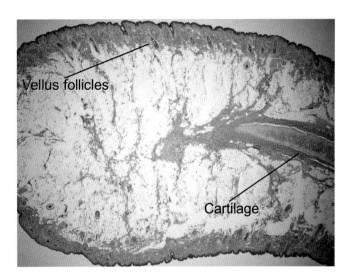

Fig. 21.20 Accessory tragus, scanning magnification

Chondroma

Key Features

- Circumscribed mass of mature hyaline cartilage
- Single or grouped chondrocytes in lacunae

Soft tissue chondromas typically occur on the fingers of middle-aged adults. Calcification can be seen.

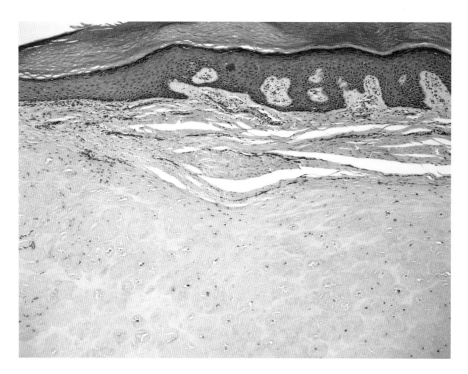

Fig. 21.21 Chondroma

Chordoma

Key Features

- Lobules separated by fibrous bands
- Sheets, cords, or individual cells in chondroid stroma
- Abundant, pale, bubbly cytoplasm (physaliphorous)
- No lacunae like chondroma or ducts like chondroid syringoma

These tumors originate from a remnant of the notochord and thus are typically seen along the axial spine, especially the sacrococcygeal area. Cutaneous involvement can occur directly or via metastasis. There is triple positivity with S100, vimentin, and keratin. Parachordomas are similar histologically but develop on the extremities adjacent to tendons, synovium, or bone. Cutaneous parachordomas are related to cutaneous myoepitheliomas.

Subungual exostosis

Key Features

- Bony stalk with fibrocartilaginous cap

This lesion occurs under the nail plate, resulting in subungual hyperkeratosis, onycholysis, or nail deformity. The great toe is the most common site. There is no cortical or medullary continuity with the underlying bone.

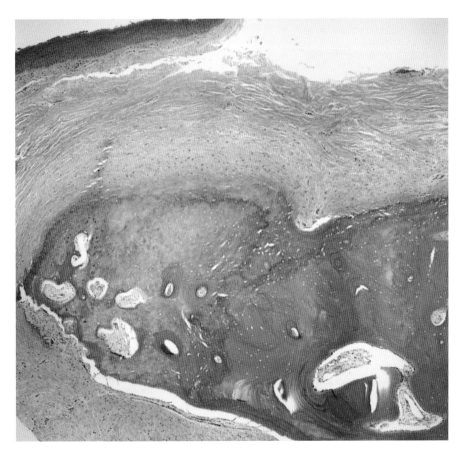

Fig. 21.22 Subungual exostosis

Further reading

Clay MR, Martinez AP, Weiss SW, et al. MDM2 Amplification in Problematic Lipomatous tumors: analysis of FISH testing criteria. Am J Surg Pathol 2015;39(10):1433–9.

Dixon AY, McGregor DH, Lee SH. Angiolipomas: an ultrastructural and clinicopathological study. Hum Pathol 1981;12(8):739–47.

Ferringer T. Immunohistology and molecular studies of smooth muscle and neural cutaneous tumors. *In*: Plaza JA, Prieto V, editors. Applied immunohistochemistry in the evaluation of skin neoplasms. Switzerland: Springer; 2016.

Fields JP, Helwig EB. Leiomyosarcoma of the skin and subcutaneous tissue. Cancer 1981;47(1):156–69.

Fletcher CD, Martin-Bates E. Spindle cell lipoma: a clinicopathological study with some original observations. Histopathology 1987;11(8):803–17.

Hamilton J, Tan J, Mudhar HS. Unilateral pleomorphic lipoma of the eyebrow. Ocul Oncol Pathol 2015;2(1):20–3.

Hurt MA, Santa Cruz DJ. Nodular-cystic fat necrosis. A reevaluation of the so-called mobile encapsulated lipoma. J Am Acad Dermatol 1989;21(3 Pt 1):493–8.

Jansen T, Romiti R, Altmeyer P. Accessory tragus: report of two cases and review of the literature. Pediatr Dermatol 2000;17(5):391–4.

Jensen ML, Jensen OM, Michalski W, et al. Intradermal and subcutaneous leiomyosarcoma: a clinicopathological and immunohistochemical study of 41 cases. J Cutan Pathol 1996;23(5):458–63.

Lee SK, Jung MS, Lee YH, et al. Two distinctive subungual pathologies: subungual exostosis and subungual osteochondroma. Foot Ankle Int 2007;28(5):595–601.

Mehregan AH, Tavafoghi V, Ghandchi A. Nevus lipomatosus cutaneus superficialis (Hoffmann-Zurhelle). J Cutan Pathol 1975;2(6):307–13.

Mehregan DA, Mehregan DR, Mehregan AH. Angiomyolipoma. J Am Acad Dermatol 1992;27(2 Pt 2):331–3.

Newman PL, Fletcher CD. Smooth muscle tumours of the external genitalia: clinicopathological analysis of a series. Histopathology 1991;18(6):523–9.

Raj S, Calonje E, Kraus M, et al. Cutaneous pilar leiomyoma: clinicopathologic analysis of 53 lesions in 45 patients. Am J Dermatopathol 1997;19(1):2–9.

Shen J, Shrestha S, Rao PN, et al. Pericytic mimicry in well-differentiated liposarcoma/atypical lipomatous tumor. Hum Pathol 2016;54:92–4.

Shmookler BM, Enzinger FM. Pleomorphic lipoma: a benign tumor simulating liposarcoma. A clinicopathologic analysis of 48 cases. Cancer 1981;47(1):126–33.

Svoboda RM, Mackay D, Welsch MJ, et al. Multiple cutaneous metastatic chordomas from the sacrum. J Am Acad Dermatol 2012;66(6):e246–7.

Thompson J, Squires S, Machan M, et al. Cutaneous mixed tumor with extensive chondroid metaplasia: a potential mimic of cutaneous chondroma. Dermatol Online J 2012;18(3):9.

Neural tumors

Tammie Ferringer

Neurofibroma

Key Features

- Loose arrangement with pale myxoid stroma
- Haphazard spindle cells with small wavy or S-shaped nuclei
- Mast cells are numerous

Neurofibromas may occur as solitary lesions. Multiple widespread neurofibromas characterize neurofibromatosis (von Recklinghausen disease) in which they are seen in association with café-au-lait macules, axillary freckling, and pigmented hamartomas of the iris (Lisch nodules).

Diffuse neurofibroma

Key Features

- At scanning magnification, diffuse replacement of dermis and infiltration of fat
- Higher magnification shows features typical of neurofibroma

Differential Diagnosis

Dermatofibrosarcoma protuberans has a similar growth pattern and can be myxoid, bearing a considerable resemblance to diffuse neurofibroma. Both may be CD34 positive, but S100 staining of the neurofibroma can distinguish the two. Spindle cell lipoma can appear similar, but occurs as an encapsulated nodule.

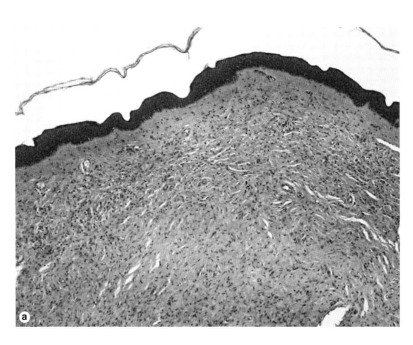

Fig. 22.1 Neurofibroma

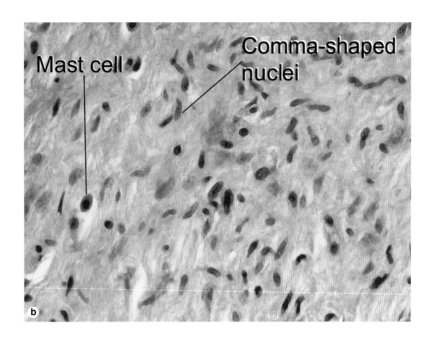

Fig. 22.1, cont'd

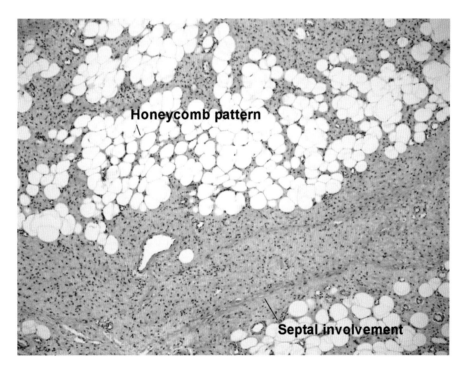

Fig. 22.2 Diffuse neurofibroma

Plexiform neurofibroma

Key Features

- Large fascicles of neurofibroma surrounded by perineurium
- Often embedded within a diffuse neurofibroma

Plexiform neurofibroma clinically resembles a "bag of worms" and is considered pathognomonic of neurofibromatosis. Both diffuse and plexiform neurofibromas probably result from loss of heterozygosity, where segmental loss of the remaining normal allele for the *NF1* gene results in a localized complete lack of tumor suppressor protein.

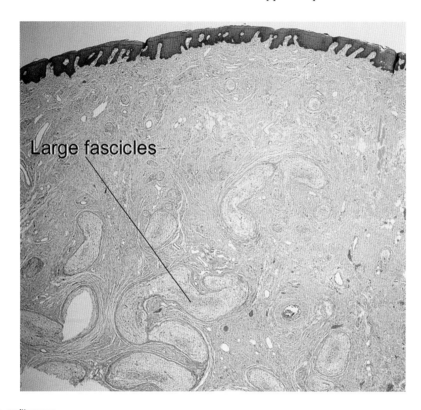

Fig. 22.3 Plexiform neurofibroma

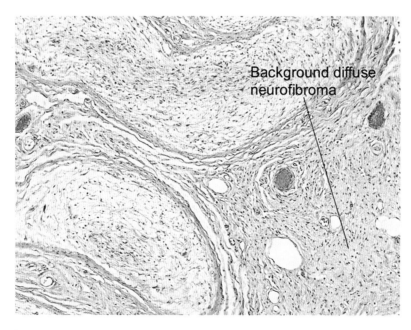

Fig. 22.4 Plexiform neurofibroma

Schwannoma (neurilemmoma)

Key Features

- Deep dermal or subcutaneous tumors with perineural capsule
- Arise within a nerve, displacing axons to the periphery, causing pain
- Antoni A tissue contains parallel rows of nuclei separated by acellular areas (Verocay bodies)
- Hard schwannomas are composed almost entirely of Antoni A tissue
- Antoni B tissue represents a degenerative change with edematous stroma, typically just below the capsule
- Soft schwannomas are composed almost entirely of Antoni B tissue

Schwannomas present as round to oval encapsulated tumors with a subcapsular crescentic zone of edema. Hard schwannomas typically demonstrate many Verocay bodies, whereas soft schwannomas are encapsulated neoplasms composed of loose edematous tissue with widely dilated hyalinized blood vessels.

Psammomatous melanotic schwannoma is a variant with psammoma bodies and melanin. It is associated with Carney complex (myxomas, spotty pigmentation, and endocrinopathy).

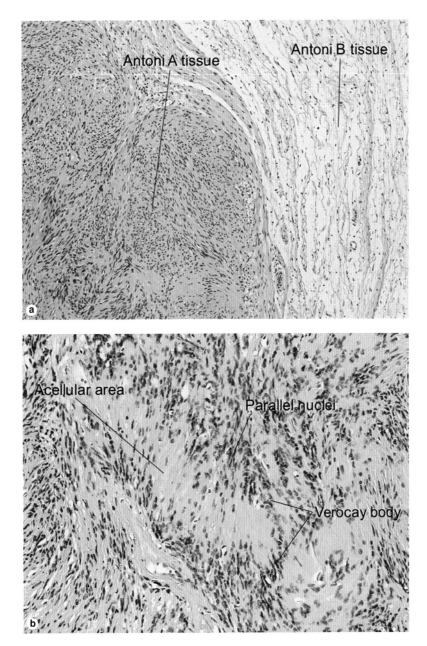

Fig. 22.5 (A) Schwannoma. **(B)** Schwannoma (Verocay bodies)

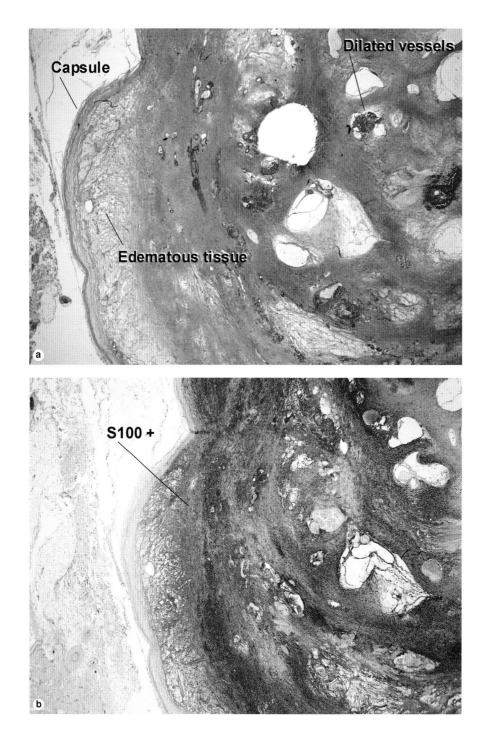

Fig. 22.6 (A) Soft schwannoma (predominantly Antoni B tissue). **(B)** Soft schwannoma (S100 immunostain)

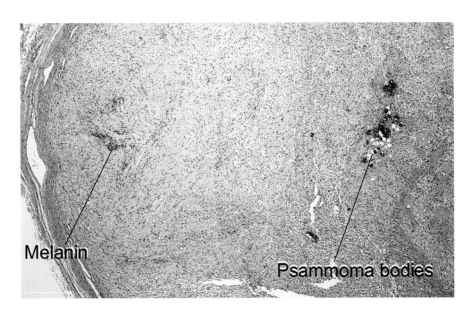

Fig. 22.7 Psammomatous melanotic schwannoma

"Ancient" schwannoma

Key Features

- Benign schwannoma with hyperchromatic pleomorphic nuclei
- No mitoses are present

These "ancient" changes in schwannomas represent a degenerative phenomenon. The absence of mitotic figures and absence of an expansile growth pattern distinguish benign ancient schwannoma from malignant peripheral nerve sheath tumors (MPNST). Typically, MPNSTs arise from neurofibromas, rather than schwannomas.

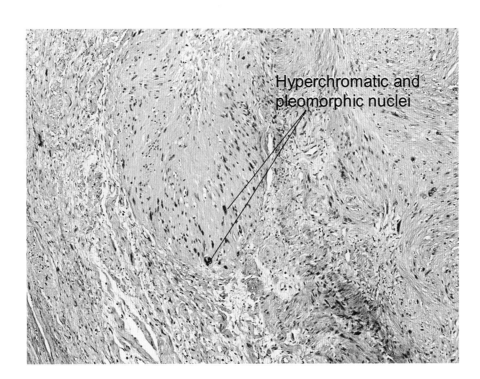

Fig. 22.8 Ancient schwannoma

Neuromas

Neuromas are nerve sheath tumors with a roughly 1:1 ratio of axons to Schwann cells.

Traumatic neuroma

Key Features

- Multiple nerve fascicles embedded within a fibrous scar
- Clefts between fascicles

Traumatic neuromas occur most commonly on the extremities where mechanical injuries are most frequent. Longitudinal growth of the regenerating nerve trunk results in complex folding. In cross-section, this appears as multiple discrete nerve fascicles.

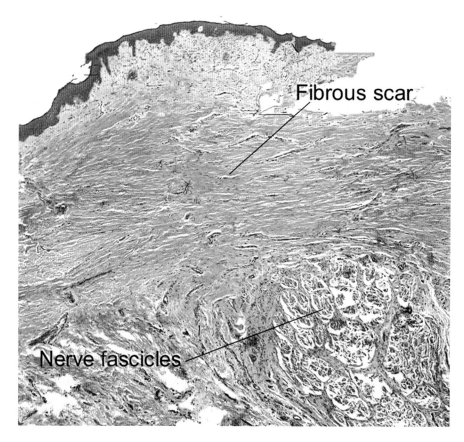

Fig. 22.9 Traumatic neuroma

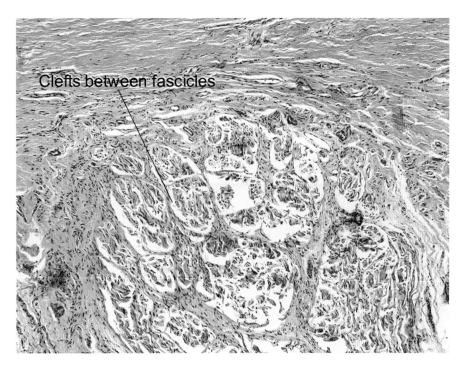

Fig. 22.10 Traumatic neuroma

Epithelial sheath neuroma

Key Features

- Large nerves within the superficial dermis
- Perineural squamous epithelial sheath

Epithelial sheath neuroma mimics perineural invasion of squamous cell carcinoma. The two are distinguished by the bland nature of the epithelium, as well as the presence of large nerves within the superficial dermis where nerves of this size would usually not be found. The epithelial sheath represents benign pseudoepitheliomatous hyperplasia and squamous metaplasia of eccrine ducts.

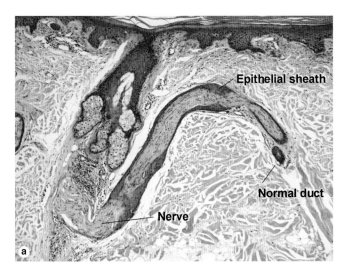

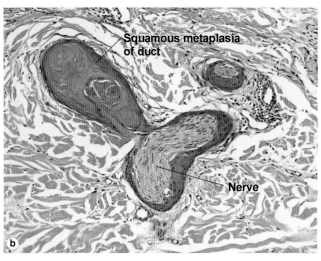

Fig. 22.11 Epithelial sheath neuroma

Palisaded encapsulated neuroma

Key Features

- Superficial dermal tumors with a thin, delicate capsule
- Fascicles of spindle cells separated by clefts

Palisaded encapsulated neuromas are solitary painless papules that occur most commonly on the lower central face. The name is somewhat of a misnomer, as there is usually no palisading and only an inconspicuous capsule. Histologically, they resemble the mucosal neuromas of multiple endocrine neoplasia syndrome type 2b, an autosomal-dominant syndrome caused by a mutation of the *RET* proto-oncogene. In addition to the multiple mucosal neuromas, the syndrome is characterized by a marfanoid habitus, medullary carcinoma of the thyroid, pheochromocytoma, and hyperparathyroidism.

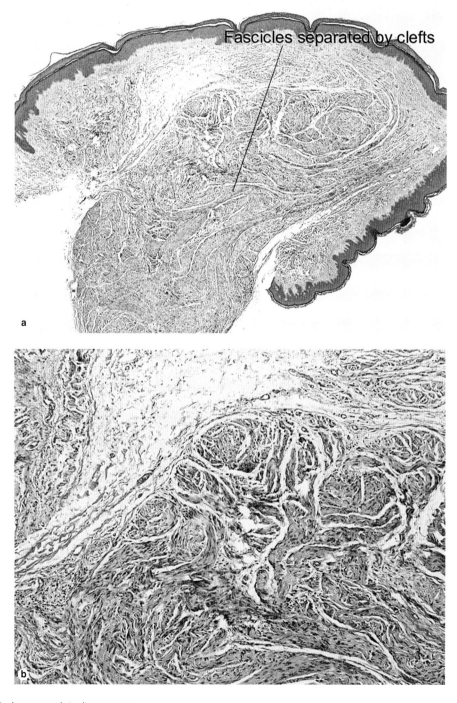

Fig. 22.12 Palisaded encapsulated neuroma

Differential Diagnosis

Unlike schwannomas, palisaded encapsulated neuromas are superficial tumors with adjacent sebaceous glands and small vellus follicles typical of facial skin. Schwannomas lack the fascicles with clefts seen in palisaded encapsulated neuromas.

Supernumerary digit (rudimentary polydactyly)

Key Features

- Acral papule with nerve bundles
- Bone or cartilage may be present

Supernumerary digit presents as a congenital papule, typically located at the base of the fifth digit along the ulnar border.

Differential Diagnosis

Acquired digital fibrokeratoma is also an acral papule; however, there are no nerve bundles and large stellate factor XIIIa-positive dendrocytes may be present. There is often longitudinal streaking of collagen.

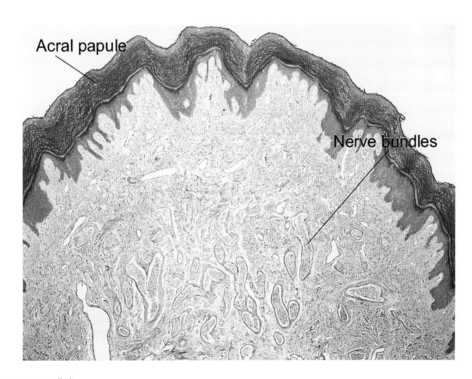

Fig. 22.13 Supernumerary digit

Merkel cell carcinoma (primary neuroendocrine carcinoma of the skin, trabecular carcinoma)

Key Features

- Composed of small blue cells with scant cytoplasm and tightly packed nuclei in sheets or a trabecular array
- Nuclear molding, apoptotic cells, and mitoses are often present
- Synaptophysin, chromogranin, neurofilament protein, and neuron-specific enolase+
- CK20+ in a paranuclear dot pattern

Membrane-bound dense core granules on electron microscopy are characteristic. Metastatic small (oat) cell carcinoma of the lung also consists of small blue cells, but CK20 is typically negative and thyroid transcription factor (TTF-1) is positive. Also in the differential diagnosis of small blue cell tumors is lymphoma, which can be distinguished by positivity for hematopoietic markers. Melanoma is S100 positive. Neuroblastoma often demonstrates elongated, angulated, "carrot-shaped" blue cells and may form rosettes. Merkel cell polyomavirus has been identified in 80% of Merkel cell carcinomas.

Differential Diagnosis

The microscopic differential diagnosis for "small blue cell" tumors can be remembered by the mnemonic "LEMONS":

- Lymphoma
- Ewing sarcoma
- Merkel cell carcinoma/melanoma
- Oat cell carcinoma of the lung
- Neuroblastoma
- Small cell endocrine carcinoma

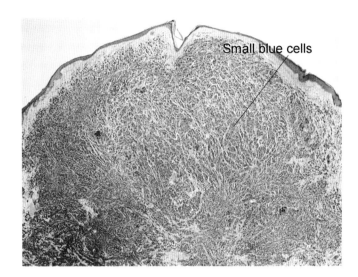

Fig. 22.14 Merkel cell carcinoma

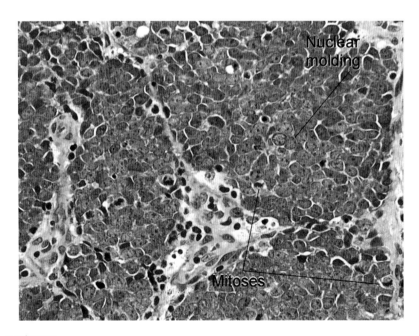

Fig. 22.15 Merkel cell carcinoma

Granular cell tumor

Key Features

- Sheets of large polygonal cells with abundant eosinophilic granular cytoplasm with central nucleus
- Discrete round, eosinophilic, giant lysosomal granules (pustulo-ovoid bodies of Milian)
- Overlying pseudoepitheliomatous hyperplasia can be mistaken for squamous cell carcinoma
- S100 and Sox-10+

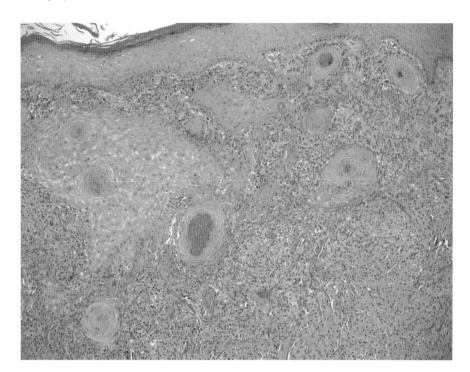

Fig. 22.16 Granular cell tumor with pseudoepitheliomatous hyperplasia

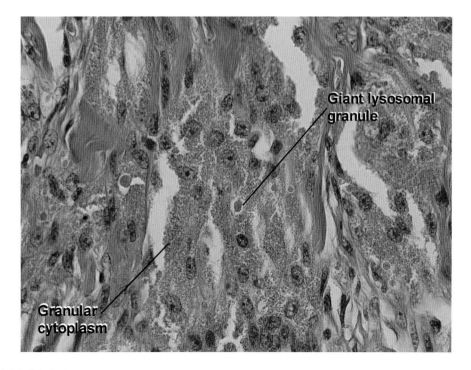

Fig. 22.17 Granular cell tumor

Granular cell tumors are Schwann cell–derived tumors that can occur anywhere, but most commonly on the tongue. The granules within the cytoplasm are phagolysosomes. Bland cytology can be a poor predictor of biologic behavior, and large tumors should be regarded as potentially malignant.

Neurothekeoma

Neurothekeomas are benign neoplasms that are divided into myxoid, mixed, and cellular types. The myxoid type is strongly S100 positive, whereas those on the cellular end of the spectrum are composed of undifferentiated cells with partial features of Schwann cells, smooth muscle cells, myofibroblasts, and fibroblasts. Cellular neurothekeoma may be closely related to plexiform fibrohistiocytic tumor.

Myxoid neurothekeoma (nerve sheath myxoma)

Key Features

- Multiple myxoid lobules containing sparse stellate cells
- S100+

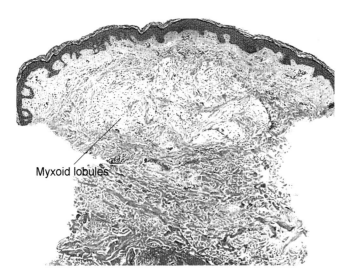

Fig. 22.18 Myxoid neurothekeoma

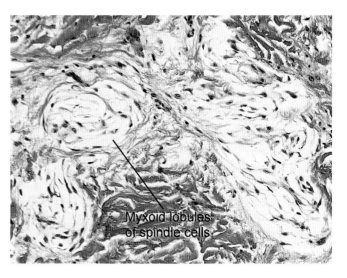

Fig. 22.19 Myxoid neurothekeoma

Cellular neurothekeoma

Key Features

- Nests and fascicles of epithelioid or spindled cells
- Moderate cellular pleomorphism and nuclear hyperchromasia
- Myxoid stroma is absent or sparse
- S100– but S100A6+, PGP9.5+, and NKI/C3+

The cellular variant is negative for S100 and desmin, but sometimes positive for smooth muscle actin, neuron-specific enolase, and factor XIIIa. It is frequently positive for NK1/C-3, S100A6, and PGP9.5 with antigen retrieval. S100A6 also stains histiocytic tumors, including atypical fibroxanthoma, as well as Spitz nevi.

Differential Diagnosis

Histologically, cellular neurothekeomas may be confused with melanocytic lesions such as dermal Spitz nevi. S100 positivity strongly favors the melanocytic lesion. The variable reactivity for factor XIIIa in cellular neurothekeoma can result in confusion with epithelioid fibrous histiocytoma. S100A6 positivity can lead to confusion with spindled atypical fibroxanthoma. Of the two, atypical fibroxanthoma is less likely to demonstrate fascicles of tumor cells. Epithelioid pilar leiomyomas may also be considered in the differential diagnosis due to the variable smooth muscle actin positivity in cellular neurothekeomas. However, the absence of desmin in cellular neurothekeoma aids in the distinction.

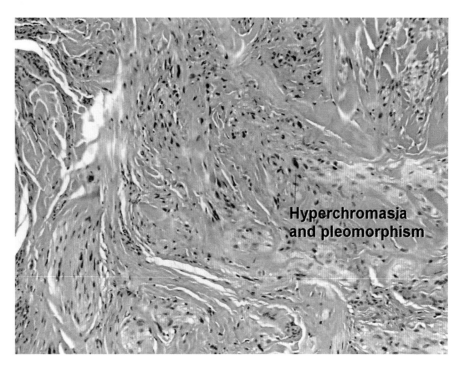

Fig. 22.20 Cellular neurothekeoma

Malignant peripheral nerve sheath tumor (MPNST) (neurofibrosarcoma, malignant schwannoma)

Key Features

- Malignant transformation of neurofibromas, especially plexiform neurofibromas
- Intersecting fascicles of spindle cells
- Expansile growth pattern
- Hypercellularity is more characteristic than atypia
- Mitoses are present but not always frequent

Foci of divergent differentiation may be present, including osseous, chondroid, and rhabdoid foci, as well as foci of adenocarcinoma or angiosarcoma. Malignant peripheral nerve sheath tumor with focal rhabdomyosarcoma is known as *malignant Triton tumor*. S100 staining is usually focal and weak in MPNSTs but diffusely positive in its mimicker: desmoplastic melanoma.

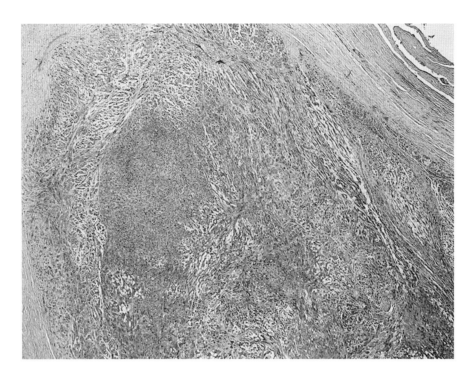

Fig. 22.21 Malignant peripheral nerve sheath tumor

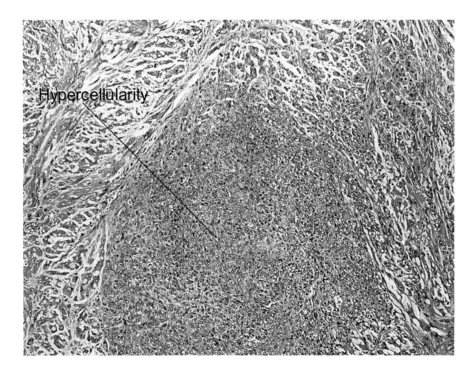

Fig. 22.22 Malignant peripheral nerve sheath tumor

Cutaneous ganglioneuroma

Key Features

- Localized dermal collection of Schwann cells with uniform, wavy, buckled nuclei
- Admixed large polygonal ganglion cells with eccentric large, round nucleus with prominent nucleolus

The ganglion cells are positive with glial fibrillary acidic protein. Ganglioneuroma has mature ganglion cells scattered in a Schwann cell background, in contrast to ganglion cell choristoma, which contains only a proliferation of ganglion cells without supporting neuromatous elements.

Perineurioma

Key Features

- Circumscribed tumor of spindle cells with elongate bipolar cytoplasmic processes
- Fascicle of cells parallel to each other or in concentric onion-skin–like whorls

Variants of perineurioma include intraneural, soft tissue, sclerosing, and cutaneous. The sclerosing variant, seen most on the hands of young adults, is characterized by prominent hyalinized stroma. Soft tissue perineuriomas are generally more cellular. Occasionally, the perineural cells are more epithelioid. These tumors are EMA, GLUT1, and claudin-1 positive and S100 negative.

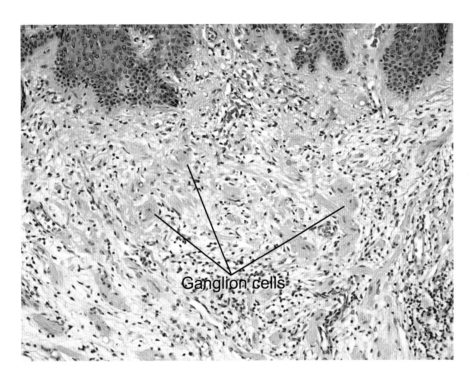

Fig. 22.23 Cutaneous ganglioneuroma

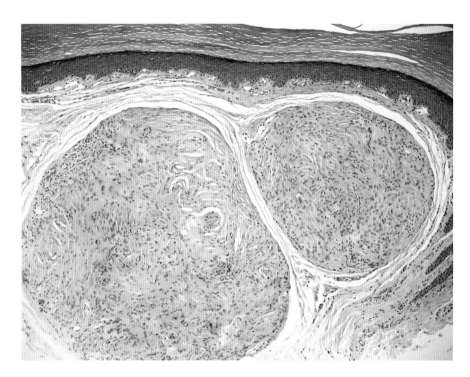

Fig. 22.24 Sclerosing perineurioma

Glial heterotopia (nasal glioma)

Key Features

- Astrocytes with round, vesicular nuclei in a loose neurofibrillary stroma

This congenital nodule or polyp typically presents in or around the nose, thus the "nasal" designation. Connection with the frontal lobe must be excluded with neuroimaging studies preoperatively. Oligodendrocytes with small hyperchromatic nuclei may be focally identified. S100 and GFAP are positive.

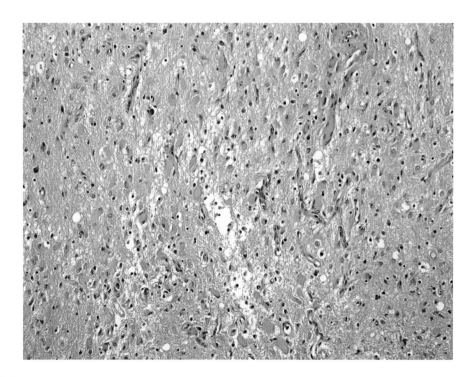

Fig. 22.25 Nasal glioma

Meningeal heterotopia (rudimentary meningocele)

Key Features

- Pseudovascular spaces dissect through collagen bundles
- Spaces are lined by small, round, epithelioid meningothelial cells
- Meningothelial cells wrap around collagen bundles
- Psammoma bodies may be present

Meningeal lesions in the skin are often referred to as *cutaneous meningiomas;* however, only type III lesions are an extension or metastasis from intracranial meningioma. Type I and type II are probably developmental and lack bone defects. Type I is the most common meningeal heterotopia. It is congenital and is also known as *ectopic meningothelial hamartoma* and *rudimentary or sequestered meningocele.* Meningothelial cells are EMA positive.

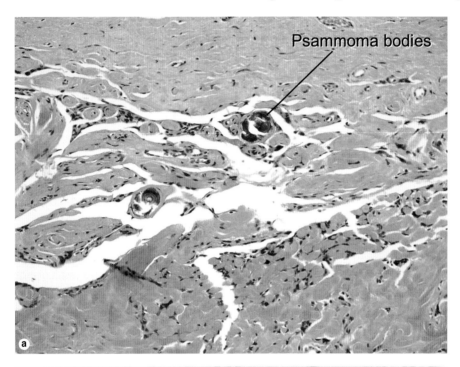

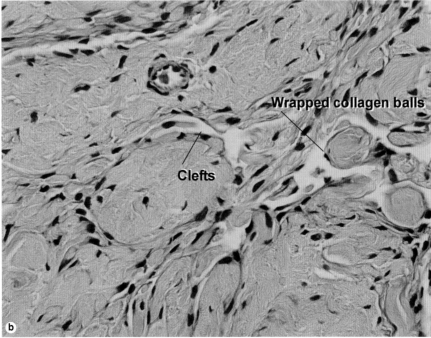

Fig. 22.26 Rudimentary meningocele

continued

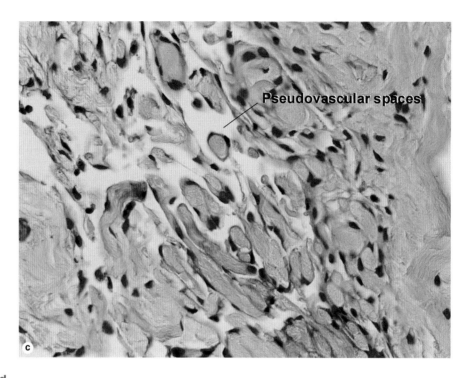

Fig. 22.26, cont'd

Meningioma

Key Features

- Most common primary brain tumor, with many histologic variants

- Grades range from benign to high-grade malignancy
- May appear in skin as a result of erosion through the skull
- Meningothelial whorls and psammoma bodies prominent in meningothelial type

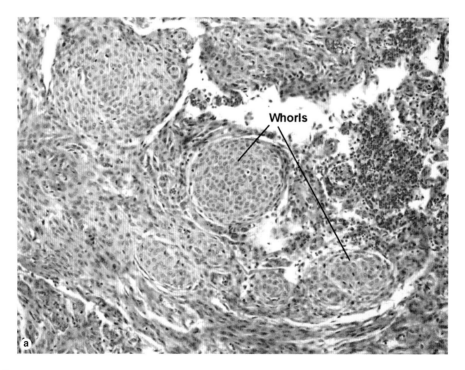

Fig. 22.27 Meningioma

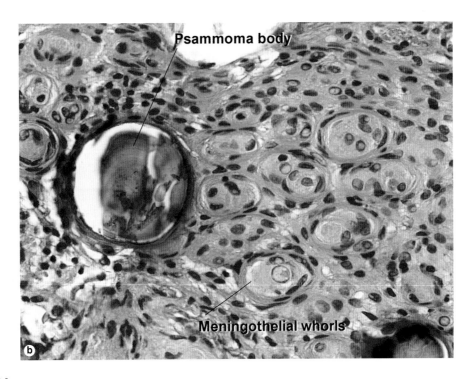

Fig. 22.27, cont'd

Neuroblastoma

Key Features

- Primitive neoplasm of neuroectodermal origin
- Composed of immature neuroblasts
- Small, round, blue cell tumor, often with salt and pepper chromatin
- Compressed, elongated "carrot cells"
- May form rosettes
- Prognostic factors include histologic subtype, grade of tumor differentiation, stage, age at diagnosis, and *MYCN* status

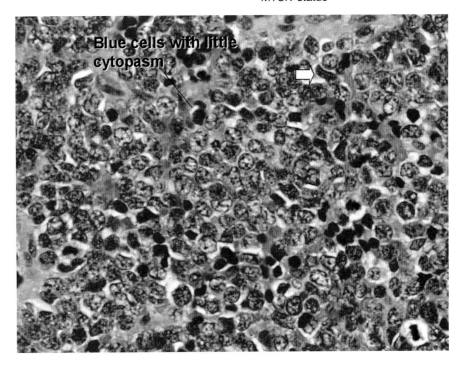

Fig. 22.28 Neuroblastoma

Further reading

Argenyi ZB. Cutaneous neural heterotopias and related tumors relevant for the dermatopathologist. Semin Diagn Pathol 1996;13(1):60–71.

Argenyi ZB, Balogh K, Abraham AA. Degenerative ("ancient") changes in benign cutaneous schwannoma. A light microscopic, histochemical and immunohistochemical study. J Cutan Pathol 1993;20(2):148–53.

Argenyi ZB, Kutzner H, Seaba MM. Ultrastructural spectrum of cutaneous nerve sheath myxoma/cellular neurothekeoma. J Cutan Pathol 1995;22(2):137–45.

Calonje E, Wilson-Jones E, Smith NP, et al. Cellular "neurothekeoma": an epithelioid variant of pilar leiomyoma? Morphological and immunohistochemical analysis of a series. Histopathology 1992;20(5):397–404.

Carney JA, Stratakis CA. Epithelioid blue nevus and psammomatous melanotic schwannoma: the unusual pigmented skin tumors of the Carney complex. Semin Diagn Pathol 1998;15(3):216–24.

Chambers PW, Schwinn CP. Chordoma. A clinicopathologic study of metastasis. Am J Clin Pathol 1979;72(5):765–76.

Dewit L, Albus-Lutter CE, de Jong AS, et al. Malignant schwannoma with a rhabdomyoblastic component, a so-called triton tumor. A clinicopathologic study. Cancer 1986;58(6):1350–6.

Ducatman BS, Scheithauer BW. Malignant peripheral nerve sheath tumors with divergent differentiation. Cancer 1984;54(6):1049–57.

Ferringer T. Immunohistology and Molecular Studies of Smooth Muscle and Neural Cutaneous Tumors. In: Plaza JA, Prieto V, editors. Applied Immunohistochemistry in the Evaluation of Skin Neoplasms. Switzerland: Springer; 2016.

Hirano-Ali SA, Bryant EA, Warren SJ. Epithelial sheath neuroma: evidence supporting a hyperplastic etiology and epidermal origin. J Cutan Pathol 2016;43(6):531–4.

Kluwe L, Friedrich RE, Mautner VF. Allelic loss of the NF1 gene in NF1-associated plexiform neurofibromas. Cancer Genet Cytogenet 1999;113(1):65–9.

Macarenco RS, Ellinger F, Oliveira AM. Perineurioma: a distinctive and underrecognized peripheral nerve sheath neoplasm. Arch Pathol Lab Med 2007;131(4):625–36.

Miedema JR, Zedek D. Cutaneous meningioma. Arch Pathol Lab Med 2012;136(2):208–11.

Wallace CA, Hallman JR, Sangueza OP. Primary cutaneous ganglioneuroma: a report of two cases and literature review. Am J Dermatopathol 2003;25(3):239–42.

Wang AR, May D, Bourne P, et al. PGP9.5: a marker for cellular neurothekeoma. Am J Surg Pathol 1999;23(11):1401–7.

CHAPTER 23

Vascular tumors

Dirk M. Elston

Angiokeratoma

Key Features

- Hyperkeratosis
- Acanthosis
- Ectatic, thin-walled vessels in contact with the epidermis
- Resembles a "bloody seborrheic keratosis"

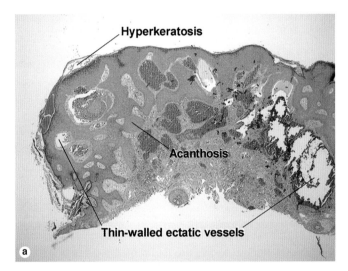

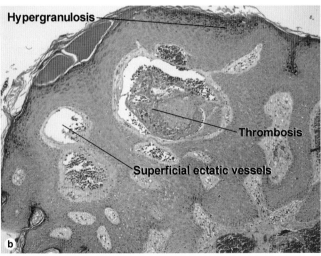

Fig. 23.1 Angiokeratoma

Lymphangioma

Key Features

- "Frog spawn" clinically
- Similar to angiokeratoma with lymph in vessels, but few erythrocytes
- D2-40+

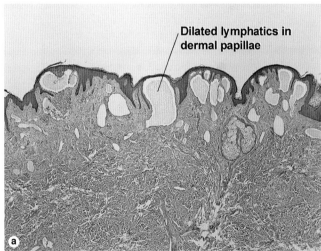

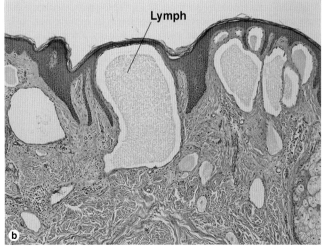

Fig. 23.2 Lymphangioma

Nevus flammeus

Key Features

- Dilated capillary-sized vessels

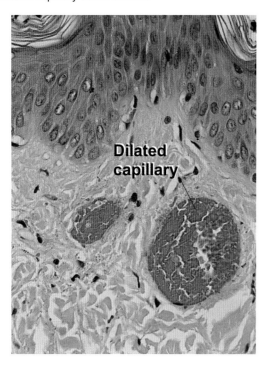

Fig. 23.3 Nevus flammeus

Angioma serpiginosum

Key Features

- Dilated tortuous capillaries in dermal papillae and the upper dermis
- Vessels lack alkaline phosphatase activity

Angioma serpiginosum presents as a progressive vascular lesion on a woman's leg. The ectatic vessels begin as minute puncta in clusters, but merge to form a serpiginous array. They often bleed freely when traumatized.

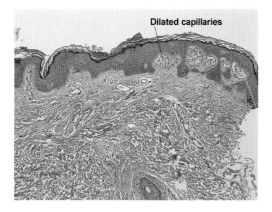

Fig. 23.4 Angioma serpiginosum

Venous lake

Key Features

- Irregular, thin-walled, ectatic vessel
- Usually collapses after biopsy

Venous lakes are common on the lips and ears of older patients. They may appear very dark, but blanch easily when compressed.

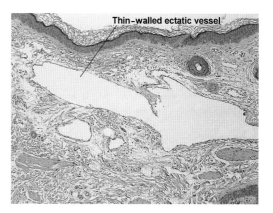

Fig. 23.5 Venous lake

Glomus tumor

Key Features

- Rows of round, dark nuclei with little cytoplasm ("string of black pearls")
- Glomus cells surround delicate vascular spaces
- Commonly tender

PEARL

- Normal glomus bodies are found on the sides of digits. A large physiologic glomus coccygeum is present in the sacral area.
- Glomus cells are modified smooth muscle cells (SMA+/CD31–).
- In general, vascular smooth muscle stains reliably with vimentin and smooth muscle actin, but not with desmin.

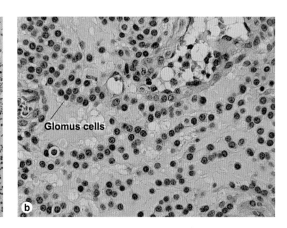

Fig. 23.6 Glomus tumor

Glomangioma

Key Features

- Commonly multiple
- One to two layers of glomus cells around prominent vessels

The vessels usually have thicker walls than the vessels in a glomus tumor. Glomangiomas have been described as vascular malformations with a few glomus cells, whereas glomus tumors have been described as tumors of glomus cells surrounding inconspicuous vessels.

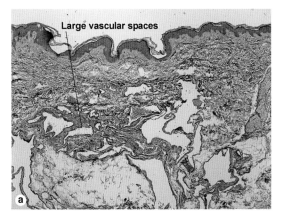

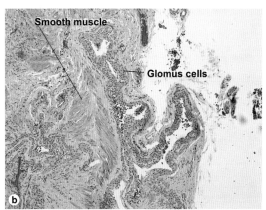

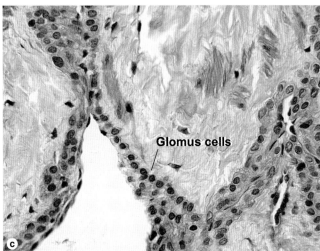

Fig. 23.7 Glomangioma

Pyogenic granuloma

Key Features

- Eruptive lobular capillary hemangioma
- Early lesions show solidly packed endothelial cells
- Later lesions show more ectatic vessels, erosion, and crusting
- Epidermal collarette common
- Commonly impetiginized on the surface

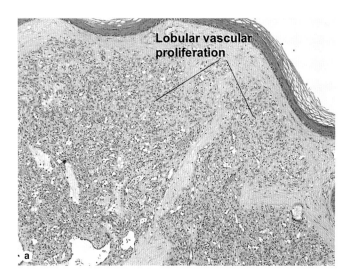

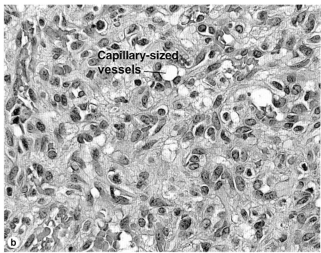

Fig. 23.8 Pyogenic granuloma

Bacillary angiomatosis

Key Features

- Usually not distinctly lobular
- Clusters of neutrophils within lesion
- Amphophilic collections of organisms

Differential Diagnosis

Pyogenic granulomas are distinctly lobular. Although surface crusting is common in pyogenic granulomas, they lack the deep clusters of neutrophils that characterize bacillary angiomatosis.

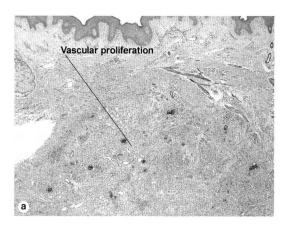

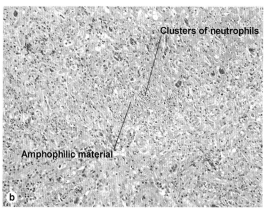

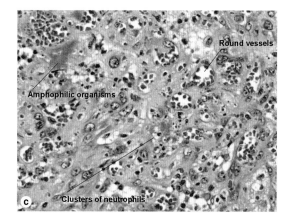

Fig. 23.9 Bacillary angiomatosis

Cherry angioma

Key Features

- Capillary hemangioma
- Pink, hyalinized vessel walls

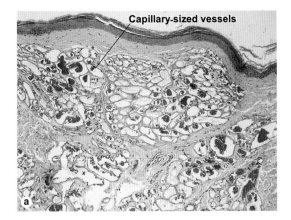

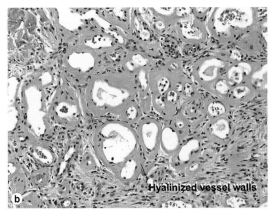

Fig. 23.10 Cherry angioma

Infantile hemangioma

Key Features

- Early lesions show solidly packed endothelial cells
- Later lesions show more ectatic vessels
- Glucose transporter 1 (GLUT1)+

Differential Diagnosis

Rapidly involuting congenital hemangioma (RICH) and noninvoluting congenital hemangioma (NICH) are fully grown at birth and are GLUT1 negative.

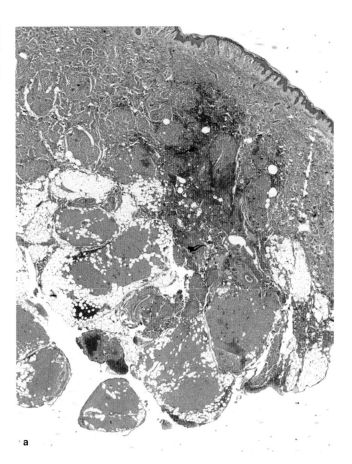

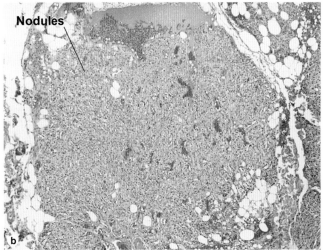

Fig. 23.11 Infantile hemangioma.

continued

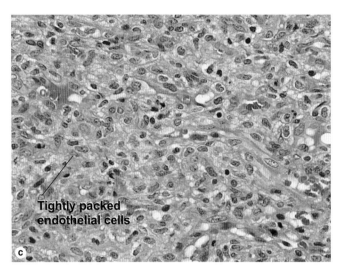

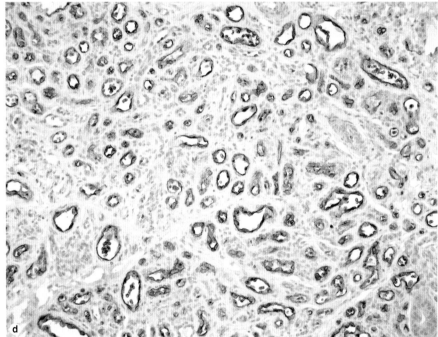

Fig. 23.11, cont'd (D) GLUT1 staining

Angiolymphoid hyperplasia with eosinophilia

Key Features

- Central thick-walled vessels with hobnail endothelium
- Peripheral proliferation of smaller vessels
- Nodular lymphoid aggregates with eosinophils

Subtypes include histiocytoid and epithelioid hemangioma. Histiocytoid endothelial cells are common.

Kimura disease

Key Features

- Lacks central thick-walled vessels with hobnail endothelium
- Deep lymphoid nodules with eosinophils
- Peripheral eosinophilia
- Elevated immunoglobulin E
- East and Southeast Asia
- Large subcutaneous lymphoid nodules
- Lymphadenopathy

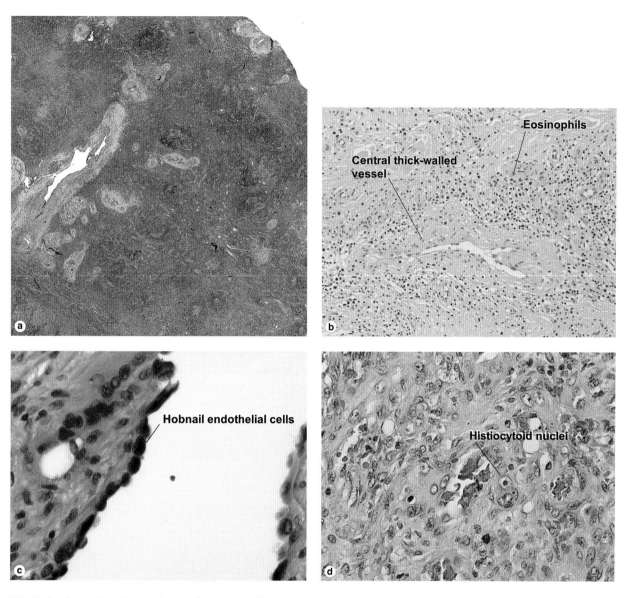

Fig. 23.12 Angiolymphoid hyperplasia with eosinophilia

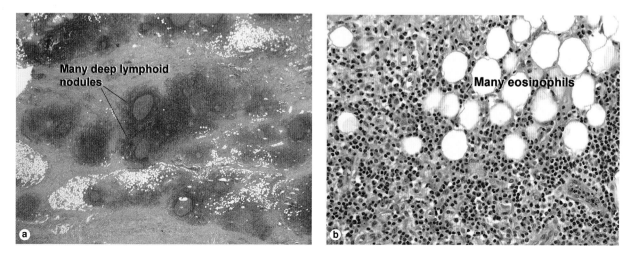

Fig. 23.13 Kimura disease (courtesy of James Fitzpatrick, MD.)

Intravascular papillary endothelial hyperplasia of Masson (IPEH)

Key Features

- Recanalizing thrombus within a vascular space
- Fibrin in thrombus
- Papillary projections with hyalinized cores

IPEH can occur in any vascular space. It is common in angiokeratomas.

Arteriovenous malformation (arteriovenous hemangioma)

Key Features

- Thick- and thin-walled vessels
- Thick-walled vessels tend to be central

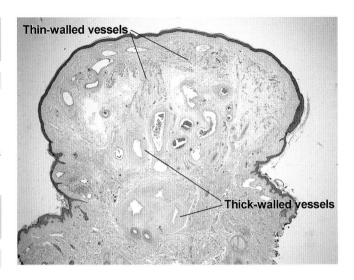

Fig. 23.15 Arteriovenous malformation

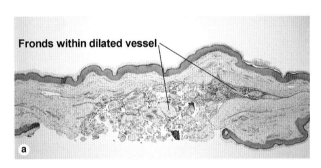

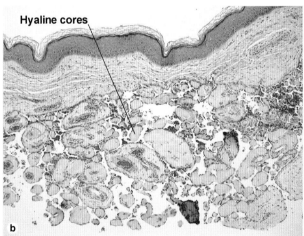

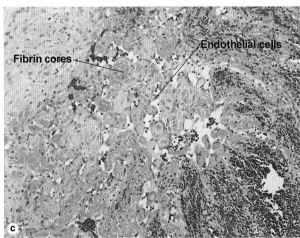

Fig. 23.14 Intravascular papillary endothelial hyperplasia

Targetoid hemosiderotic hemangioma (hobnail hemangioma)

Key Features

- Central superficial dilated vessels with hobnail nuclei
- Peripheral proliferation of small vessels
- Peripheral vascular proliferation tends to surround preexisting vessels and adnexae (like Kaposi sarcoma)
- Hemosiderin

Targetoid hemosiderotic hemangiomas probably arise as a result of trauma to a preexisting hemangioma.

Eccrine angiomatous hamartoma

Key Features

- Discrete lobules
- Each composed of capillaries, mature eccrine glands, and ducts

Usually a solitary bluish nodule. Often involves acral sites, although the example shown was on the back. May be tender.

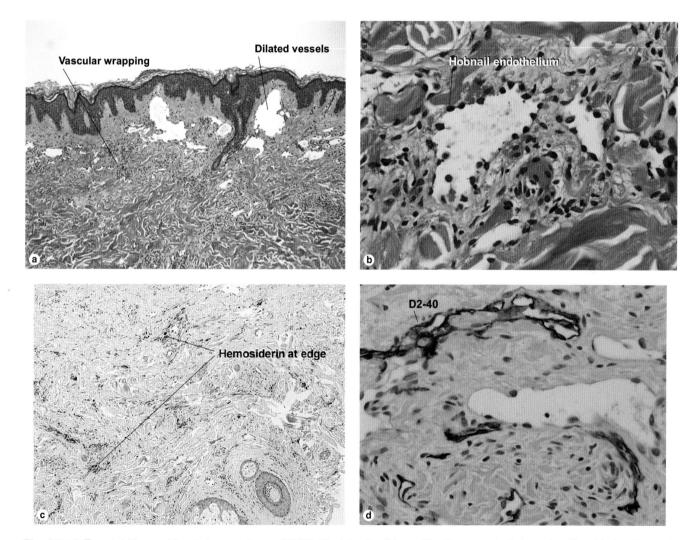

Fig. 23.16 Targetoid hemosiderotic hemangioma. **(D)** D2-40 stains the thin proliferating vessels, but not the dilated hobnail vessels

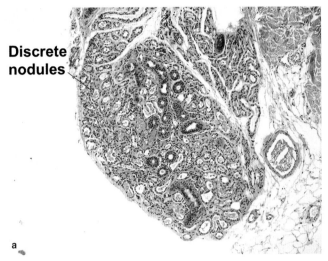

Discrete nodules

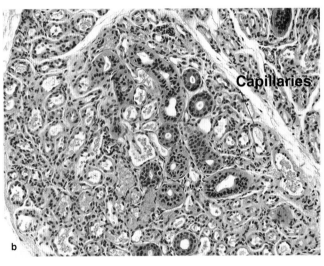

Capillaries

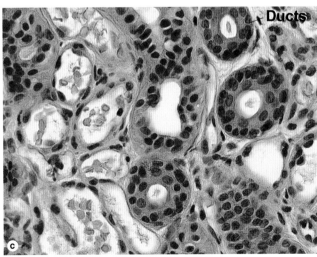

Ducts

Fig. 23.17 Eccrine angiomatous hamartoma

Glomeruloid hemangioma

Key Features

- Capillary loops within a dilated vascular space, resembling a glomerulus
- Sequestered degenerating erythrocytes

Glomeruloid hemangioma is associated with POEMS syndrome (Crow–Fukase syndrome, polyneuropathy, organomegaly, endocrinopathy, M protein, and skin changes) and Castleman disease. Two types of endothelial cell have been noted: cells with large vesicular nuclei, an open chromatin pattern, and large amount of cytoplasm, and a second population with small basal nuclei, a dense chromatin pattern, and scant cytoplasm. Lesions not associated with POEMS syndrome have been referred to as *papillary hemangioma*.

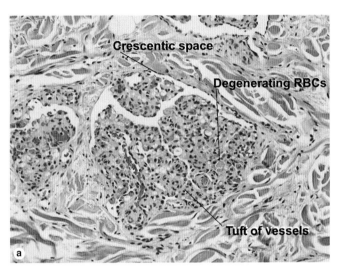

Crescentic space

Degenerating RBCs

Tuft of vessels

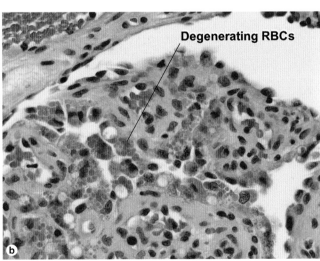

Degenerating RBCs

Fig. 23.18 Glomeruloid hemangioma

Microvenular hemangioma

Key Features

- Monomorphous, elongated blood vessels with small lumens
- Surrounding pericytes

Sometimes occurs in POEMS syndrome.

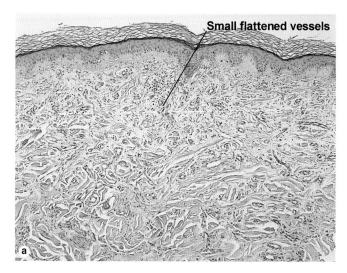

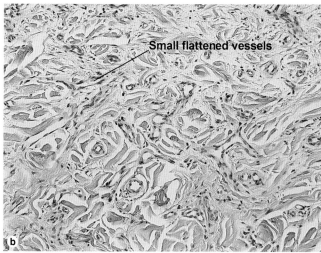

Fig. 23.19 Microvenular hemangioma

Tufted angioma (angioblastoma)

Key Features

- "Cannonball" tufts of capillary-sized vessels in the dermis
- Slowly expanding plaque clinically, often on the shoulder of a child

Differential Diagnosis

- Glomeruloid hemangioma has sequestered degenerating erythrocytes and tufts protruding into a crescentlike space
- Dermal pyogenic granuloma has fibrous septae with ropey collagen between lobules

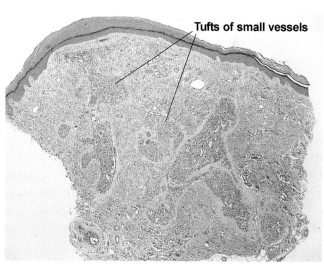

Fig. 23.20 Tufted angioma

Myopericytoma (perivascular myoid tumor)

Key Features

- Round to ovoid cells with amphophilic cytoplasm
- Concentric onion-skin–like layers surrounding vascular channels
- May have hemangiopericytoma-like staghorn vessels

Tumor cells express SMA, calponin, and caldesmon but desmin only rarely and focally. Myopericytomas have overlapping features with myofibroma, glomus tumor, hemangiopericytoma, and angioleiomyoma. The cells are larger than glomus cells with more cytoplasm.

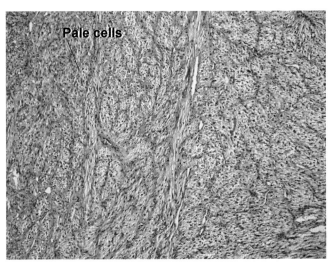

Fig. 23.22 PEComa

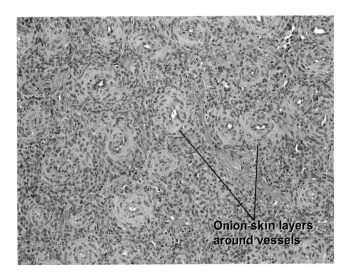

Fig. 23.21 Myopericytoma

PEComa (perivascular epithelioid cell tumor)

Key Features

- Mesenchymal tumor with perivascular clear cell and epithelioid features that coexpress melanocytic and muscle markers
- Perivascular clear cells range from epithelioid to spindled
- S100–, HMB-45+, Mart-1+

PEComas include perivascular clear cell tumors, clear cell sugar tumors, and angiomyolipomas of tuberous sclerosis. Their behavior is usually benign, although some high-grade tumors occur.

Kaposiform hemangioendothelioma

Key Features

- Large lobules
- Less well circumscribed than tufted angioma
- Involves deeper tissues
- Spindled endothelial cells
- Slitlike, cracklike, and staghorn vascular spaces
- Deep extension to soft tissue and bone

Kasabach–Merritt coagulopathy is usually associated with kaposiform hemangioendothelioma or tufted angioma, and hybrid tumors have been described.

PEARL

Kaposiform hemangioendothelioma shows CD34 staining restricted to luminal endothelial cells, tufted angiomas show a proliferation of CD34-positive endothelial cells with few actin-positive cells, and infantile hemangiomas show actin-positive cells outnumbering CD34-positive cells.

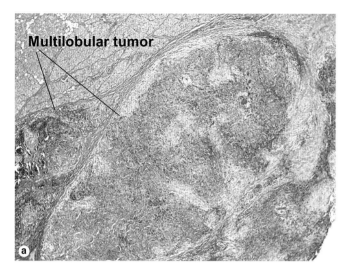

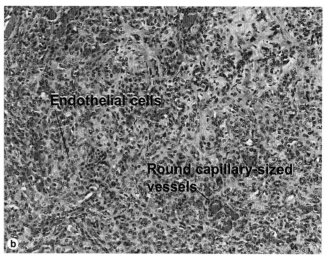

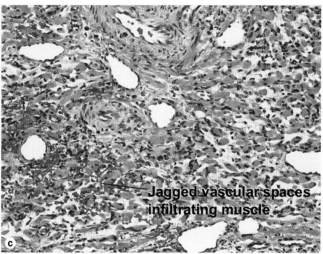

Fig. 23.23 Kaposiform hemangioendothelioma

Pleomorphic hyalinizing angiectatic tumor (PHAT)

Key Features

- Prominent dilated hyalinized vessels
- Spindle and pleomorphic cells with hyperchromatic nuclei
- Low mitotic index
- Occasional nuclear pseudoinclusions
- Hemosiderin in the cytoplasm of lesional cells

Part fibrous tumor, part vascular, PHATs are best recognized by the characteristic hyalinized vessels, so we have placed them in this chapter. PHATs are found in a wide age range (10–89 years, median 51), most commonly on the lower extremity. They often recur and have been classified as borderline neoplasms or low-grade sarcomas. PHAT is strongly positive for CD34 but negative for S100, CD31, desmin, SMA, cytokeratin, and EMA. CD99 and VEGF reactivity has been reported.

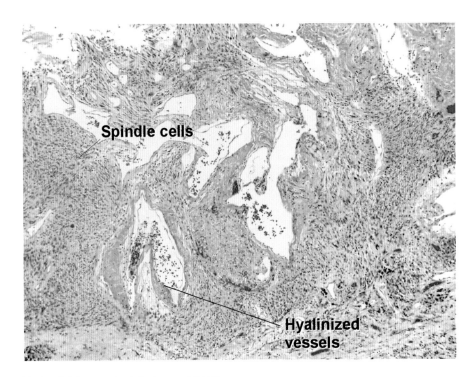

Fig. 23.24 Pleomorphic hyalinizing angiectatic tumor (PHAT)

Hemangiopericytoma

Key Features

- Endothelial-lined vessels surrounded by a proliferation of pericytes
- Concentric or curlicue pattern of spindle cells
- Staghorn ectatic vascular spaces
- Most represent examples of solitary fibrous tumor with staghorn vessels

Hemangiopericytomas occur in the skin and soft tissues. It may be difficult to distinguish between benign and malignant hemangiopericytoma histologically. Large size and higher mitotic rate suggest a malignant potential. Infantile tumors are typically cutaneous, with a good prognosis.

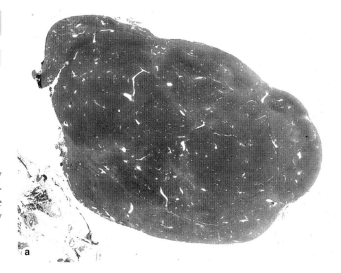

Fig. 23.25 Hemangiopericytoma

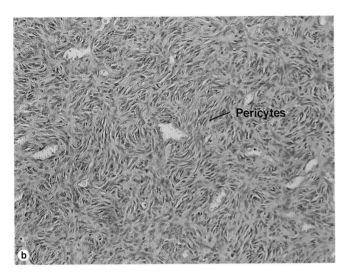

Pericytes

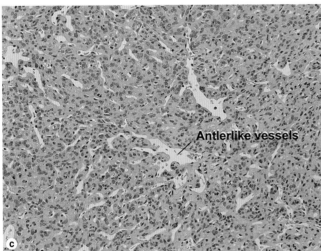

Antlerlike vessels

Fig. 23.25, cont'd

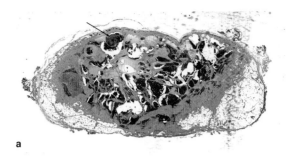

a

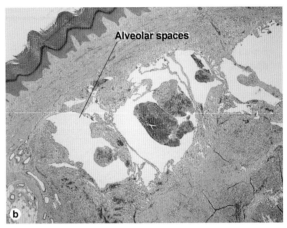

Alveolar spaces

b

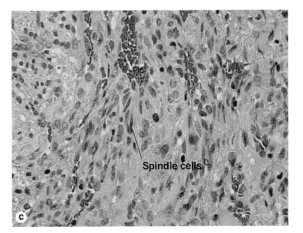

Spindle cells

c

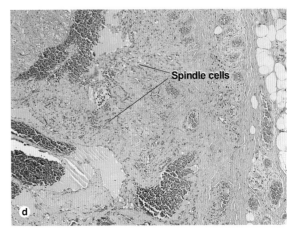

Spindle cells

d

Spindle cell hemangioma (spindle cell hemangioendothelioma)

Key Features

- At scanning power, resembles "hemorrhagic lung" with alveolar spaces
- Solid areas of spindle cells
- Phleboliths

Fig. 23.26 Spindle cell hemangioendothelioma. **(A)** Arrow points to phlebolith

Epithelioid hemangioendothelioma

Key Features

- Dilated vascular channels with solid epithelioid and spindle cell areas
- Intracytoplasmic lumens
- Variable pleomorphism and mitotic activity

Epithelioid hemangioendotheliomas tend to occur on the extremities of young people. They are best regarded as low-grade malignancies.

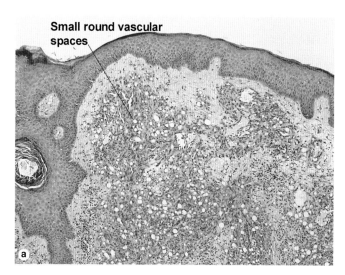

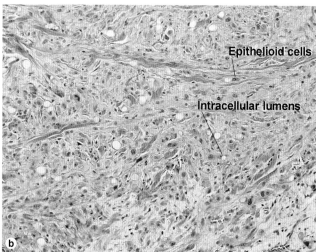

Fig. 23.27 Epithelioid hemangioendothelioma

Retiform hemangioendothelioma

Key Features

- Arborizing blood vessels reminiscent of rete testis

Retiform hemangioendothelioma is a low-grade angiosarcoma that occurs mostly on the extremities of young adults.

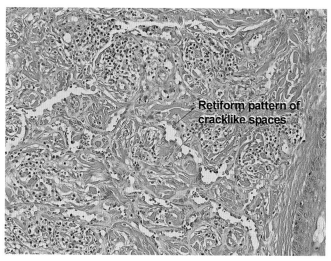

Fig. 23.28 Retiform hemangioendothelioma

Angiosarcoma

Key Features

- Cracklike spaces between collagen bundles
- Spaces lined by hyperchromatic endothelial cells
- Nodular areas commonly epithelioid with more pronounced atypia

Angiosarcomas typically appear as bruiselike lesions on the forehead or scalp of an older patient. Epithelioid variants may be nodular. Stewart–Treves syndrome is angiosarcoma in the setting of a lymphedematous limb. Often, there is a history of radiation therapy.

PEARL

Immunostaining for angiosarcoma:
- Factor VIII (unreliable)
- CD34 (clean stain, little background, not specific)
- CD31 (very specific, but background staining common)
- ERG-1 (nuclear stain)
- *Ulex europaeus* lectin (clean staining, marks endothelium and epithelium)
- D2-40 (stains lymphatic vessels, most angiosarcomas, and most tumors associated with Kasabach–Merritt syndrome)
- MYC is amplified in postradiation angiosarcoma, but not in atypical vascular lesion (AVL) occurring after radiation therapy.

Differential Diagnosis

Diffuse dermal angiomatosis is an acquired benign vascular proliferation in response to stasis or ischemia. It occurs in association with arteriovenous fistulae or in large pendulous breasts. The patients are often heavy smokers. It is characterized by poorly circumscribed, violaceous plaques with frequent ulceration. New vessels dissect between collagen bundles, but atypia and mitoses are absent.

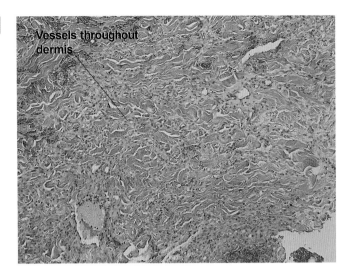

Fig. 23.30 Diffuse dermal angiomatosis

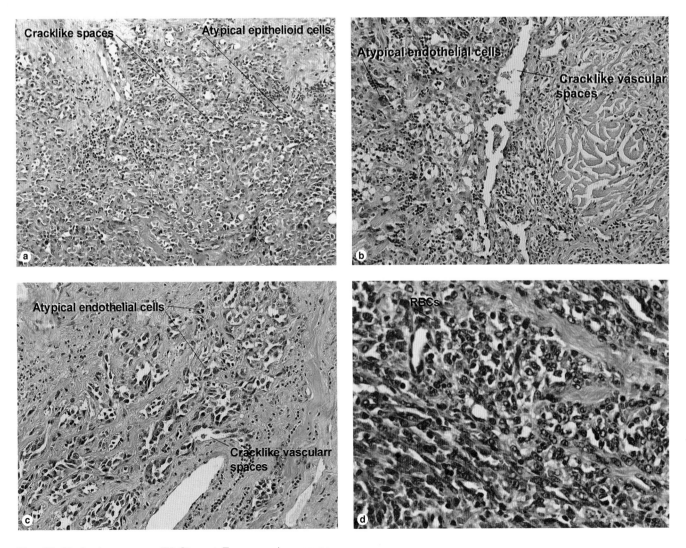

Fig. 23.29 Angiosarcoma. **(D)** Stewart–Treves angiosarcoma

Atypical vascular lesion (AVL)

Key Features

- Proliferation of thin-walled, irregular to stag-horn vessels, with minimal anastomosis, and a single layer of non–atypical-appearing endothelial cells
- Generally limited to the dermis

Atypical vascular lesion is generally located on the breast and appears several years after irradiation. Clinically, the lesions are initially small, purple-pink to red-brown, multifocal papules that are well circumscribed histopathologically. Although initially described as benign (acquired progressive lymphangioma or benign lymphangiomatous papules of the skin), many authors now consider these lesions to be potential precursors of angiosarcoma. Thus, close clinical follow-up or sometimes complete excision has been recommended. Amplification of MYC suggests a diagnosis of angiosarcoma rather than AVL. Angiosarcoma shows deeper, infiltrative involvement of the dermis with anastomosing vessels, cytologic atypia, and multilayering of endothelial cells.

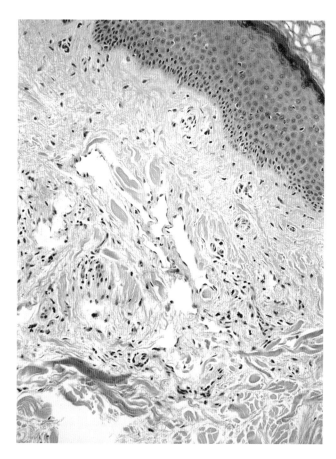

Fig. 23.31 Atypical vascular lesion

Kaposi sarcoma

Key Features

- HHV-8 associated
- Patch, plaque, and tumor stages

Early-patch-stage Kaposi sarcoma

Key Features

- Bizarre staghorn, ectatic, lymphatic-like vessels
- Plasma cells

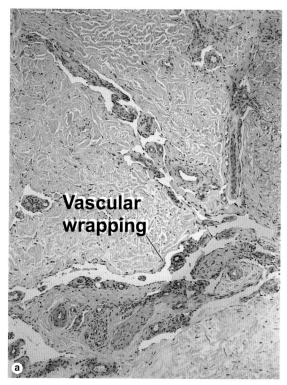

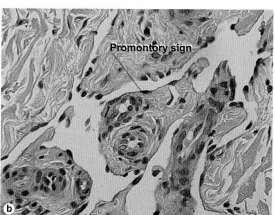

Fig. 23.32 Early-patch Kaposi sarcoma

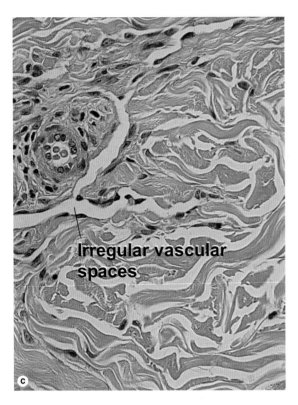

Fig. 23.32, cont'd

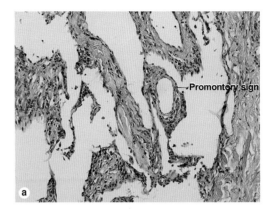

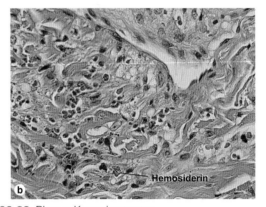

Fig. 23.33 Plaque Kaposi sarcoma

Later-patch/plaque Kaposi sarcoma

Key Features

- Busy dermis surrounding adnexal structures and preexisting vessels
- Pale appearance of busy area (appears understained)
- Promontory sign

Plaque lesions of Kaposi sarcoma are characterized by "vascular wrapping." New vessels wrap and surround preexisting vascular and adnexal structures. The preexisting structure commonly protrudes into a lakelike ectatic space (promontory sign).

Nodular Kaposi sarcoma

Key Features

- Nodule composed of fascicles of parallel spindle cells
- Erythrocytes between spindle cells
- Eosinophilic globules
- Mitoses
- Hemosiderin

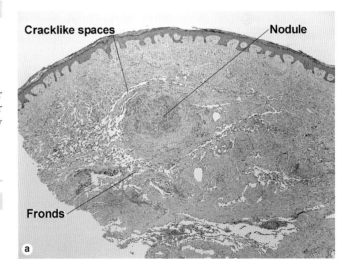

Fig. 23.34 (A-B) Nodular Kaposi sarcoma.

continued

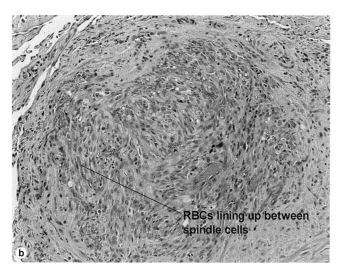

RBCs lining up between spindle cells

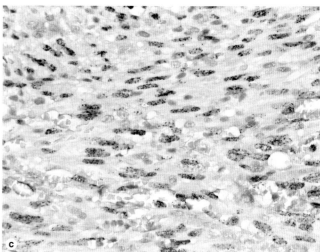

Fig. 23.34, cont'd (C) HHV-8 immunostain

Further reading

Alvarez-Mendoza A, Lourdes TS, Ridaura-Sanz C, et al. Histopathology of vascular lesions found in Kasabach-Merritt syndrome: review based on 13 cases. Pediatr Dev Pathol 2000;3(6):556–60.

Ayturk UM, Couto JA, Hann S, et al. Somatic activating mutations in GNAQ and GNA11 are associated with congenital hemangioma. Am J Hum Genet 2016;98(4):789–95.

Berenguer B, Mulliken JB, Enjolras O, et al. Rapidly involuting congenital hemangioma: clinical and histopathologic features. Pediatr Dev Pathol 2003;6(6):495–510.

Billings SD, Folpe AL, Weiss SW. Epithelioid sarcoma-like hemangioendothelioma. Am J Surg Pathol 2003;27(1):48–57.

Chu CY, Hsiao CH, Chiu HC. Transformation between Kaposiform hemangioendothelioma and tufted angioma. Dermatology 2003;206(4):334–7.

Kishimoto S, Takenaka H, Shibagaki R, et al. Glomeruloid hemangioma in POEMS syndrome shows two different immunophenotypic endothelial cells. J Cutan Pathol 2000;27(2):87–92.

Liu Q, Jiang L, Wu D, et al. Clinicopathological features of Kaposiform hemangioendothelioma. Int J Clin Exp Pathol 2015;8(10):13711–18. eCollection 2015.

Mentzel T, Partanen TA, Kutzner H. Hobnail hemangioma ("targetoid hemosiderotic hemangioma"): clinicopathologic and immunohistochemical analysis of 62 cases. J Cutan Pathol 1999;26(6):279–86.

Nayler SJ, Rubin BP, Calonje E, et al. Composite hemangioendothelioma: a complex, low-grade vascular lesion mimicking angiosarcoma. Am J Surg Pathol 2000;24(3):352–61.

Reis-Filho JS, Paiva ME, Lopes JM. Congenital composite hemangioendothelioma: case report and reappraisal of the hemangioendothelioma spectrum. J Cutan Pathol 2002;29(4):226–31.

Requena L, Kutzner H. Hemangioendothelioma. Semin Diagn Pathol 2013;30(1):29–44.

Requena L, Sangueza OP. Cutaneous vascular neoplasms. Part II. J Am Acad Dermatol 1997;37:887.

Requena L, Sangueza OP. Cutaneous vascular neoplasms. Part III. J Am Acad Dermatol 1998;38:143.

Sangüeza OP. Update on vascular neoplasms. Dermatol Clin 2012;30(4):657–65.

Cutaneous T-cell lymphoma, NK-cell lymphoma, and myeloid leukemia

David J. DiCaudo

Cutaneous T-cell lymphoma and NK-cell lymphoma

Mycosis fungoides

Patch stage

Key Features

- Lymphocytes "line up" along the dermal–epidermal junction (simulates vacuolar interface dermatitis, with a "lymphocyte in every hole")
- Large dark lymphocytes with irregular nuclear contours and perinuclear haloes ("lump of coal on a pillow")
- Pautrier microabscesses (intraepidermal clusters of atypical lymphocytes, larger than the benign recruited dermal lymphocytes)
- Mild bandlike infiltrate in superficial dermis
- Sclerosis of the papillary dermis
- Eosinophils and necrotic keratinocytes are rarely present

Mycosis fungoides (MF) is the most common type of cutaneous lymphoma. In most cases, the disease is indolent and slowly progressive over a period of years or decades. Three main stages of the lymphoma are recognized: patch, plaque, and tumor. In the patch stage of MF, patients typically present with broad pink or tan, oval-shaped patches with a predilection for the bathing trunk area. The patches may be asymptomatic or pruritic. Both clinically and histopathologically, distinction from eczematous dermatitis is sometimes difficult in the earliest stages of the lymphoma. In the evaluation of patch-stage MF, multiple shave biopsies are often helpful, because the shave technique provides a broad area of epidermis for examination. The typical immunophenotype is CD3+, CD4+, CD8–, CD30–. Aberrant immunophenotypes (with loss of normal T-cell markers, such as CD7) can frequently be demonstrated. Clonal rearrangement of the T-cell receptor gene is helpful in supporting the diagnosis, although the earliest cases may sometimes not have a detectable clone.

Differential Diagnosis

- Dermatitis generally has more spongiosis and fewer intraepidermal lymphocytes.
- Lichenoid drug eruption typically has more apoptotic keratinocytes and eosinophils.
- Lymphomatoid drug eruption may look nearly identical. Pautrier microabscesses favor MF.

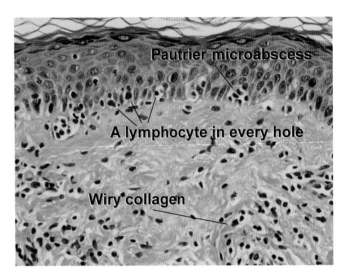

Fig. 24.1 Patch-stage mycosis fungoides

Table 24.1 Mature T and NK neoplasms characteristically involving the skin in the 2016 revision of the WHO classification of lymphoid neoplasms.

Mycosis fungoides
Sézary syndrome
Adult T-cell leukemia/lymphoma
Primary cutaneous CD30+ T-cell lymphoproliferative disorders
    Lymphomatoid papulosis
    Primary cutaneous anaplastic large cell lymphoma
Subcutaneous panniculitis-like T-cell lymphoma
Extranodal NK/T-cell lymphoma, nasal type
Peripheral T-cell lymphoma, NOS
Primary cutaneous aggressive epidermotropic CD8+ cytotoxic T-cell lymphoma*
Primary cutaneous gamma–delta T-cell lymphoma
Primary cutaneous CD4+ small/medium T-cell lymphoproliferative disorder*
Follicular T-cell lymphoma*
Angioimmunoblastic T-cell lymphoma
Primary cutaneous acral CD8+ T-cell lymphoma*
Hydroa vacciniforme-like lymphoproliferative disorder

*Asterisk indicates provisional entities.
Data from Swerdlow SH, Campo E, Pileri SA, et al. The 2016 revision of the World Health Organization classification of lymphoid neoplasms. Blood. 2016;127(20):2375–2390.*

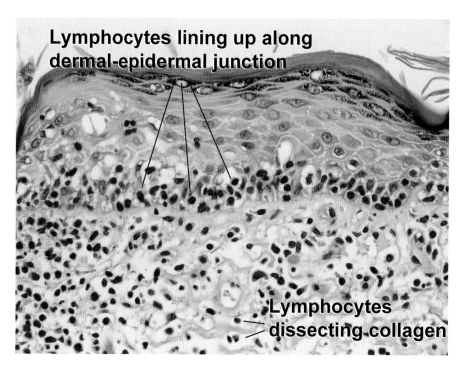

Fig. 24.2 Patch-stage mycosis fungoides

Plaque stage

Key Features

- Like patch stage, but with a denser, bandlike infiltrate in the upper dermis
- Atypical lymphocytes present in the dermal band

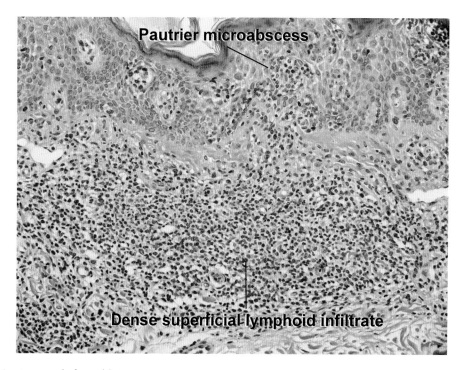

Fig. 24.3 Plaque-stage mycosis fungoides

Tumor stage

Key Features

- Dense, nodular lymphocytic infiltrate in the superficial and deep dermis
- Many atypical lymphocytes present in the dermal infiltrate

- Transformation to large-sized lymphocytes in some cases
- Acquisition of CD30 expression in some cases
- Loss of epidermotropism with progression

Over time, patients with MF may progress to develop thicker plaques and tumors. Whereas patch-stage MF is usually associated with long survival, the prognosis is poorer for those patients who progress to the tumor stage.

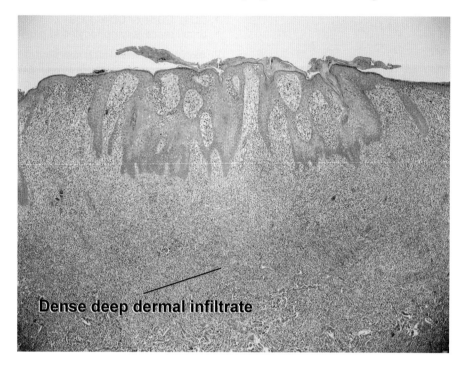

Fig. 24.4 Tumor-stage mycosis fungoides

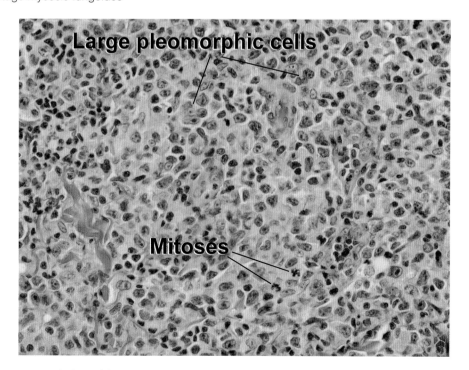

Fig. 24.5 Tumor-stage mycosis fungoides

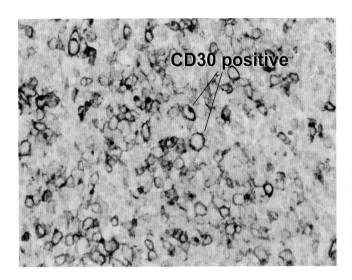

Fig. 24.6 Tumor-stage mycosis fungoides

Pagetoid reticulosis variant

Key Features

- Solitary or multiple patches or plaques on distal extremities
- Atypical large lymphocytes extensively infiltrating the epidermis
- CD3+
- CD4+ CD8− or CD4− CD8+
- Small reactive lymphocytes in papillary dermis

The term *pagetoid reticulosis* is now limited to the Woringer–Kolopp type, which presents as one or several patches or plaques on the distal extremities. This type of lymphoma is associated with an excellent prognosis. The disseminated Ketron–Goodman type of pagetoid reticulosis has been reclassified into several other types of cutaneous T-cell lymphoma.

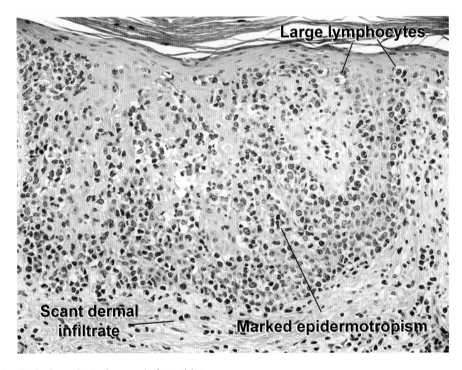

Fig. 24.7 Pagetoid reticulosis variant of mycosis fungoides

Folliculotropic variant

Key Features

- Atypical lymphocytes infiltrate the follicular epithelium
- Basaloid induction and hyperplasia of follicular epithelium
- Eosinophils common
- *Follicular mucinosis* (pools of mucin in the follicular epithelium)
- Epidermis usually spared
- CD3+, CD4+, and CD8− in most cases

The folliculotropic variant of MF presents with follicular papules and boggy plaques, most frequently involving the head and neck. Follicular mucinosis is often present. Folliculotropic MF is generally associated with earlier progression than conventional MF.

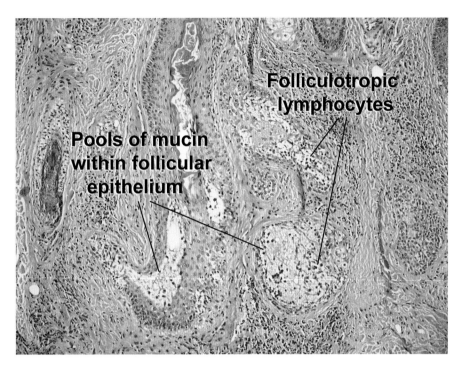

Fig. 24.8 Folliculotropic variant of mycosis fungoides

Granulomatous slack skin

Key Features

- Pendulous folds in intertriginous regions
- Preceded by insidious onset of patches, papules, and plaques
- Massive dermal and subcutaneous infiltrate ± epidermal involvement
- Small T lymphocytes with epidermotropism and mild cytologic atypia
- Huge multinucleate giant cells with numerous nuclei, often in wreathlike arrangement
- Phagocytosis of lymphocytes by multinucleate cells
- Dermal edema or fibrosis
- Loss of dermal elastic tissue fibers
- CD3+, CD4+, and CD8− immunophenotype

Granulomatous slack skin syndrome is an extremely rare variant of MF with a slowly progressive clinical course. The clinical presentation is striking. In fully developed cases, massive folds of skin extend from flexural areas, such as the axillae or groin. An association with nodal Hodgkin lymphoma has been documented in multiple cases.

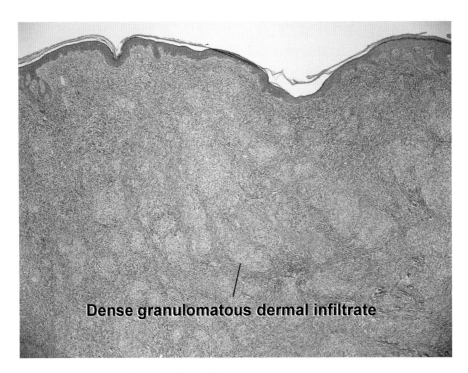

Fig. 24.9 Granulomatous slack skin variant of mycosis fungoides

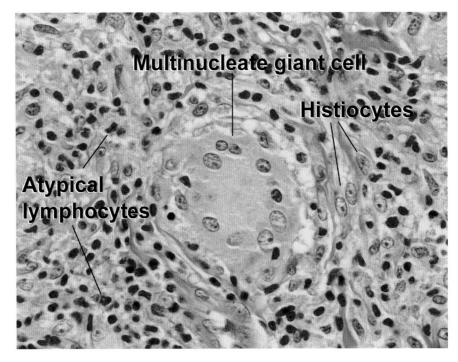

Fig. 24.10 Granulomatous slack skin variant of mycosis fungoides

Sézary syndrome

Key Features

- Erythroderma with generalized pruritus
- Palmoplantar keratoderma
- Generalized lymphadenopathy
- Peripheral blood Sézary cell count of ≥1000 cells/microliter
- Peripheral blood lymphocytes with aberrant phenotype or CD4/CD8 ratio >10
- Clonal rearrangement of T-cell receptor genes in blood and/or skin
- Histopathology like MF, or may show only nonspecific dermatitis

Although previously believed to be a leukemic variant of MF, Sézary syndrome is now considered to originate from a different subset of T cells (central memory T cell in Sézary syndrome versus skin resident memory T cell in MF). In contrast to MF, Sézary syndrome has a rapidly progressive clinical course and a poor prognosis. The diagnosis is confirmed by evaluation of the peripheral blood. Skin biopsy is sometimes useful in demonstrating a histopathologic pattern similar to MF. It should be recognized, however, that skin biopsy findings may be nondiagnostic in some cases of Sézary syndrome. In an erythrodermic patient, nonspecific biopsy findings (such as spongiotic dermatitis) do not exclude the diagnosis. It is important to evaluate the peripheral blood if there is clinical suspicion for Sézary syndrome.

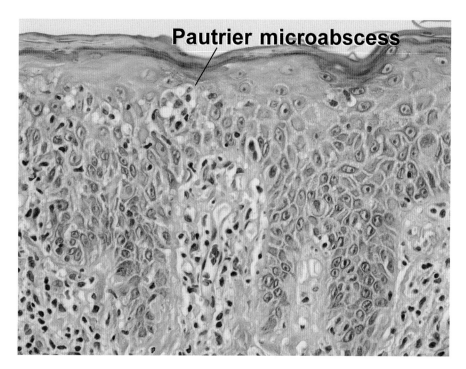

Pautrier microabscess

Fig. 24.11 Sézary syndrome

Adult T-cell leukemia/lymphoma (ATCLL)

Key Features

- Endemic in Japan, Caribbean, southeastern United States, and central Africa
- Hypercalcemia
- Osteolytic bone lesions
- Organomegaly
- Lymphadenopathy
- Dermal and/or subcutaneous lymphoid infiltrates
- T cells with multilobed nuclei
- Epidermotropism in some cases
- CD3+, CD4+, CD8–, and CD25+ neoplastic cell population in blood, nodes, and skin
- Peripheral blood flower cells with multilobed nuclei
- Clonal integration of the HTLV-1 genome within neoplastic cells
- Clonal rearrangement of T-cell receptor genes

Adult T-cell leukemia/lymphoma is remarkable for its well-established viral etiology, that is, human T-cell leukemia virus type 1 (HTLV-1). HTLV-1 infection is transmitted by sexual contact, blood transfusion, and mother-to-child vertical transmission. In areas with the highest rates of HTLV-1 infection, such as southwestern Japan, only a relatively small percentage of infected individuals eventually develop the lymphoma or leukemia. ATCLL may occur as an acute or smoldering disease. The skin is involved in up to 50% of patients. Nodules, papules, and plaques may occur. The most specific diagnostic finding is the clonal integration of the HTLV-1 genome within lymphoma cells. This feature is helpful in distinguishing the smoldering variant of ATCLL from MF.

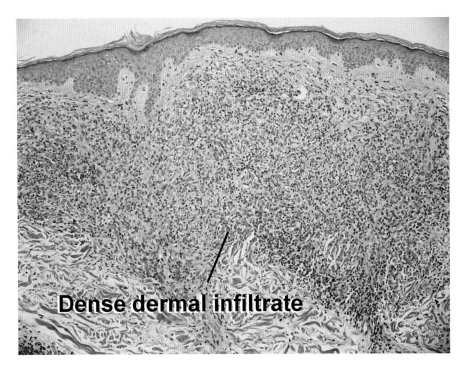

Fig. 24.12 Adult T-cell leukemia/lymphoma

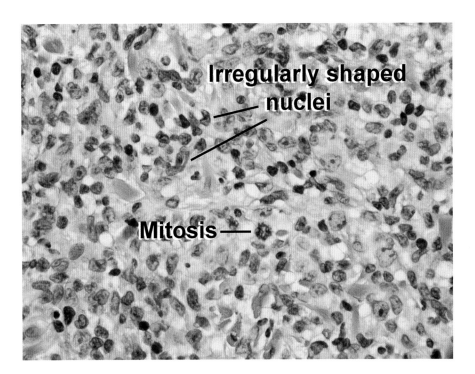

Fig. 24.13 Adult T-cell leukemia/lymphoma

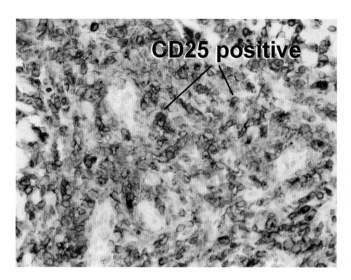

Fig. 24.14 Adult T-cell leukemia/lymphoma

Primary cutaneous CD30+ lymphoproliferative disorders

Lymphomatoid papulosis

Key Features

Type A
- Wedge-shaped dermal infiltrate with mixed population of cells
- CD30+ Reed–Sternberg-like cells with large nuclei, prominent nucleoli, and abundant cytoplasm
- Neutrophils, eosinophils, and small lymphocytes in background

Type B
- Epidermotropic infiltrate of CD3+ small lymphocytes, often CD30–

Type C
- Diffuse sheets of CD30+ Reed–Sternberg-like cells in dermis

Type D
- Markedly epidermotropic CD8+ and CD30+ lymphocytes, often TIA-1+ or granzyme B+

Type E
- Angioinvasive CD30+, Beta F1+ lymphocytes, often CD8+ and/or TIA-1+

LyP with chromosomal rearrangement of *DUSP22-IRF4* on 6p25.3
- Biphasic pattern
- Small cerebriform lymphocytes infiltrating epidermis

- Larger atypical lymphocytes forming dense nodule in dermis
- CD30 strongly and diffusely positive in dermis; weakly positive in epidermis
- Fluorescence in situ hybridization (FISH) confirms 6p25.3 rearrangement at *DUSP22-IRF4* locus

Clinicopathologic correlation is particularly important in the diagnosis of lymphomatoid papulosis (LyP). Patients present with crops of ulcerated nodules and papules most frequently involving the trunk and limbs. Lesions regress spontaneously, while new lesions erupt at other sites. Different lesions from an individual patient may simultaneously demonstrate a single or multiple histologic subtypes. Type A is the most common and characteristic type of LyP.

LyP is a spontaneously regressing lymphoproliferative disorder. Clonal rearrangement of the T-cell receptor genes is detectable in many cases. LyP itself is a nonfatal disease, but it can be associated with other more aggressive lymphoproliferative disorders. In 10%–20% of cases, it is associated with MF, cutaneous or systemic anaplastic large cell lymphoma, or Hodgkin lymphoma. These associated lymphomas may precede, accompany, or follow the diagnosis of LyP.

Differential Diagnosis

Type B LyP may histologically mimic MF. The clinical features distinguish the two entities. Spontaneously regressing papules or nodules favor LyP. Persistent patches or plaques favor MF.

Type C LyP may be histologically indistinguishable from anaplastic large cell lymphoma (ALCL). Crops of spontaneously regressing papules or nodules favor LyP. Persistent, solitary, or localized nodules or tumors favor ALCL. The two are closely related and may in fact represent a spectrum of a single disorder.

Type D LyP histologically mimics primary cutaneous aggressive epidermotropic CD8+ cytotoxic T-cell lymphoma, but is CD30+ and has the typical course of LyP with crops of self-resolving ulcerative papulonodules.

Type E LyP histologically mimics extranodal NK/T-cell lymphoma, nasal type, which is similarly angioinvasive and angiodestructive. The two entities are distinguished by the clinical course and the presence or absence of Epstein–Barr virus (EBV) within the tumor cells. NK/T-cell lymphoma has an aggressive clinical course; lesions of type E LyP regress spontaneously. The tumor cells of NK/T-cell lymphoma are EBV positive by in situ hybridization and usually CD56 positive by immunohistochemistry; the cells of type E LyP are EBV negative and usually CD56 negative.

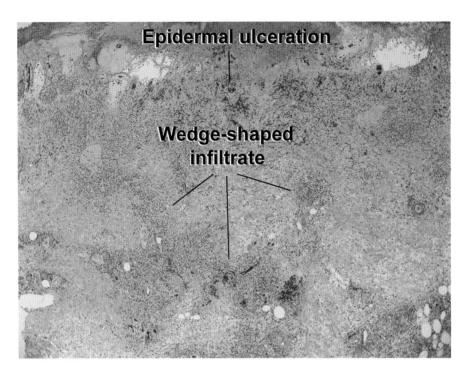

Fig. 24.15 Lymphomatoid papulosis

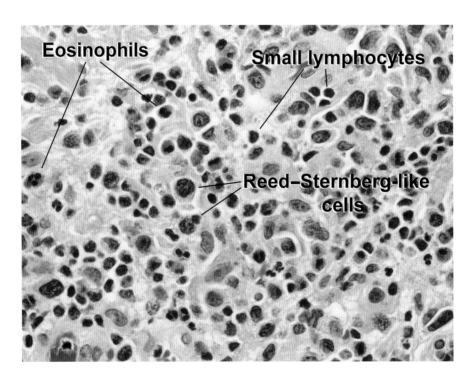

Fig. 24.16 Lymphomatoid papulosis, type A

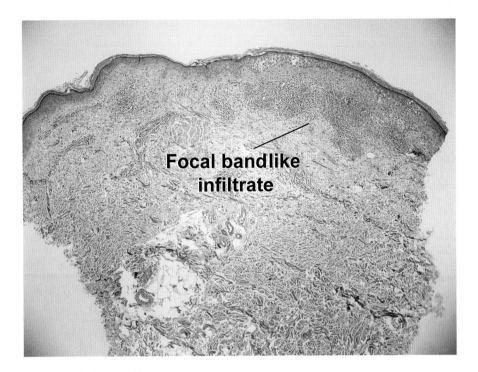

Fig. 24.17 Lymphomatoid papulosis, type B

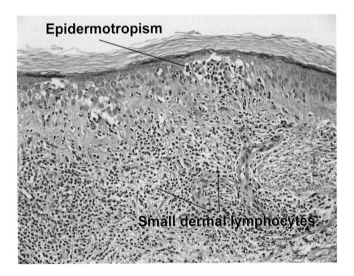

Fig. 24.18 Lymphomatoid papulosis, type B

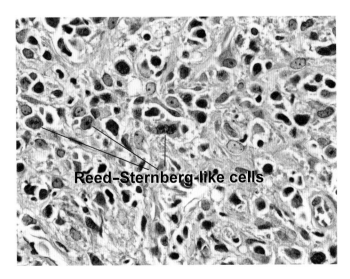

Fig. 24.19 Lymphomatoid papulosis, type C

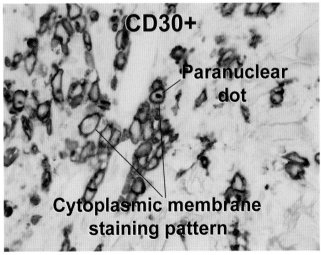

Fig. 24.20 Lymphomatoid papulosis

Primary cutaneous anaplastic large cell lymphoma

Key Features

- Sheets of large Reed–Sternberg-like cells in dermis ± subcutaneous fat
- Reactive small lymphocytes, histiocytes, and eosinophils variably present in background
- CD30 expression by >75% of large cells in infiltrate

Primary cutaneous ALCL most often presents with solitary or localized tumors or nodules. Spontaneous regression occasionally occurs. Extracutaneous dissemination is uncommon. The prognosis is generally favorable with 5-year survival rates of ≥90%.

Differential Diagnosis

ALCL may also originate in lymph nodes and spread secondarily to the skin. By routine microscopy, primary cutaneous ALCL is virtually indistinguishable from nodal ALCL. The distinction is important because nodal ALCL has a much worse prognosis. Immunohistochemistry can provide useful clues to distinguish the two. Nodal ALCL has a chromosomal translocation t(2;5), which results in expression of anaplastic lymphoma–related tyrosine kinase (ALK-1). ALK-1 expression can be demonstrated by immunohistochemistry in most cases of nodal ALCL, but ALK-1 is generally absent in primary cutaneous ALCL. Nevertheless, staging is mandatory in all cases and is ultimately more important than immunohistochemistry in distinguishing primary cutaneous ALCL from its nodal counterpart.

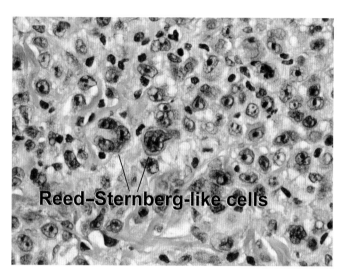

Fig. 24.22 Primary cutaneous anaplastic large cell lymphoma

Subcutaneous panniculitis-like T-cell lymphoma

Key Features

- Lacelike pattern of infiltration in the fat
- No significant involvement of the dermis or epidermis
- Variable cytologic atypia, minimal to marked
- Cytophagocytosis: beanbag cells—macrophages filled with karyorrhectic debris
- CD8+ and Ki67+ T-cells rimming the individual adipocytes
- T-cell receptor beta (Beta F1) immunostain+, T-cell receptor delta immunostain–
- Cytotoxic phenotype: granzyme B+, TIA-1+, and perforin+

Patients with subcutaneous panniculitis-like T-cell lymphoma (SPTCL) typically present with deep indurated nodules and plaques. The legs are a common site of involvement. Survival rates are approximately 80% at 5 years. SPTCL is sometimes associated with a potentially fatal hemophagocytic syndrome, consisting of pancytopenia, hepatosplenomegaly, and fever. In hemophagocytic syndrome, blood cells are engulfed by macrophages in the bone marrow and lymphoid organs.

Differential Diagnosis

Lupus panniculitis may be very difficult to distinguish from early SPTCL. Interface vacuolization, dermal mucin, and hyaline necrosis are all typical of lupus panniculitis but may sometimes be seen in SPTCL. Rimming of adipocytes by CD8+ and Ki67+ T cells is characteristic of SPTCL and is helpful in the distinction from lupus panniculitis. Clonal rearrangement of T-cell receptor genes also generally supports the diagnosis of SPTCL. Nevertheless, definitive diagnosis may be challenging in some cases, and rare reports in the literature describe well-documented cases of lupus panniculitis that have later apparently evolved to SPTCL.

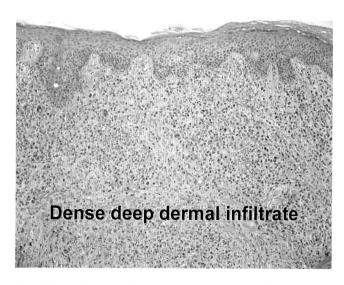

Fig. 24.21 Primary cutaneous anaplastic large cell lymphoma

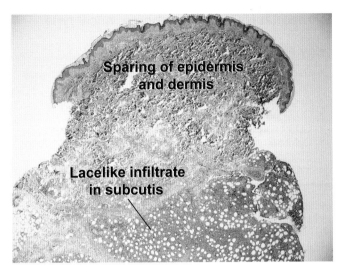

Fig. 24.23 Subcutaneous panniculitis-like T-cell lymphoma

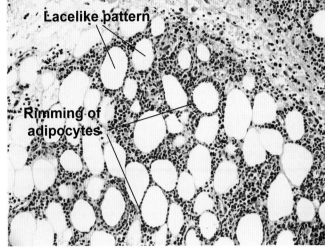

Fig. 24.24 Subcutaneous panniculitis-like T-cell lymphoma

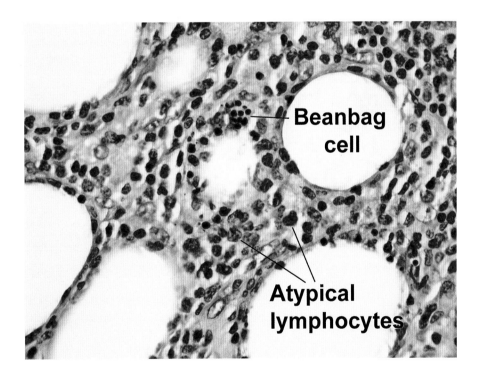

Fig. 24.25 Subcutaneous panniculitis-like T-cell lymphoma

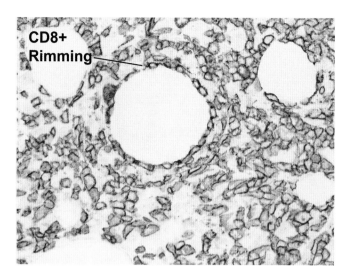

Fig. 24.26 Subcutaneous panniculitis-like T-cell lymphoma

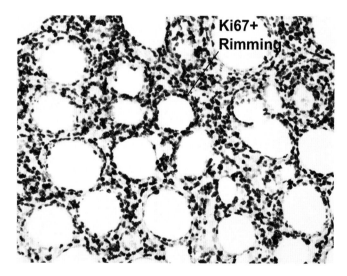

Fig. 24.27 Subcutaneous panniculitis-like T-cell lymphoma

Extranodal NK/T-cell lymphoma, nasal type

Key Features

- Dense lymphoid infiltrates in dermis and subcutaneous fat ± epidermis
- Angiocentricity, angiodestruction, and zonal necrosis
- CD2+ and CD3epsilon+, usually CD56+ (NK-cell marker)
- CD3 expression variable
- Cytotoxic phenotype: granzyme B+, TIA-1+, and perforin+
- EBV detected within lymphoma cells by in situ hybridization

Extranodal NK/T-cell lymphoma, nasal type (ENKTCL), develops within the nasal cavity or skin. It is most commonly seen in Asia and Latin America. The nasal cavity and palate can be infiltrated and destroyed by the lymphoma. Cases previously described as lethal midline granuloma included some examples of ENKTCL. This lymphoma is associated with an aggressive clinical course. Hemophagocytic syndrome occurs in a subset of patients. In most cases, no clonal rearrangement of the T-cell receptor can be demonstrated. The oncogenic role of EBV is an important feature of this lymphoma.

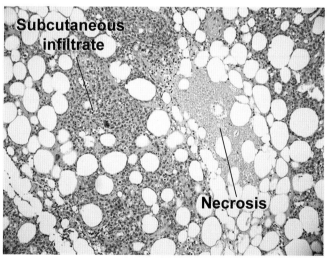

Fig. 24.28 Extranodal NK/T-cell lymphoma, nasal type

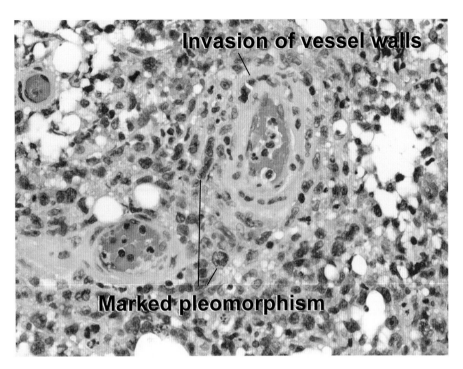

Fig. 24.29 Extranodal NK/T-cell lymphoma, nasal type

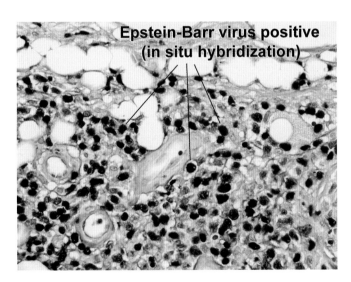

Fig. 24.30 Extranodal NK/T-cell lymphoma, nasal type

Primary cutaneous peripheral T-cell lymphoma, NOS

Peripheral T-cell lymphoma, NOS (not otherwise specified), is a heterogeneous category of lymphomas. Several distinctive, cutaneous variants of peripheral T-cell lymphoma are recognized, as described in the following sections.

Primary cutaneous aggressive epidermotropic CD8+ cytotoxic T-cell lymphoma (provisional entity)

Key Features

- Bandlike, lichenoid lymphoid infiltrate with marked epidermotropism
- Beta F1+, CD3+, and CD8+
- Cytotoxic phenotype: granzyme B+, TIA-1+, and perforin+

Primary cutaneous aggressive epidermotropic CD8+ T-cell lymphoma presents with patches, papules, nodules, or tumors. Ulceration and hemorrhage are frequent. As the name implies, the clinical course is rapidly progressive.

Differential Diagnosis

Distinguished from pagetoid reticulosis and type D LyP by the clinical features, especially the aggressive clinical course.

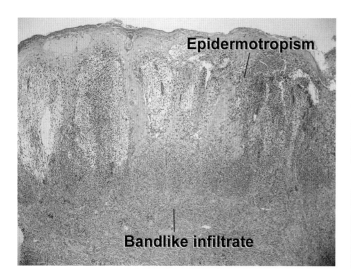

Epidermotropism

Bandlike infiltrate

Fig. 24.31 Primary cutaneous aggressive epidermotropic CD8+ cytotoxic T-cell lymphoma

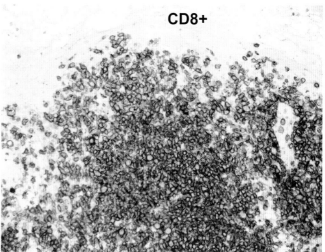

CD8+

CD8+

Fig. 24.33 Primary cutaneous aggressive epidermotropic CD8+ cytotoxic T-cell lymphoma

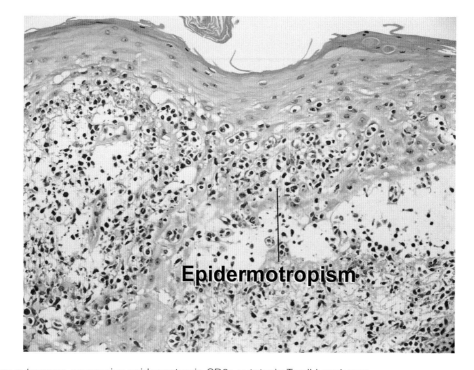

Epidermotropism

Fig. 24.32 Primary cutaneous aggressive epidermotropic CD8+ cytotoxic T-cell lymphoma

Primary cutaneous gamma–delta T-cell lymphoma

Key Features

- Location of infiltrate: subcutaneous, dermal, epidermal
- T-cell receptor delta immunostain+, T-cell receptor beta (Beta F1) immunostain−, CD3+, CD56+, and CD4−
- Cytotoxic phenotype: granzyme B+, TIA-1+, and perforin+
- Clonal rearrangement of T-cell receptor genes

Patients with primary cutaneous gamma–delta T-cell lymphoma develop plaques, ulcerated nodules, and tumors, most frequently involving the extremities. This lymphoma is sometimes associated with hemophagocytic syndrome. The clinical course is usually rapidly progressive.

Differential Diagnosis

Subcutaneous cases of gamma–delta T-cell lymphoma may be histologically similar to subcutaneous panniculitis-like T-cell lymphoma, but the gamma–delta lymphomas have a much worse prognosis. Distinguishing the two entities is important. In contrast to SPTCL, gamma–delta lymphomas often extend into the dermis and sometimes into the epidermis. By immunohistochemistry, SPTCL is positive with the T-cell receptor beta immunostain (Beta F1) and negative with the T-cell receptor delta immunostain. Gamma–delta lymphoma has the opposite staining pattern.

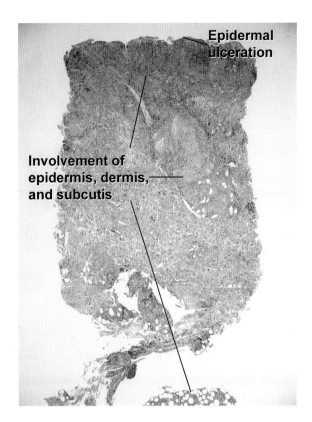

Fig. 24.34 Primary cutaneous gamma–delta T-cell lymphoma

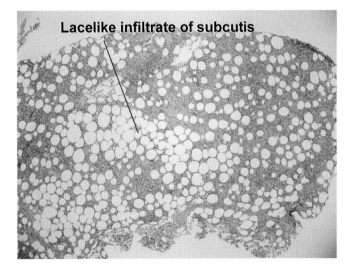

Fig. 24.35 Primary cutaneous gamma–delta T-cell lymphoma

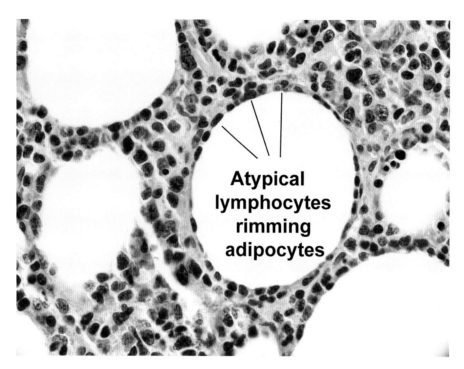

Fig. 24.36 Primary cutaneous gamma–delta T-cell lymphoma

Primary cutaneous CD4+ small/medium T-cell lymphoproliferative disorder (provisional entity)

Key Features

- Plaque, nodule or tumor, typically solitary
- Dermal infiltrate ± involvement of subcutaneous fat and epidermis
- CD3+, CD4+, CD8–, and CD30–
- Aberrant immunophenotype (variably present) with loss of some T-cell markers
- Pseudo-rosettes of PD-1+ cells surrounding large reactive B cells (variably present)
- Clonal rearrangement of T-cell receptor genes

Primary cutaneous CD4+ small/medium T-cell lymphoproliferative disorder (SMPTCL) is a provisional entity in the 2016 revision of the World Health Organization (WHO) classification. SMPTCL is remarkable for its localized distribution and indolent clinical behavior. The entity was renamed as a lymphoproliferative disorder (formerly termed a *lymphoma*) because the published cases do not appear to fulfill clinical criteria for malignancy. Diagnosis requires clinical correlation to exclude MF and peripheral T-cell lymphoma, NOS. In contrast to MF, no preceding patches are noted by history. By histology, epidermotropism is less conspicuous than that seen in early MF.

Some reports suggest that this provisional category may represent a heterogeneous group of lymphoproliferative disorders. Primary cutaneous follicular T-cell lymphoma may partially overlap with SMPTCL. Follicular helper T cells commonly express CD10, BCL-6, and CXCL-13. Expression of these markers has been variable in reported cases of SMPTCL.

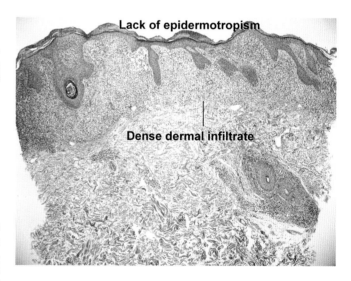

Fig. 24.37 Primary cutaneous CD4+ small/medium T-cell lymphoproliferative disorder

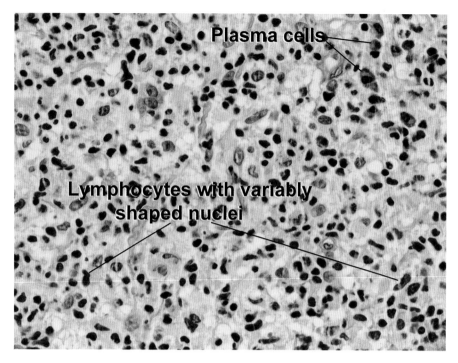

Fig. 24.38 Primary cutaneous CD4+ small/medium T-cell lymphoproliferative disorder

Follicular T-cell lymphoma (provisional entity)

Key Features

- Nodular dermal infiltrate
- No epidermotropism
- Monomorphous small to medium-sized T cells
- Follicular helper T-cell markers: BCL-6+, PD-1+, and CD10+
- Numerous reactive B cells and histiocytes, variable numbers of eosinophils
- May represent a monomorphous variant of SMPTCL

Follicular T-cell lymphoma (FTCL) is a rare, recently described lymphoma with expression of follicular helper T-cell markers. It is designated as a provisional entity in the 2016 revision of the WHO classification. FTCL may be nodal or may originate in the skin. Patients with primary cutaneous FTCL present typically with multiple papules, nodules, and plaques, sometimes localizing to intertriginous sites such as the axilla and inguinal region. Most primary cutaneous cases remain localized to the skin, but are relatively resistant to therapy.

Angioimmunoblastic T-cell lymphoma

Key Features

- Systemic lymphoma that may involve the skin
- Lymph nodes are primary site
- Older patients

- Generalized lymphadenopathy and multiorgan involvement typical
- Neoplastic follicular T-helper cells drive B-cell expansion
- PD-1+, CXCL13+, and BCL-6+ (variable) in T cells
- Reactive B cells with variable positivity for EBV

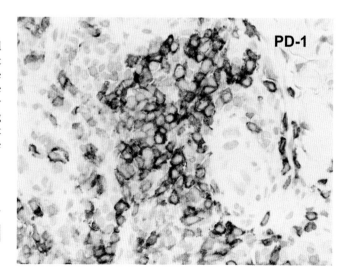

Fig. 24.39 Angioimmunoblastic T-cell lymphoma

Angioimmunoblastic T-cell lymphoma (AITL) is usually diagnosed by lymph node biopsy. The skin is secondarily involved in about half of patients. Occasionally the cutaneous lesions may be the initial sign of disease. The eruption often involves the trunk, limbs, or neck. Cutaneous lesions range from macules and papules to plaques and nodules. In early maculopapular lesions, skin biopsy findings are frequently subtle and nonspecific, and in some cases, may not be readily identifiable as a malignant infiltrate. A drug eruption or connective tissue disease may be suspected both clinically and histopathologically. Follicular T-helper markers, particularly PD-1 and CXCL13, may be helpful in identifying the neoplastic cells.

Differential Diagnosis

AITL, follicular T-cell lymphoma, and some cases of primary cutaneous CD4+ small/medium T-cell lymphoproliferative disorder share the feature of expressing follicular T-helper markers, such as PD-1, CXCL13, and BCL-6. All three may also have numerous reactive B cells within the infiltrate. However, the three generally differ in their clinical features. In addition, EBV-positive, reactive B-cells are common in AITL, uncommon in follicular T-cell lymphoma, and absent in SMPTCL.

Primary cutaneous acral CD8+ T-cell lymphoma (provisional entity)

Key Features

- Characteristic location on the ear
- Dense, diffuse dermal lymphoid infiltrate with grenz zone
- No epidermotropism
- Small- to medium-sized monomorphic CD8+ T cells
- Indolent behavior

Primary cutaneous acral CD8+T-cell lymphoma is a recently recognized lymphoproliferative disorder that is designated as a provisional entity in the 2016 revision of the WHO classification. This lymphoma has also been described in the literature as *indolent CD8+ lymphoid proliferation of the ear*. Involvement of the ear may be unilateral or bilateral. A few reports describe similar CD8+ infiltrates occurring as an isolated nodule on the nose. Multiple published cases have responded to radiation therapy. Systemic dissemination has not been described.

Hydroa vacciniforme–like lymphoproliferative disorder

Key Features

- Asian, Mexican, and Central and South American children
- Ulcerative papulovesicles with scarring
- Face and extremities
- Hypersensitivity to mosquito bites
- Angiocentric infiltrates of small- or medium-sized lymphocytes
- EBV detected within lymphoid cells by in situ hybridization
- TIA-1+, CD2+, CD8 variable, and CD56 variable

Hydroa vacciniforme–like lymphoproliferative disorder is an EBV-associated disease of childhood. Early in the course, the clinical presentation mimics hydroa vacciniforme, although the disease activity is often independent of sun exposure. Disordered immune regulation confers severe sensitivity to mosquito bites. Over a period of years, the lymphoproliferative disorder may progress to systemic involvement with fever, lymphadenopathy, and organomegaly. When systemic involvement occurs, the clinical course is aggressive.

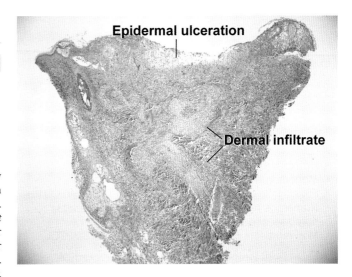

Fig. 24.40 Hydroa vacciniforme-like lymphoproliferative disorder

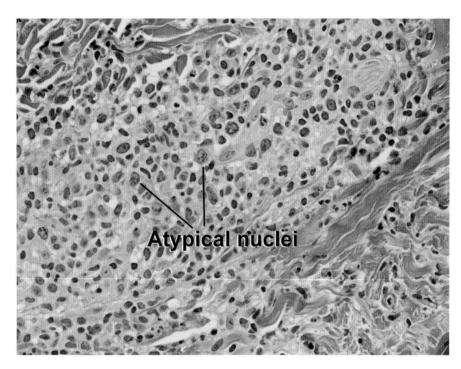

Fig. 24.41 Hydroa vacciniforme-like lymphoproliferative disorder

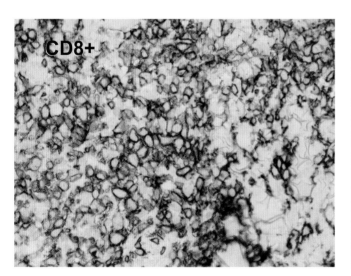

Fig. 24.42 Hydroa vacciniforme–like lymphoproliferative disorder

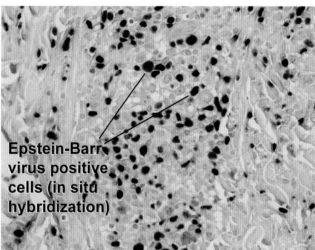

Fig. 24.43 Hydroa vacciniforme–like lymphoproliferative disorder

Myeloid neoplasms

Blastic plasmacytoid dendritic cell neoplasm

Key Features

- Monomorphous or polymorphous infiltrate in the dermis and subcutis
- No epidermotropism
- CD4+, CD56+, and CD123+
- CD3–, CD20–, lysozyme–, and myeloperoxidase–
- Cytotoxic markers negative
- No clonal rearrangement of the T-cell receptor genes
- Negative in situ hybridization for EBV

Previous names for this entity include *CD4+/CD56+ hematodermic neoplasm* and *blastic NK-cell lymphoma*. The cell of origin is a precursor of CD123-positive plasmacytoid dendritic cells. Patients present with solitary or multiple nodules or tumors. Tumor cells rapidly disseminate to the lymph nodes, bone marrow, and blood. The prognosis is poor. T-cell markers are negative, and there is no clonal rearrangement of the T-cell receptor genes. An association with acute myeloid leukemia (AML) occurs in about 10%–20% of patients.

Differential Diagnosis

See "Myeloid leukemia" next.

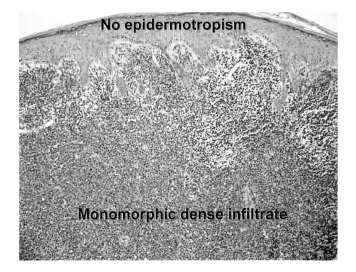

Fig. 24.44 Blastic plasmacytoid dendritic cell neoplasm

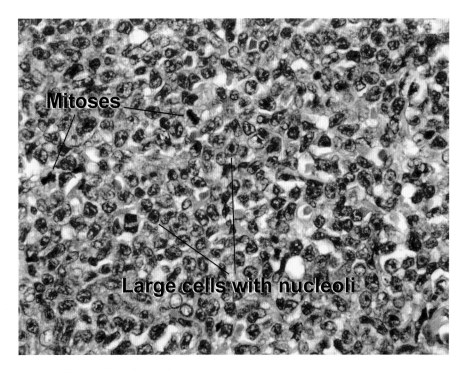

Fig. 24.45 Blastic plasmacytoid dendritic cell neoplasm

Myeloid leukemia

Key Features

- Diffuse interstitial, perivascular, and periadnexal infiltrate in dermis and subcutis
- No epidermotropism
- Grenz zone separates the infiltrate from the epidermis
- Single filing of cells splaying dermal collagen (variable)
- Mononuclear cells (blasts) ranging from large to small
- Prominent nucleoli (variable)
- Eosinophilic cytoplasm (variable)
- Scattered bilobed cells resembling neutrophilic "bands" sometimes present
- Lysozyme+, myeloperoxidase+, and chloroacetate esterase+

Cutaneous infiltrates of leukemic cells occur frequently in AML and rarely in chronic myelogenous leukemia. Direct involvement of the skin is particularly common in acute monocytic and myelomonocytic leukemia. Infiltration of the gingivae is also common in these two subtypes. Patients present with papules, nodules, plaques, purpura, or ulcers. Unusual presentations include a generalized maculopapular eruption clinically resembling an allergic drug eruption or viral exanthem. In skin biopsy specimens, AML and chronic myelogenous leukemia may have similar morphologic features. Some types of acute leukemia are associated with specific chromosomal translocations, such as t(15;17) in promyelocytic leukemia (M3).

PEARL

Myeloid leukemia and blastic plasmacytoid dendritic cell neoplasm (BPDCN) should be considered when a malignant hematologic infiltrate is negative for CD3, CD20, and CD30.

Differential Diagnosis

Lysozyme and myeloperoxidase are typically positive in myeloid leukemia and are negative in blastic plasmacytoid dendritic cell neoplasm. Occasional cases of myeloid leukemia lack expression of lysozyme and myeloperoxidase and may be particularly difficult to differentiate from BPDCN. Both neoplasms frequently express CD4 and CD56. In contrast to myeloid leukemia, BPDCN is more likely to express CD123, TCL-1, TdT, and myxovirus A. Myeloid leukemia expresses myeloid cell nuclear differentiation antigen, whereas BPDCN is negative.

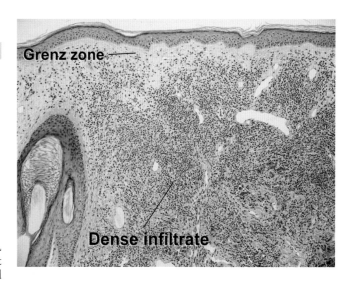

Fig. 24.46 Acute myeloid leukemia

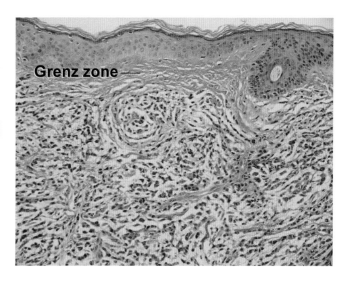

Fig. 24.47 Acute myeloid leukemia

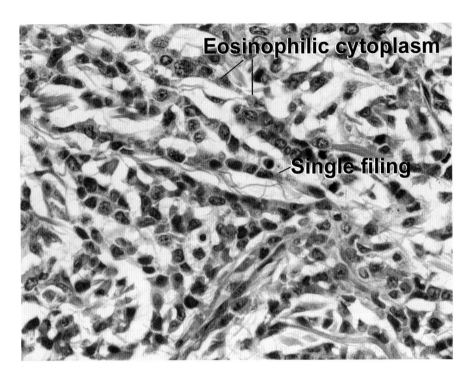

Eosinophilic cytoplasm

Single filing

Fig. 24.48 Acute myeloid leukemia

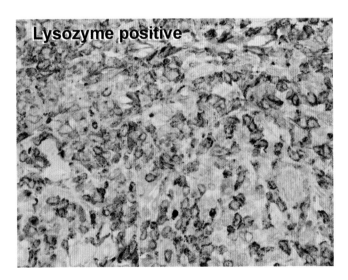

Lysozyme positive

Fig. 24.49 Acute myeloid leukemia

Further reading

Battistella M, Beylot-Barry M, Bachelez H, et al. Primary cutaneous follicular helper T-cell lymphoma: a new subtype of cutaneous T-cell lymphoma reported in a series of 5 cases. Arch Dermatol 2012;148:832–9.

Beltraminelli H, Leinweber B, Kerl H, et al. Primary cutaneous CD4+ small-/medium-sized pleomorphic T-cell lymphoma: a cutaneous nodular proliferation of pleomorphic T lymphocytes of undetermined significance? A study of 136 cases. Am J Dermatopathol 2009;31:317–22.

Botros N, Cerroni L, Shawwa A, et al. Cutaneous manifestations of angioimmunoblastic T-cell lymphoma: clinical and pathological characteristics. Am J Dermatopathol 2015;37(4):274–83.

Campbell JJ, Clark RA, Watanabe R, et al. Sezary syndrome and mycosis fungoides arise from distinct T-cell subsets: a biologic rationale for their distinct clinical behaviors. Blood 2010;116:767–71.

Cronin DM, George TI, Reichard KK, et al. Immunophenotypic analysis of myeloperoxidase-negative leukemia cutis and blastic plasmacytoid dendritic cell neoplasm. Am J Clin Pathol 2012;137(3):367–76.

Devata S, Wilcox RA. Cutaneous T-cell lymphoma: a review with a focus on targeted agents. Am J Clin Dermatol 2016;17(3):225–37.

El Shabrawi-Caelen L, Kerl H, Cerroni L. Lymphomatoid papulosis: reappraisal of clinicopathologic presentation and classification into subtypes A, B, and C. Arch Dermatol 2004;140:441–7.

Fernandez-Flores A. Comments on cutaneous lymphomas: since the WHO-2008 classification to present. Am J Dermatopathol 2012;34:274–84.

Gammon B, Guitart J. Intertriginous mycosis fungoides: a distinct presentation of cutaneous T-cell lymphoma that may be caused by malignant follicular helper T cells. Arch Dermatol 2012;148(9):1040–4.

Karai LJ, Kadin ME, Hsi ED, et al. Chromosomal rearrangements of 6p25.3 define a new subtype of lymphomatoid papulosis. Am J Surg Pathol 2013;37(8):1173–81.

Kempf W, Kazakov DV, Schärer L, et al. Angioinvasive lymphomatoid papulosis: a new variant simulating aggressive lymphomas. Am J Surg Pathol 2013;37:1–13.

Kempf W, Ostheeren-Michaelis S, Paulli M, et al. Granulomatous mycosis fungoides and granulomatous slack skin. Arch Dermatol 2008;144:1609–17.

Kluk J, Kai A, Koch D, et al. Indolent CD8-positive lymphoid proliferation of acral sites: three further cases of a rare entity and an update on a unique patient. J Cutan Pathol 2016;43(2):125–36.

Lan TT, Brown NA, Hristov AC. Controversies and considerations in the diagnosis of primary cutaneous CD4+ small/medium T-cell lymphoma. Arch Pathol Lab Med 2014;138(10):1307–18.

LeBlanc RE, Tavallaee M, Kim YH, et al. Useful parameters for distinguishing subcutaneous panniculitis-like T-cell lymphoma from lupus erythematosus panniculitis. Am J Surg Pathol 2016;40(6):745–54.

Marchetti MA, Pulitzer MP, Myskowski PL, et al. Cutaneous manifestations of human T-cell lymphotrophic virus type-1-associated adult T-cell leukemia/lymphoma: a single-center, retrospective study. J Am Acad Dermatol 2015;72(2):293–301.

Massone C, El-Shabrawi-Caelen L, Kerl H, et al. The morphologic spectrum of primary cutaneous anaplastic large T-cell lymphoma: a histopathologic study on 66 biopsy specimens from 47 patients with report of rare variants. J Cutan Pathol 2008;35:46–53.

Nofal A, Abdel-Mawla MY, Assaf M, et al. Primary cutaneous aggressive epidermotropic CD8+ T-cell lymphoma: proposed diagnostic criteria and therapeutic evaluation. J Am Acad Dermatol 2012;67:48–59.

Olsen EA. Evaluation, diagnosis, and staging of cutaneous lymphoma. Dermatol Clin 2015;33(4):643–54.

Rovner R, Smith HL, Katz PJ, et al. Influence of clinical and pathologic features on the pathologist's diagnosis of mycosis fungoides: a pilot study. J Cutan Pathol 2015;42(7):471–9.

Sangle NA, Schmidt RL, Patel JL, et al. Optimized immunohistochemical panel to differentiate myeloid sarcoma from blastic plasmacytoid dendritic cell neoplasm. Mod Pathol 2014;27(8):1137–43.

Shi Y, Wang E. Blastic plasmacytoid dendritic cell neoplasm: a clinicopathologic review. Arch Pathol Lab Med 2014;138(4):564–9.

Swerdlow SH, Campo E, Pileri SA, et al. The 2016 revision of the World Health Organization classification of lymphoid neoplasms. Blood 2016;127(20):2375–90.

Wang JY, Nguyen GH, Ruan J, et al. Primary cutaneous follicular helper T-cell lymphoma: a case series and review of the literature. Am J Dermatopathol 2017;39(5):374–83.

Willemze R, Jansen PM, Cerroni L, et al. Subcutaneous panniculitis-like T-cell lymphoma: definition, classification, and prognostic factors: an EORTC cutaneous lymphoma group study of 83 cases. Blood 2008;111:838–45.

CHAPTER

25

B-cell lymphoma and lymphocytic leukemia

Steven Peckham

A more detailed table on the WHO Classification of B-cell Tumors of Hematopoietic and Lymphoid Tissues and a lymphoma atlas can be found in the online content for this book.

Cutaneous B-cell lymphoproliferative disorders

The primary cutaneous B-cell lymphomas share some histologic features with their nodal counterparts, but in many cases represent distinct clinicopathologic entities with significant clinical, immunophenotypic, molecular, and prognostic differences from their extracutaneous counterparts. In general, primary cutaneous B-cell lymphomas have a better prognosis than their nodal-based counterparts, and treatment strategies for them may be different. The classification system used in this chapter reflects the 2016 revision of the 2008 World Health Organization (WHO) classification of lymphoid neoplasms. Note that not all entities included here are necessarily of primary cutaneous origin (e.g., chronic lymphocytic leukemia/small lymphocytic lymphoma, mantle cell lymphoma, Burkitt lymphoma, intravascular large B-cell lymphoma, lymphomatoid granulomatosis) but may frequently involve the skin.

Normal lymph node and benign reactive lymphoid hyperplasia

Key features

- Germinal center >90% MIB-positive
- Follicle center cells express BCL-6 and CD10
- CD21 and CD23 demonstrate a well-defined dendritic network within the germinal center
- Mantle zone of small lymphocytes that normally express BCL-2
- Kappa:lambda ratio 2:1
- Marginal zone is inconspicuous

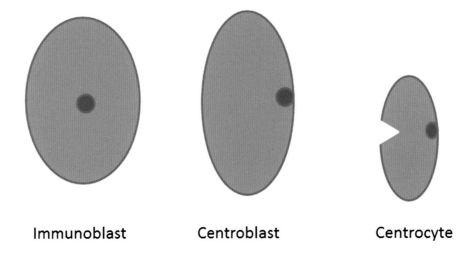

Fig. 25.1 Nuclear features of an immunoblast, centroblast, and centrocyte

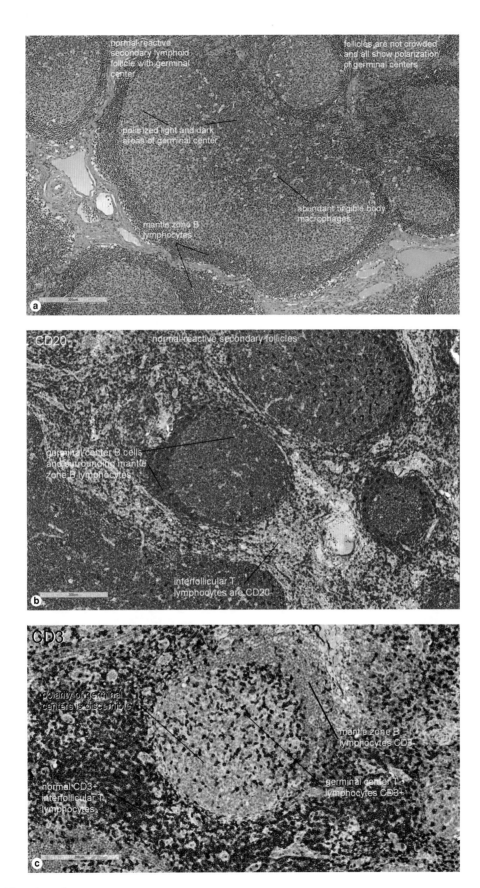

Fig. 25.2 Normal lymph node

continued

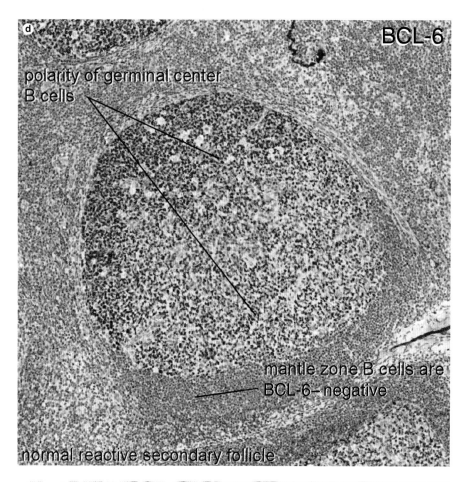

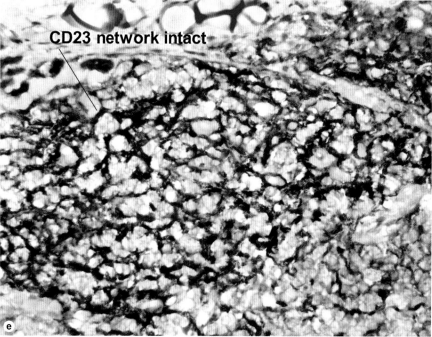

Fig. 25.2, cont'd

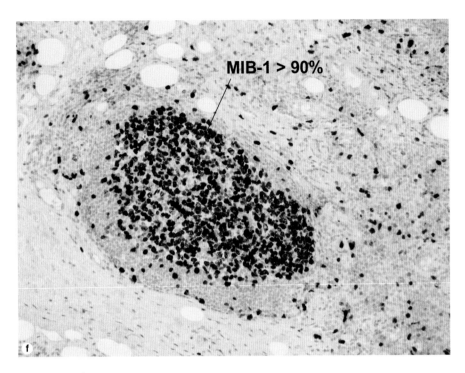

MIB-1 > 90%

Fig. 25.2, cont'd

Primary cutaneous marginal zone lymphoma

Key Features

- Patchy, nodular, or diffuse infiltrate of lymphoid cells in the dermis and superficial panniculus
- Characteristic "inverse" pattern of central darker, benign reactive lymphocytes with surrounding neoplastic cells with paler abundant cytoplasm (marginal zone cells)
- Lack of epidermotropism
- Small lymphocytes may surround or invade eccrine coils
- Surrounding benign reactive follicles may be colonized by neoplastic cells
- Neoplastic marginal zone cells often comprise only a minority of lymphoid cells in the lesions
- CD20+, CD79+, CD5−, CD10−, CD43−, BCL-6−, and BCL-2+
- Clonal rearrangement of immunoglobulin (Ig) H gene in >70% of cases
- t(14;18)(q32;q21) present in a minority of cases
- Intracytoplasmic monoclonal immunoglobulin (kappa or lambda) restriction

Primary cutaneous marginal zone B-cell lymphoma is an indolent lymphoma of small lymphocytes of B-cell origin, including centrocyte (marginal zone)-like cells with small- to medium-sized slightly irregular nuclei with inconspicuous nucleoli, admixed with plasmacytoid lymphocytes and occasional centroblast-like cells. Marginal zone lymphoma is one of the most common types of cutaneous B-cell lymphoma. The prognosis is excellent, with 5-year survival rates approaching 100%. The lesions usually present as violaceous nodules or plaques preferentially on the trunk and extremities, with upper extremities more commonly involved than lower extremities. The lesions have a nodular or diffuse architecture, often with a characteristic "inverse" pattern relative to benign reactive lymphoid follicles, i.e., they show a dense, darker-staining central nodular portion of benign reactive lymphocytes, which may contain germinal centers, surrounded by neoplastic lymphoid cells with slightly irregular nuclei and more abundant paler cytoplasm (monocytoid or marginal zone B cells). Often, the neoplastic lymphoid population only represents a minority of the cells in the lesion. The epidermis is spared, without epidermotropism of lymphocytes. Surrounding benign reactive germinal centers may be present, and are often colonized by tumor cells. In some cases, the neoplastic cells may surround and infiltrate eccrine coils, similar to the lymphoepithelial lesions seen in extranodal marginal zone lymphomas of the gastrointestinal tract (MALTomas). Primary cutaneous marginal zone B-cell lymphoma includes cases designated as primary cutaneous immunocytoma in earlier classification systems. Primary cutaneous immunocytomas are often associated with *Borrelia* and demonstrate high numbers of monotypic (i.e., they demonstrate monoclonal intracytoplasmic immunoglobulin) plasma cells and lymphoplasmacytoid lymphocytes, some of which may contain intranuclear immunoglobulin deposits (Dutcher bodies).

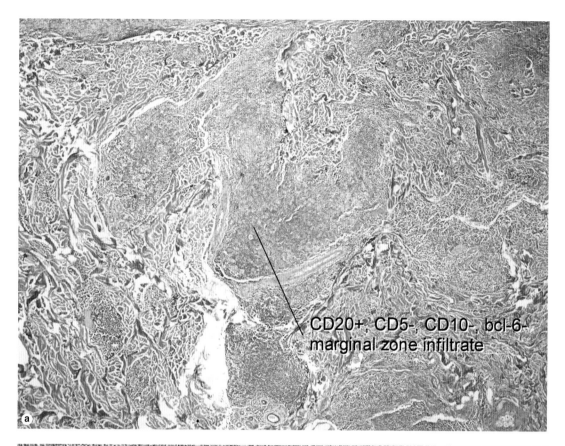

CD20+, CD5-, CD10-, bcl-6-
marginal zone infiltrate

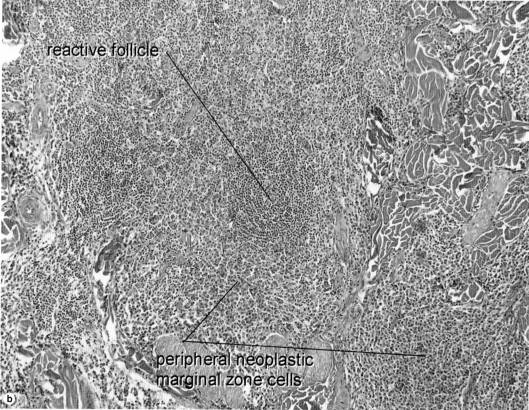

reactive follicle

peripheral neoplastic
marginal zone cells

Fig. 25.3 Primary cutaneous marginal zone lymphoma

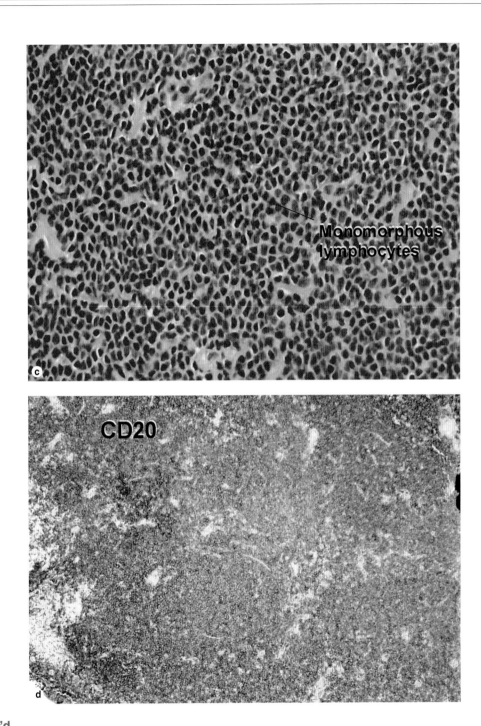

Fig. 25.3, cont'd

Primary cutaneous follicle center cell lymphoma

Key Features

- Diffuse, nodular and diffuse, or nodular lymphoid proliferation
- If mixed architecture, lesions tend to have neoplastic follicles at the periphery of a central diffuse neoplastic infiltrate
- Follicles have reduced or absent mantle zones
- Follicles have decreased to absent tingible body macrophages
- Lack of polarity of follicles (i.e., absent light and darker zones of polarity in follicle germinal centers)
- CD20+ and CD79+
- CD10+ (follicular pattern, most cases) or CD10– (diffuse pattern, most cases)
- BCL-6+, BCL-2–, CD5–, CD43–, most cases are FOXP1– and IgM–
- Reduced proliferative fraction by MIB-1 compared with benign reactive germinal centers

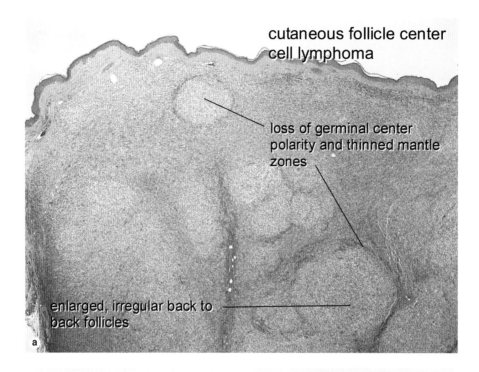

cutaneous follicle center
cell lymphoma

loss of germinal center
polarity and thinned mantle
zones

enlarged, irregular back to
back follicles

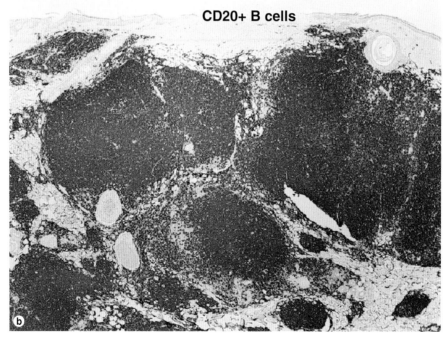

CD20+ B cells

Fig. 25.4 Primary cutaneous follicle center cell lymphoma

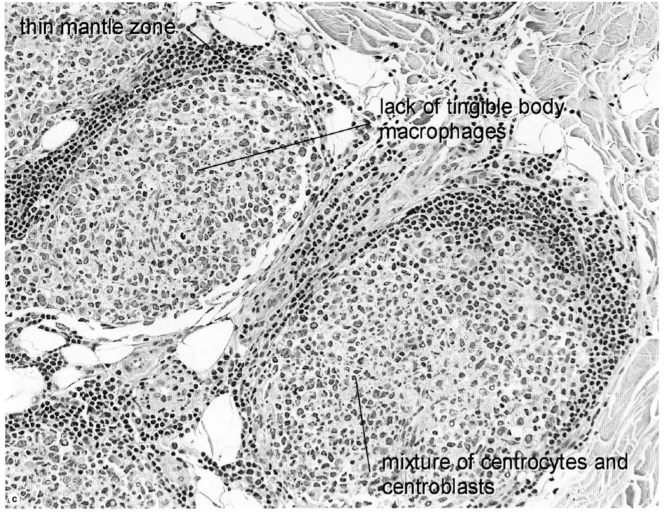

thin mantle zone

lack of tingible body macrophages

mixture of centrocytes and centroblasts

c

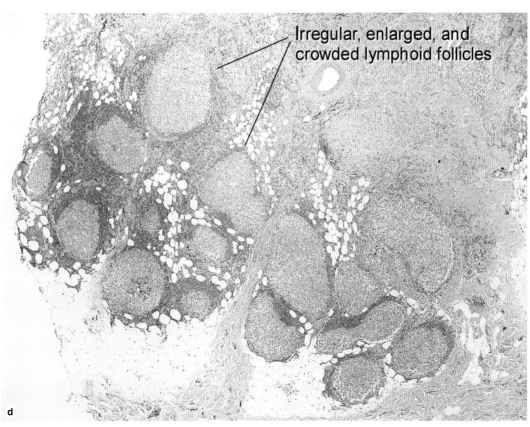

Irregular, enlarged, and crowded lymphoid follicles

d

Fig. 25.4, cont'd

continued

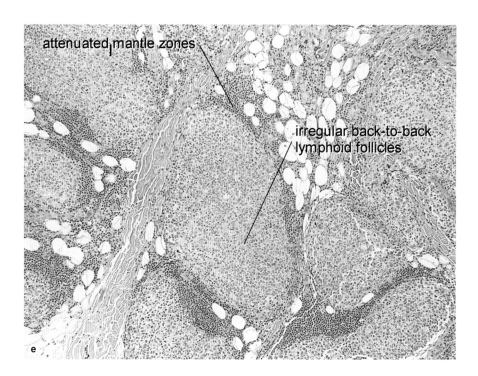

attenuated mantle zones

irregular back-to-back lymphoid follicles

Fig. 25.4, cont'd

- Monoclonal rearrangement of immunoglobulin heavy chain J gene
- t(14;18) translocation is very uncommon in primary cutaneous follicle center cell lymphoma lesions

Primary cutaneous follicle center cell lymphoma is also an indolent mature B-cell lymphoma that exhibits a predilection for the head and trunk. In contrast to its nodal counterpart (primary nodal follicle center cell lymphoma), primary cutaneous follicle center cell lymphoma has a more favorable prognosis, with 5-year survival rates >90%. As with their nodal counterparts, these lesions may have a follicular, follicular and diffuse, or diffuse architecture, most commonly diffuse. However, it must be emphasized again that, despite similar appearances by hematoxylin and eosin, these lesions have different immunohistochemical, genetic, and prognostic features from primary nodal follicle center cell lymphomas. Histology shows a nodular or diffuse proliferation of centrocyte-like lymphocytes with small, slightly irregular nuclei and variable numbers of larger centroblast-like cells with larger, rounded vesicular nuclei and one or a few prominent nucleoli. In nodular lesions, the follicles appear monomorphous, with a loss of the normal polarity of light and dark zones of the germinal centers, an attenuated mantle zone around germinal centers, and lack of tingible body macrophages in the germinal centers. In larger lesions, the center may show a diffuse architecture, with residual monomorphous neoplastic follicles at the periphery. Unlike primary nodal follicle center cell lymphoma, primary cutaneous follicle center cell lymphoma is not graded at the current time.

PEARL

In primary cutaneous follicle center cell lymphoma, the BCL-6–positive cells typically stray outside of the follicle. BCL-2 expression is characteristic of follicle center cell lymphoma in lymph nodes, but is rare in the primary cutaneous variety. At cutaneous sites, BCL-2 positivity in a follicle center cell lymphoma should raise suspicion for a nodal primary with secondary involvement of the skin.

Cutaneous diffuse large B-cell lymphoma, leg type

Key Features

- Predominantly affects older patients (>70), with a predilection for females
- Usual location is one or more red to brown nodules on one distal extremity, although lesions can present as multiple nodules and at other sites
- Five-year survival of approximately 50%
- Histology reveals a dense, diffuse infiltrate of predominantly large, round immunoblast-type cells with prominent nucleoli; occasional large cleaved, multilobated, or anaplastic cells may also be seen
- Centrocytes are largely absent
- Grenz zone may be present, and adnexal structures are often destroyed

- Epidermotropism of neoplastic lymphoid cells may closely simulate the epidermotropism characteristic of T-cell lymphomas
- CD20+, CD79a+, and BCL-2+ in great majority; most cases also express BCL-6 and/or CD10 and IgM (most cases of primary follicle center cell lymphoma are IgM–)
- MUM-1/IRF4 strong positive staining is very important to distinguish from diffuse form of follicle center cell lymphoma (MUM-1–), which may look similar by routine hematoxylin and eosin staining; FOX P1+ staining is also useful for this differential (only rarely expressed in primary cutaneous follicle center cell lymphoma)
- Rare variant is positive for CD30 and must not be mistaken for anaplastic large cell lymphoma
- Monoclonal rearrangement of J heavy gene is present; no specific chromosomal alterations

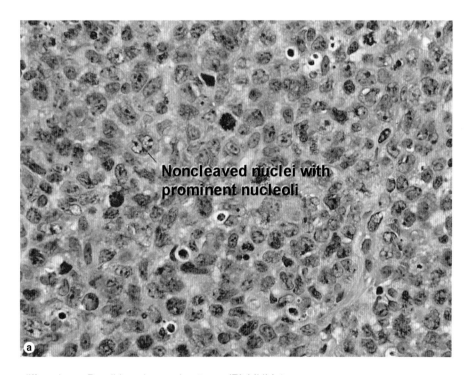

Fig. 25.5 Cutaneous diffuse large B-cell lymphoma, leg type. **(B)** MUM-1

continued

MUM-1 (nuclear stain)

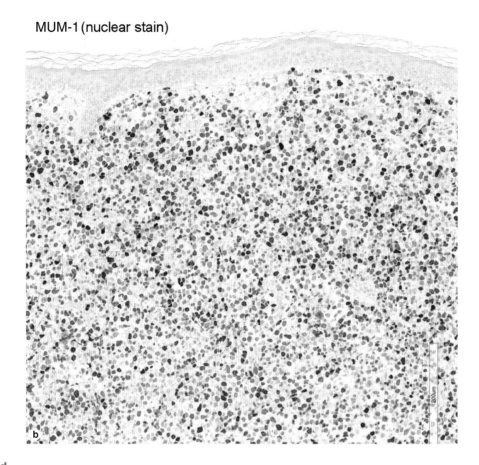

Fig. 25.5, cont'd

Cutaneous diffuse large B-cell lymphoma, other than leg type

Key Features

- Very rare
- May involve head, trunk, or extremities
- B-cell lymphoma showing a diffuse growth pattern composed of large transformed B cells, which lack the typical features of the previously described diffuse large B-cell lymphoma of the leg type or the diffuse pattern of follicle center cell lymphoma
- Histology shows a monomorphous population of centroblast-like cells with a benign mixed background of lymphoid cells
- Usually BCL-6+, may be BCL-2–; otherwise, express typical pan–B-cell markers

Intravascular large B-cell lymphoma

Key Features

- Highly malignant, rare neoplasm of large atypical B cells that presents within the lumens of small vessels, particularly capillaries and venules
- May produce neurologic deficits through involvement of central nervous system
- Neoplastic cells are large with round or oval vesicular nuclei, prominent nucleoli, and frequent mitoses
- Tumor cells may appear to be attached to endothelium, giving a hobnail appearance
- Partial occlusion of vessels by tumor cells and fibrin causes a pattern of reticular erythema seen clinically
- Extravascular involvement may be present
- Must distinguish from reactive angioendotheliomatosis and intravascular lymphomas of other lineages
- Cells express CD20 and CD79a, and may aberrantly coexpress CD5, CD10, and CD11a

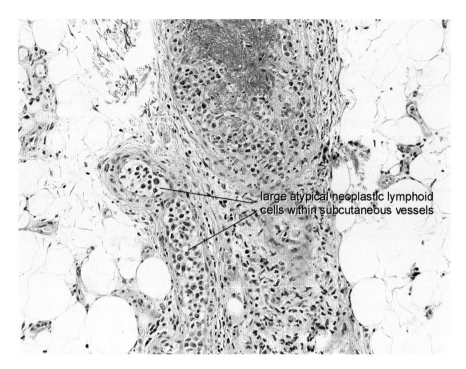

Fig. 25.6 Intravascular B cell lymphoma

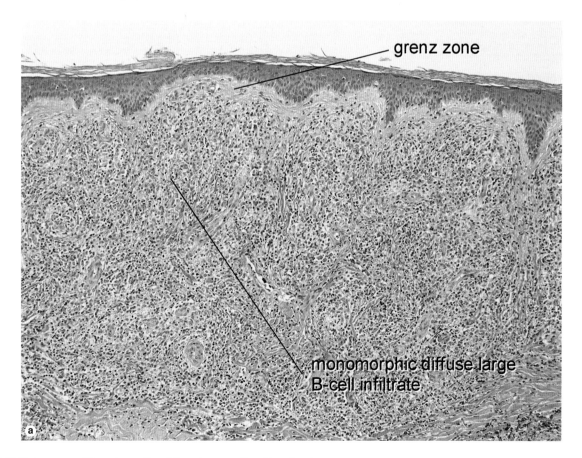

Fig. 25.7 Cutaneous diffuse large B cell lymphoma, other than leg type

continued

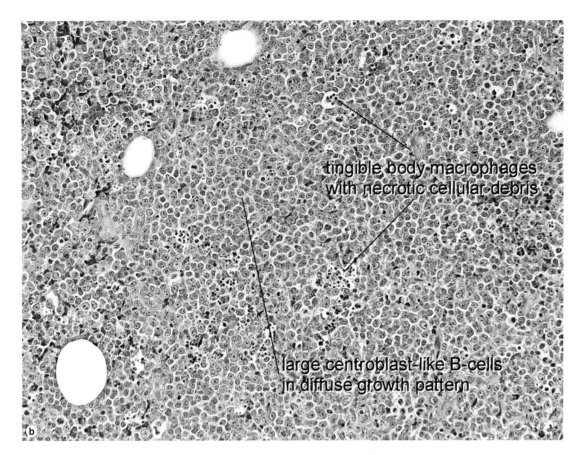

tingible body macrophages with necrotic cellular debris

large centroblast-like B-cells in diffuse growth pattern

Fig. 25.7, cont'd

Lymphomatoid granulomatosis

Key Features

- B-cell lymphoproliferative disorder associated with Epstein–Barr virus (EBV) infection
- Involves lungs, central nervous system (CNS), and skin most often; histology shows a variable infiltrate of large atypical perivascular lymphoid cells and areas of necrosis
- Presence of an angiocentric and angiodestructive mixed polymorphous mononuclear infiltrate with variable numbers of large EBV+ lymphocytes; granulomatous inflammation may also be present
- Lesions are graded histologically from 1 to 3, based upon the increasing proportion of EBV+ cells relative to the population of background reactive mixed infiltrate
- CD20+ and EBV+ large B lymphocytes in a background of reactive T cells
- Important to recognize benign reactive T cells constitute the majority of cells of the lesions

Chronic lymphocytic leukemia/small lymphocytic lymphoma

Key Features

- Most common leukemia in adults in the Western hemisphere
- Proliferation of mature round lymphocytes of B-cell origin
- Same disease process as small lymphocytic lymphoma; difference is determined by the presence of tumor in blood/bone marrow for chronic lymphocytic leukemia versus malignant lymphoid cells in other tissues/organs for small lymphocytic lymphoma (without evidence of leukemia)
- Nodular and/or diffuse infiltration of the dermis with dark, small, round, mature-appearing lymphoid cells
- May have occasional larger cells with vesicular nuclei with a single nucleolus (prolymphocytes)
- Grenz zone is often present
- CD19+, CD20+ (usually weak), CD5+, CD23+, CD43+, CD10–, and cyclin D1–
- Proliferation centers are not seen as commonly as in lymph nodes

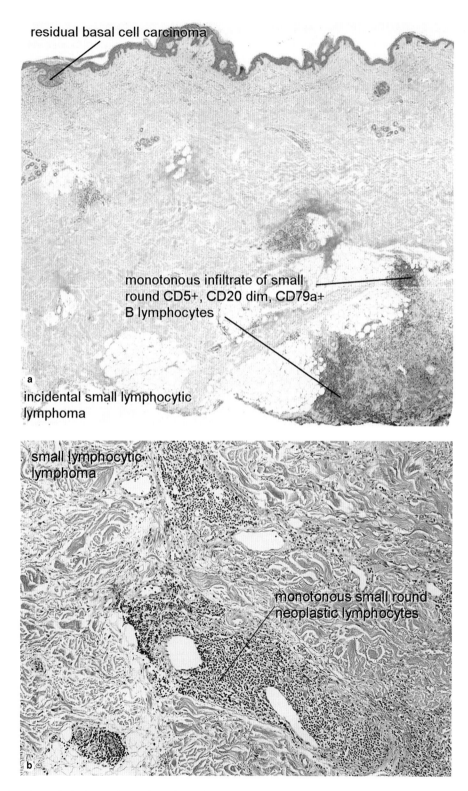

residual basal cell carcinoma

monotonous infiltrate of small round CD5+, CD20 dim, CD79a+ B lymphocytes

a

incidental small lymphocytic lymphoma

small lymphocytic lymphoma

monotonous small round neoplastic lymphocytes

b

Fig. 25.8 Chronic lymphocytic leukemia/small lymphocytic lymphoma

Mantle cell lymphoma

Key Features

- Rare B-cell lymphoma that resembles mantle zone of lymphoid follicle
- Usually the result of nodal-based lymphoma with skin involvement; rare cases of putative primary cutaneous mantle cell lymphoma are of doubtful validity

- Histology shows diffuse monomorphous infiltrates of intermediate-sized lymphocytes with irregular nuclei and nucleoli frequently
- CD20+, CD5+, CD43+, BCL-2+, and CD23–
- Cyclin D1 is an important marker; positive staining results from overexpression of gene product due to t(11;14) translocation

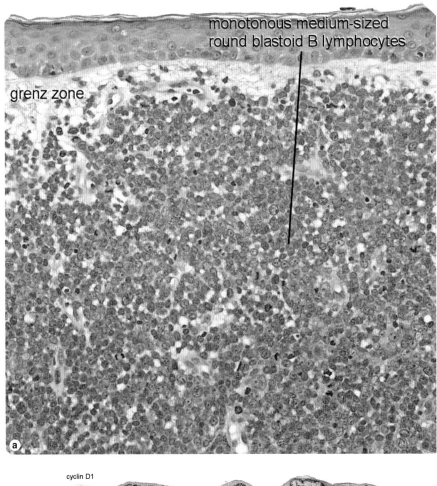

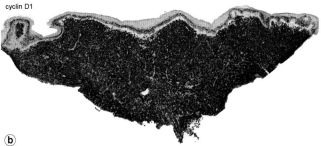

Fig. 25.9 Blastoid mantle zone lymphoma. **(B)** Cyclin D1

Burkitt lymphoma

Key Features

- Not a primary cutaneous entity but infrequently shows cutaneous involvement
- Various clinical forms recognized (endemic form in Africa and sporadic in other regions)
- Most common in first two decades, but can occur at any age
- Monomorphic, diffuse growth of medium-sized cells with round (noncleaved) vesicular nuclei, multiple nucleoli, and moderate amount of basophilic cytoplasm that often contains multiple clear (lipid-filled) vacuoles
- "Starry-sky" pattern due to abundant benign macrophages within tumor phagocytizing necrotic tumor cells/debris
- Extremely high proliferative/mitotic index, nearly 100% observed with MIB-1
- CD19+, CD20+, CD79a+, CD22+, CD10+, CD5−, CD23−, BCL-2−, and terminal deoxyribonucleotidyl transferase (TdT)−
- Atypical variant (Burkitt-like lymphoma) shows greater cellular pleomorphism and heterogeneity than classic Burkitt lymphoma

B-cell lymphoblastic lymphoma/leukemia

Key Features

- A small proportion of patients with precursor B-cell lymphoblastic lymphoma/leukemia may present with solid tumors, most often in skin, bone, and lymph nodes
- Composed of lymphoblasts slightly larger than mature lymphocytes, but smaller than cells of large B-cell lymphoma
- Blasts contain round or convoluted nuclei and fine chromatin (paler and finer than normal mature lymphocytes), with inconspicuous nucleoli and scant basophilic cytoplasm
- Diffuse pattern with frequent mitoses and tingible body macrophages ("starry-sky" pattern)
- TdT+ (90%), CD34+ (75%), CD79a+, CD19+, CD22+, CD10+ (80–%85%), CD20± (may be dim or negative), and surface Ig−

EBV+ mucocutaneous ulcer

Key Features

- Indolent, often self-limited EBV+ B-cell proliferation with ulceration on oropharyngeal mucosa or skin (most common cutaneous sites lips, arms, chest)
- Associated with immunosuppression, iatrogenic suppression (especially due to medications, including methotrexate, azathioprine, and cyclosporine A), or immunosenescence of old age
- Most in elderly patients, 70+ years
- Segregated from EBV+ diffuse large B-cell lymphoma as it does not progress to systemic disease and in many cases spontaneously resolves; in fact, it may not even be neoplastic
- Sharply circumscribed ulcer with polymorphous infiltrate of variable numbers of medium to large immunoblast-like cells and pleomorphic Reed–Sternberg-like EBV+ and CD30+ cells with a B-cell immunophenotype (most cases express CD79a; fewer express CD20 and CD45/LCA)
- Background of small T lymphocytes, histiocytes, eosinophils, and plasma cells with circumscribed periphery of infiltrate
- Apoptotic cells with plasmacytoid features often seen
- May show pseudoepitheliomatous epidermal hyperplasia adjacent to ulcer and necrosis

---

PEARL

EBV+ mucocutaneous ulcer may appear very similar histologically to classical Hodgkin lymphoma, given the presence of large CD30+ cells, which may also express CD15 in a minority of cases; remember primary cutaneous or mucosal Hodgkin lymphoma is vanishingly rare, and most cases of EBV+ mucocutaneous ulcer are also CD45/leukocyte common antigen positive. In addition, lesional EBV+ and CD30+ cells are of variable size, from large and pleomorphic to small, unlike classical Hodgkin lymphoma, in which neoplastic cells tend to be mostly all large.

Table 25.1 WHO classification of primary cutaneous B-cell lymphoma

Primary cutaneous follicle center lymphoma

- Most common anatomic site is head/neck (often scalp), followed by trunk
- Composed of neoplastic follicle center cells (i.e., centrocytes and centroblasts in various proportions)
- Centrocytes are small with cleaved nuclei
- Centroblasts are larger, with noncleaved nuclei and one to three nucleoli attached to inside of nuclear membrane
- If diffuse growth pattern with sheets of centroblasts, is classified as diffuse large B cell rather than follicular lymphoma
- Otherwise, numbers of centrocytes and centroblasts do not matter, as primary FCL is *not* graded
- Immunophenotype:
  - Follicular pattern
    - CD20+ CD79a+, BCL-6+, and CD10+
  - Diffuse pattern
    - CD20+ CD79a+, BCL-6+ and CD10–, FOXP1–, and IgM– usually

Primary cutaneous marginal zone lymphoma (cutaneous MALT-type lymphoma)

- Includes entities previously classified as:
- Primary cutaneous plasmacytoma without underlying myeloma
- Primary cutaneous immunocytoma
- Erythematous to purple nodules/tumors most often on trunk and extremities, often single or few lesions
- Proliferation of small marginal zone centrocyte-like B cells, usually surrounding benign reactive germinal centers
- Immunophenotype: CD20+, CD79a+, BCL-2+, CD5–, CD10–, and BCL-6–
- Approximately 70% show evidence of monoclonal light chain restriction

Primary cutaneous diffuse large B-cell lymphoma, leg type

- 80% of cases occur in patients ≥70 years
- Poorer prognosis
- Diffuse proliferation of monotonous large transformed B cells
- Activated B-cell immunophenotype, with strong BCL-2+ cells, which are MUM-1/IRF4+, CD19+, CD20+, CD79a+, BCL-6 variable, FOXP1+, and usually IgM+

Primary cutaneous diffuse large B-cell lymphoma, other

- Includes intravascular/angiotropic B-cell lymphoma and other non–leg type diffuse large B-cell lymphomas with only skin involvement

Adapted from World Health Organization Classification of Tumours of Haematopoietic and Lymphoid Tissues, 2016 revision of fourth edition.

Further reading

Ahearn IM, Hu SW, Meehan SA, et al. Primary cutaneous follicle-center lymphoma. Dermatol Online J 2014;20(12).

Bradford PT, Devessa SS, Anderson WF, et al. Cutaneous lymphoma incidence patterns in the United States: a population based study of 3884 cases. Blood 2009;113:5064–73.

Charli-Joseph Y, Cerroni L, LeBoit PE. Cutaneous spindle-cell B-cell lymphomas: most are neoplasms of follicular center cell origin. Am J Surg Pathol 2015;39(6):737–43.

De Laval L, Harris NL, Longtine J, et al. Cutaneous B-cell lymphomas of follicular and marginal zone types. Am J Surg Pathol 2001;25(6):732–41.

Demierre M, Kerl H, Willemze R. Primary cutaneous B cell lymphomas: a practical approach. Hematol Oncol Clin North Am 2003;17:1333–50.

Dewar R, Andea AA, Guitart J, et al. Best practices in diagnostic immunohistochemistry: workup of cutaneous lymphoid lesions in the diagnosis of primary cutaneous lymphoma. Arch Pathol Lab Med 2015;139(3): 338–50.

Dojcinov SD, Venkataraman G, Raffield M, et al. EBV positive mucocutaneous ulcer—a study of 26 cases associated with various sources of immunosuppression. Am J Surg Pathol 2010;34:405–17.

Hallerman C, Niermann C, Fischer R-J, et al. New prognostic relevant factors in primary cutaneous diffuse large B-cell lymphomas. J Am Acad Dermatol 2007;56:588–97.

Hart M, Thakral B, Yohe S, et al. EBV positive mucocutaneous ulcer in organ transplant recipients: a localized indolent posttransplant lymphoproliferative disorder. Am J Surg Pathol 2014;38:1522–9.

Hristow AC. Primary cutaneous diffuse large B-cell lymphoma, leg type: diagnostic considerations. Arch Pathol Lab Med 2012;136:876–81.

Koens L, Vermeer MH, Willemze R, et al. IgM expression on paraffin sections distinguishes primary cutaneous large

B-cell lymphoma, leg type from primary cutaneous follicle center lymphoma. Am J Surg Pathol 2010;34:1043–8.

Lima M. Cutaneous primary B-cell lymphomas: from diagnosis to treatment. An Bras Dermatol 2015;90(5):687–706.

Ritter J, Adesokan P, Fitzgibbon J, et al. Paraffin section immunohistochemistry as an adjunct to morphologic analysis in the diagnosis of cutaneous lymphoid infiltrates. J Cutan Pathol 1994;21:481–93.

Roglin J, Boer A. Skin manifestations of intravascular lymphoma mimic inflammatory diseases of the skin. Br J Dermatol 2007;157:16–25.

Sander C, Kaudewitz P, Schirren C, et al. Immunocytoma and marginal zone B cell lymphoma (MALT lymphoma) presenting in skin-different entities or a spectrum of disease? J Cutan Pathol 1996;23:59a.

Sokol L, Naghashpour M, Glass F. Primary cutaneous B-cell lymphomas: recent advances in diagnosis and management. Cancer Control 2012;19(3):236–44.

Swerdlow SH, Campo E, Harris NL, et al. World Health Organization (WHO) Classification of Tumors of Hematopoietic and Lymphoid Tissues. Lyon: World Health Organization; 2008.

Swerdlow SH, Campo E, Pileri SA, et al. The 2016 revision of the World Health Organization Classification of Lymphoid Neoplasms. Blood 2016;127(20):2375–90.

Wilcox RA. Cutaneous B-cell lymphomas: 2015 update on diagnosis, risk-stratification, and management. Am J Hematol 2015;90(1):73–6.

Willemze R, Jaffe ES, Burg G, et al. WHO-EORTC Classification for cutaneous lymphomas. Blood 2005;105:3768–85.

Metastatic tumors and simulators

Christine J. Ko

It is important to distinguish cutaneous metastases, particularly metastatic adenocarcinoma, from primary adnexal tumors of the skin. Adenocarcinoma metastatic to the skin is commonly of breast or lung origin. Focal areas of glandular differentiation may be highlighted with a mucicarmine stain. Most metastatic tumors are situated in the dermis, although occasionally epidermotropic metastases form intraepidermal nests.

> **PEARL**
>
> Positivity with both cytokeratin 5/6 and p63 or p40 is suggestive of a primary cutaneous adnexal tumor over adenocarcinoma metastatic to the skin.

Breast carcinoma

Key Features

- Poorly differentiated adenocarcinoma
- Various patterns: single cells infiltrating through collagen, cords and tubules of atypical cells, collections of cells with glandular formation, clusters of cells in pools of mucin, and dense sheets of atypical cells
- Occasionally, there is epidermotropism

- Gross cystic disease fluid protein (GCDFP)-15+, estrogen receptor+, and cytokeratin (CK) 7+

Breast carcinoma is the most common cause of cutaneous metastatic disease in women. In general, metastases are seen on the chest wall, sometimes as a result of direct extension of the tumor. Various clinical and histologic presentations are possible. Distinct subtypes are discussed next.

Carcinoma *en cuirasse*

Key Features

- Rectangular punch
- Busy dermis
- Dense collagen
- Single files of hyperchromatic cells with nuclear molding (black box cars)

A *cuirasse* is a suit of armor made of leather. Carcinoma *en cuirasse* presents with woody induration of the skin. The skin is infiltrated by single files of hyperchromatic nuclei with prominent nuclear molding. Dense collagen is laid down between the tumor cells. Because the dermis is sclerotic, the punch is rectangular rather than tapered.

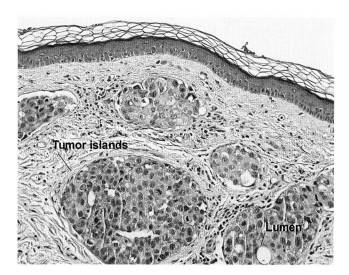

Fig. 26.1 Breast carcinoma

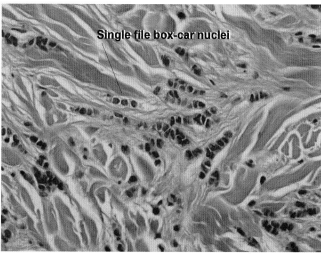

Fig. 26.2 Carcinoma *en cuirasse*

Inflammatory carcinoma (carcinoma erysipeloides)

Key Features

- Tumor cells within dilated lymphatic vessels
- Congested capillaries

Clinically, the lesions present with skin erythema that ranges from faint macular erythema to an erysipelas-like presentation. Inflammation is usually absent histologically, and the erythema is likely secondary to blood vessel congestion.

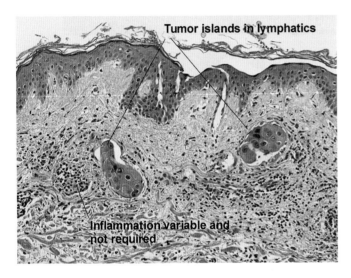

Fig. 26.3 Inflammatory carcinoma

Alopecia neoplastica

Key Features

- Sclerotic dermis
- Infiltrative cords of atypical cells
- Loss of hair follicles

Occasionally, metastatic breast carcinoma presents as skin-colored to slightly erythematous patches of alopecia on the scalp. Clinically, it is often mistaken for alopecia areata. A biopsy is performed when hair fails to regrow in response to intralesional injection of corticosteroid.

Lung carcinoma

Key Features

- Metastases from the lung may be of the small cell type, adenocarcinoma, squamous cell carcinoma, or undifferentiated
- Most are thyroid transcription factor (TTF)-1+

Lung carcinoma is the most common cause of cutaneous metastases in men. Generally, the metastases present on the trunk as a single nodule or cluster of papules.

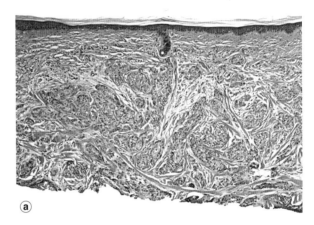

(a)

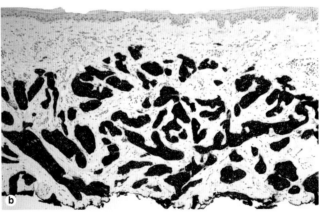

b

Fig. 26.4 Metastatic lung carcinoma. **(A–C)** Metastatic adeno-carcinoma. CK7 positive **(B)** and negative for CK5/6 **(C)** as well as p40 (not shown).

continued

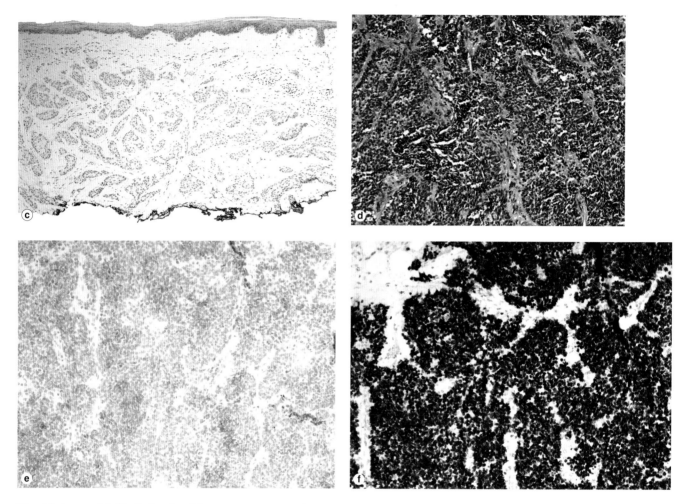

Fig. 26.4, cont'd (D–F) Small cell lung carcinoma **(E)** CK20 negative **(F)** TTF-1 positive

Small cell lung carcinoma

Key Features

- Sheets of uniform, round, blue nuclei with little cytoplasm
- Crush artifact may be prominent
- Nuclear molding may be seen
- TTF-1 positivity (and CK20-negativity) distinguishes this from Merkel cell carcinoma of the skin

Renal carcinoma

Key Features

- Tubules of clear glycogenated cells
- Prominent vascular component with hemosiderin and extravasated erythrocytes
- CD10+
- Periodic acid–Schiff (PAS)+
- RCC+

The scalp is a common site for metastatic renal cell carcinoma (RCC). The lesion is typically nodular. The vessels have a "chicken-wire" pattern.

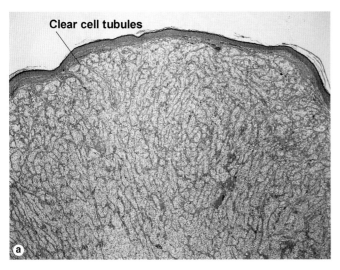

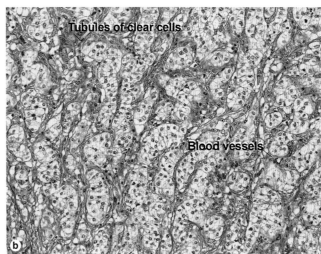

Fig. 26.5 Renal carcinoma

Colon carcinoma

Key Features

- Well-to-moderately differentiated adenocarcinoma
- May mimic mucinous carcinoma of the skin, with clusters of blue cells floating in pools of mucin

- Typically CK20+
- CDX2+

Colon carcinoma is typically CK20 positive and CK7 negative. Rectal carcinoma may stain with both or with CK7 only. Figs. 26.6C and D demonstrate this paradoxical immunostaining pattern in a rectal adenocarcinoma.

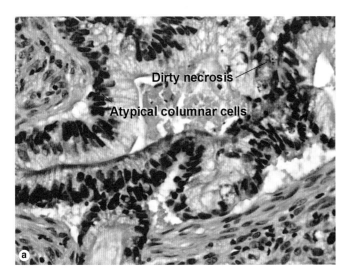

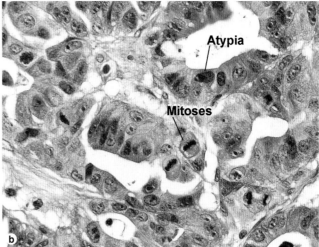

Fig. 26.6 (A and B) Colon carcinoma.

continued

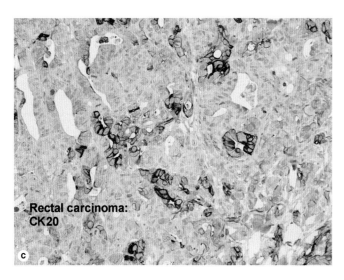

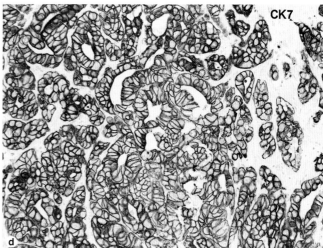

Fig. 26.6, cont'd (C and D) Paradoxical immunostaining pattern in rectal carcinoma (CK20 weak, CK7+). Colon cancer is usually CK20+ and CK7–

Ovarian carcinoma

Key Features

- Well-differentiated adenocarcinoma
- Sometimes the tumor demonstrates papillary fronding
- Psammoma bodies (concentric calcifications) may be seen
- CK7+ and CA125+ and PAX8+

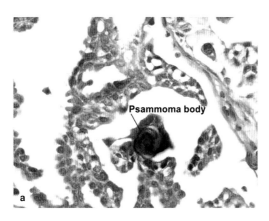

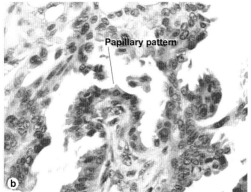

Fig. 26.7 Ovarian carcinoma

Signet-ring carcinoma

Key Features

- Atypical cells with central pale area (mucin) that compresses the nucleus to the periphery
- Loose stroma

The site of origin is most commonly gastric, although they may arise from other parts of the gastrointestinal tract or breast.

Thyroid carcinoma

Key Features

- Papillary is most common, followed by follicular
- Psammoma bodies may be seen, especially in papillary carcinoma
- "Orphan Annie" nuclei (large nuclei, a pale center) and nuclear pseudoinclusions are typical of papillary carcinoma
- Medullary carcinoma stains with calcitonin
- Thyroglobulin+ and TTF-1+

Metastases from the thyroid often spread hematogenously, allowing thyroid carcinoma to present at a variety of body sites. The scalp is a common site. Papillary thyroid carcinoma displays fronds of cells with occasional psammoma bodies and "Orphan Annie" eye nuclei. A follicular variant exists, but retains the characteristic "Orphan Annie" eye nuclei and pseudoinclusions. Follicular thyroid carcinoma is composed of thyroid follicles with colloid. Medullary thyroid carcinomas generally consist of sheets of atypical cells with amyloid; they may be sporadic but occasionally are markers for multiple endocrine neoplasia syndromes IIA (Sipple syndrome) and IIB.

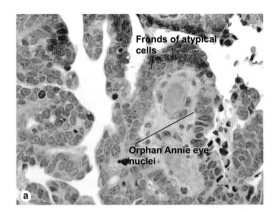

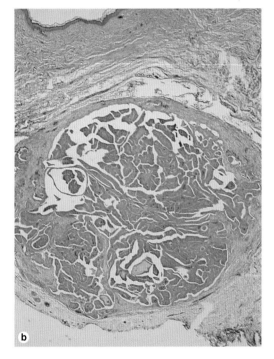

Fig. 26.8 Papillary thyroid carcinoma

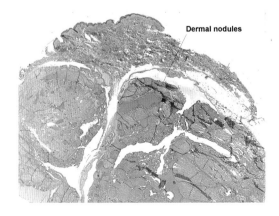

Fig. 26.9 Follicular thyroid carcinoma

Prostate carcinoma

Key Features

- Poorly differentiated adenocarcinoma
- Atypical cells infiltrating through collagen
- Prostate-specific antigen (PSA)+

Metastatic prostate carcinoma generally presents on the thighs/groin area, although it has been reported at other sites.

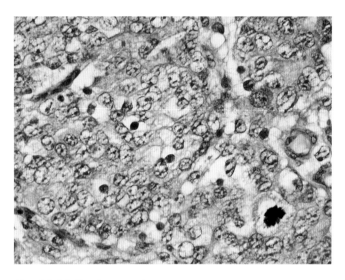

Fig. 26.10 Prostate carcinoma

Metastatic squamous cell carcinoma

Key Features

- Tumor in deeper dermis
- Generally lacks an epidermal connection
- Occasional squamous pearls present
- May be poorly differentiated; helpful positive stains include p63 or p40 and cytokeratins

Metastatic squamous cell carcinoma most commonly originates from the oral cavity, lung, esophagus, or skin. Other rare primary sites include the cervix and the male genitalia. Epidermotropic metastases may simulate primary cutaneous squamous cell carcinoma.

Cytokeratin AE1/AE3 does not always stain squamous cell carcinoma. Pankeratin cocktails, cytokeratin MNF116, or cytokeratin 34βE12 (CK903) are commonly more reliable.

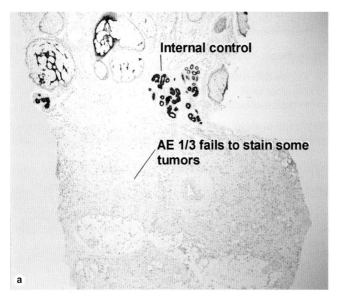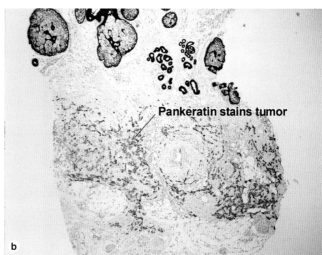

Fig. 26.11 Squamous cell carcinoma

Meningioma

Key Features

- Spindled to ovoid cells in whorls or groups
- Fibrocollagenous to loose stroma
- Cells may be in sheetlike syncytia
- Psammoma bodies may be seen
- EMA+

The cutaneous presentation of an intracranial meningioma may be secondary to direct extension of the intracranial tumor or true metastatic spread. Lesions are generally seen on the scalp.

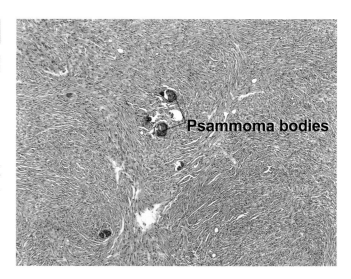

Fig. 26.12 Meningioma

Table 26.1 Keratin immunostains for metastatic adenocarcinoma					
	Breast	Colon	Lung	Urinary tract	Pancreas/biliary
Cytokeratin 7	+	–	+	+	+
Cytokeratin 20	–	+	–	+	+

Table 26.2 Immunostains for metastatic carcinoma

Adenocarcinoma	Immunostain
Breast	GCDFP-15+, CEA+, CK7+, EMA+
Gastrointestinal	CEA+, CK20+, CDX2+
Lung	TTF-1+, CEA+
Ovarian	CA125+, PAX8+
	(mucinous subtype is CK7 and CK20+)
Prostate	PSA+
Renal	CD10+
	RCC+, PAX8+
Thyroid	TTF-1+, thyroglobulin+, calcitonin+ (medullary type), PAX8+

CA, cancer antigen; *CD,* cluster of differentiation; *CEA,* carcinoembryonic antigen; *CK,* cytokeratin; *EMA,* epithelial membrane antigen; *GCDFP,* gross cystic disease fluid protein; *RCC,* renal cell carcinoma antigen; *PSA,* prostate-specific antigen; *TTF,* thyroid transcription factor.

Lesions that mimic metastatic carcinoma

Endometriosis

Key Features

- Glandular spaces
- Loose concentric fibromyxoid stroma
- RBCs ± hemosiderin in stroma
- Decidualized endometriosis has large polygonal decidual cells in the stroma

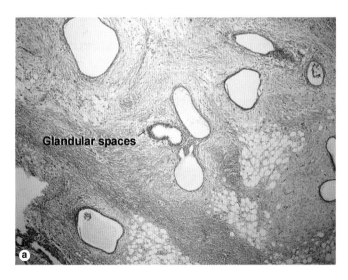

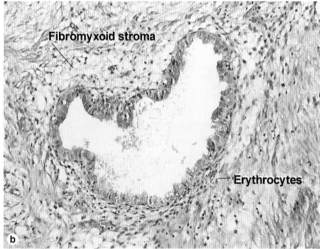

Fig. 26.13 (A and B) Endometriosis.

continued

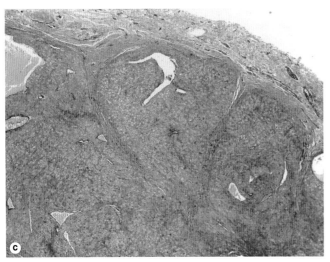

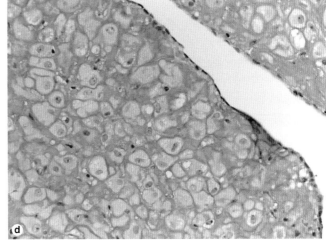

Fig. 26.13, cont'd (C and D) Decidualized endometriosis

Omphalomesenteric duct polyp

Key Features

- Polypoid tumor in umbilical area
- Surface squamous epithelium adjacent to mucosal epithelium
- Columnar epithelium with goblet cells
- Smooth muscle may be present underlying the mucosal epithelium

Columnar epithelium and goblet cells

Fig. 26.14 Omphalomesenteric duct polyp

Further reading

Abrol N, Seth A, Chattergee P. Cutaneous metastasis of prostate carcinoma to neck and upper chest. Indian J Pathol Microbiol 2011;54(2):394–5.

Amin A, Burgess EF. Skin manifestations associated with kidney cancer. Semin Oncol 2016;43(3):408–12.

Marcoval J, Penín RM, Llatjós R, et al. Cutaneous metastasis from lung cancer: retrospective analysis of 30 patients. Australas J Dermatol 2012;53(4):288–90.

Raghavan D. Cutaneous manifestations of genitourinary malignancy. Semin Oncol 2016;43(3):347–52.

Rollins-Raval M, Chivukula M, Tseng GC, et al. An immunohistochemical panel to differentiate metastatic breast carcinoma to skin from primary sweat gland carcinomas with a review of the literature. Arch Pathol Lab Med 2011;135(8):975–83.

Tan AR. Cutaneous manifestations of breast cancer. Semin Oncol 2016;43(3):331–4.

Dermatopathology mnemonics

"Neuts in the horn" = PTICSS	Eosinophilic spongiosis = HAAPPIE	PEH with pus = "Here come big green leafy veggies"
Psoriasis	**H**erpes gestationis	**H**alogenoderma
Tinea	**A**rthropod bite	**C**hromomycosis
Impetigo	**A**llergic contact dermatitis	**B**lastomycosis
Candida	**P**emphigus	**G**ranuloma inguinale
Seborrheic dermatitis	**P**emphigoid	**L**eishmaniasis
Syphilis	**I**ncontinentia pigmenti	Pemphigus **v**egetans(eosinophils predominate)
	Erythema toxicum neonatorum (spongiosis adjacent to a follicle)	

Neuts stuffed in the dermal papillae = PLAID	Subcorneal pustule = CAT PISS	Lichenoid DDX
Bullous **p**emphigoid	**C**andida	LP
Lupus (bullous)	**A**cropustulosis of infancy/AGEP	LPLK (BLK)
EB**A**	**T**ransient neonatal pustular melanosis/Tinea	Lichenoid drug
Linear **i**mmunoglobulin A	**P**ustular psoriasis	Lichenoid regression of melanocytic lesion
DH	**I**mpetigo	Lichenoid graft-versus-host disease
	Sneddon–Wilkinson	Lupus (acral – "lips and tips")
	Staphylococcal-scalded skin syndrome	

Stellate abscess (palisaded granuloma with neuts) = Stella has the "CLATS"	Parasitized histiocytes = "pH GIRL"	Busy dermis = "Busy dermis can kill grandma's sweet nieces"
Cat scratch	**P**enicillium marneffei	**B**lue nevus
LGV	**H**istoplasmosis	**D**F/**d**ermal Spitz
Atypical mycobacterial	**G**ranuloma **i**nguinale	**C**utaneous metastasis
Tularemia rarely melioidosis	**R**hinoscleroma	**K**aposi (plaque)
Sporotrichosis (plus rarely melioidosis, *Nocardia*)	**L**eishmaniasis/**l**eprosy	**G**ranuloma annulare
	Lymph in every hole	**S**cleromyxedema
	MF	**N**eurofibroma
	LPLK (BLK)	**S**yphilis
	PLEVA	
	PLC	

Vasculitis		Spindle cells *SLAM*med against the epidermis	Buckshot scatter
Big 5	**Little 5**	**S**pindle cell SCC	Paget
Granulomatosis with polyangiitis (formerly Wegener's granulomatosis) Eosinophilic granulomatosis with polyangiitis (formerly Churg-Strauss) Rheumatoid Septic Microscopic polyarteritis/ polyarteritis nodosa	HSP Cryos Drug CTD Serum sickness	**L**eiomyosarcoma **A**FX **M**elanoma (spindle cell)	Bowen Melanoma Center of acral nevus Center of Spitz Sebaceous carcinoma
Ulceroglandular infections = "Please Tell Me That Lawyers Can Get Convicted"		**Rectangular biopsy specimen = "Most Normal Skin Can't Get Really Square"**	**Paisley-tie differential = "Most MDs (wear paisley ties)"**
Plague **T**uberculosis **M**elioidosis **T**ularemia **L**ymphogranuloma venerum **C**at scratch **G**landers **C**hancroid *Courtesy of Adam Lake*		**M**orphea **N**ormal back **S**car **C**onnective tissue nevi **C**hronic Graft versus host **R**adiation treatment **S**cleroderma/Scleredema *Courtesy of Al Strickler*	**M**orpheaform basal cell carcinoma **M**icrocystic adnexal carcinoma **D**esmoplastic trichoepithelioma **S**yringoma *Courtesy of Al Strickler*
Eosinophilic panniculitis = "Many Eosinophils Are Hyper In Panniculitis"		**Spongiotic dermatitis = "Spongiotic Dermatitis Appears So DAINTY Per the Scope"**	**Dermato***M*yo**F**ibroma = "Doesn't move follicles"
Medication **E**osinophilic fasciitis **A**rthropod **H**ypereosinophilic syndrome **I**diopathic **P**arasite *Courtesy of Al Strickler*		**S**pongiotic pigmenting purpura **D**yshidrotic dermatitis **A**llergic contact dermatitis **I**D reaction **N**ummular dermatitis **T**inea **Y**east (*Candida*) **P**ityriasis rosea **S**tasis dermatitis *Courtesy of Al Strickler*	*Courtesy of Tyler Vukmer*

AGEG, acute generalized exanthematous pustulosis; *AFX*, atypical fibroxanthoma; *BLK*, benign lichenoid keratosis; *Cryos*, mixed cryoglobulinemia; *CTD*, connective tissue disease; *DDX*, differential diagnosis; *DF*, dermatofibroma; *DH*, dermatitis herpetiformis; *EBA*, epidermolysis bullosa acquisita; *HSP*, Henoch–Schönlein purpura; *LGV*, lymphogranuloma venereum; *LP*, lichen planus; *LPLK*, lichen planus–like keratosis; *MF*, mycosis fungoides; *PLC*, pityriasis lichenoides chronica; *PLEVA*, pityriasis lichenoides et varioliformis acuta; *SCC*, squamous cell carcinoma.

Skin ultrastructure

Sunita Bhuta

1. Desmosome

A classic desmosome showing the following features: (1) uniform gap of 20–30 nm between the apposed trilaminar plasma membranes with an intermediate line *(arrow)* in this gap; and (2) sharply delineated dense plaques into which tonofibrils (F) converge.

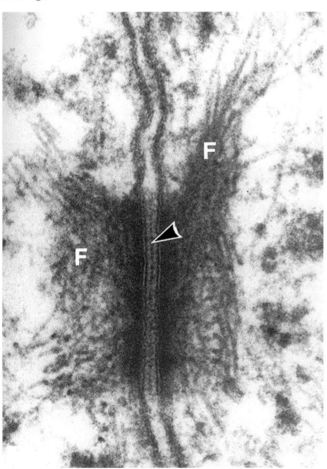

2. Langerhans cell (with Birbeck granules)

This electronmicrograph shows characteristic racket-shaped profiles of the granules in the cytoplasm (inset with higher magnification of the Birbeck granule).

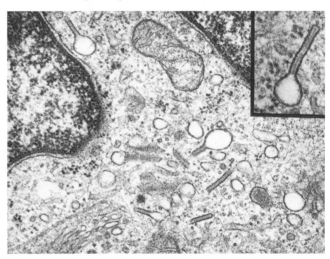

3. Premelanosome

Solitary melanosome with characteristic internal striated structure.

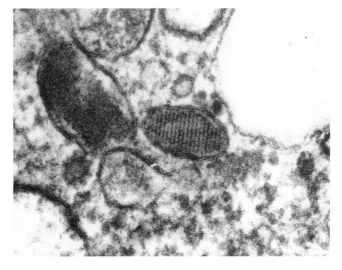

4. Tonofibrils

Tonofibrils (intermediate filaments) lying free in the cytoplasm of a squamous cell.

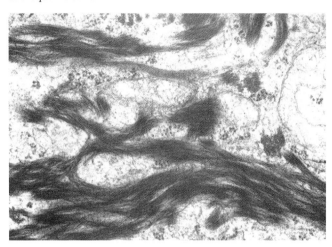

5. Eosinophil

(A) Binucleate (N) with intracytoplasmic-specific granules. **(B)** Specific granules have a finely granular matrix and a crystalline (Cr) core.

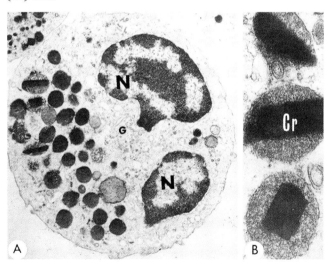

6. Mast cell

Mast cell with numerous electron-dense granules. Inset shows internal structure of granules with membranous whorls (scrolls).

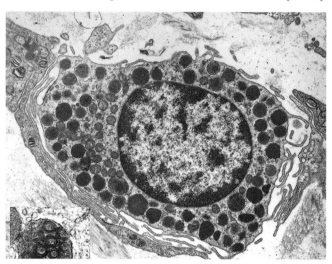

7. Merkel cell

Merkel cell with intracytoplasmic membrane-bound, electron-dense, round granules with a halo (neurosecretory granules).

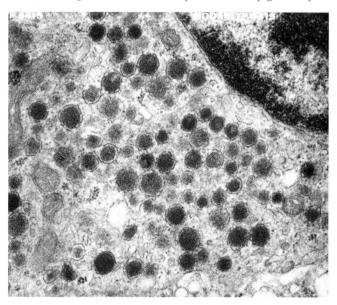

External agents and artifacts

Tammie Ferringer

1. Electrocautery

- Keratinocytes show marked parallel vertical elongation
- Homogenization of the collagen

2. Gelfoam

- Blue-purple, arabesque, netlike pattern with surrounding granulomatous reaction

3. Aluminum chloride

- Epidermal effacement and horizontal fibrosis consistent with scar and underlying light gray-blue granules, often in histiocytes, with focal calcification

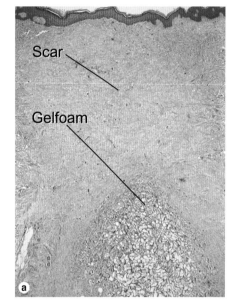

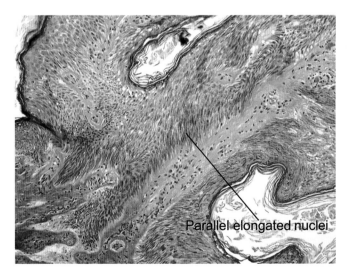

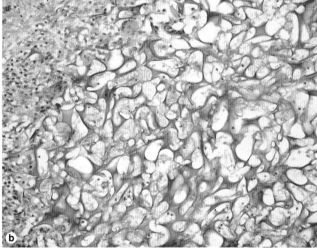

Fig. Ap3.1 Electrocautery artifact

Fig. Ap3.2 (A,B) Gelfoam

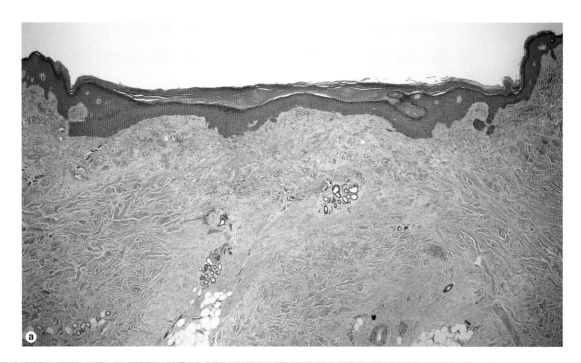

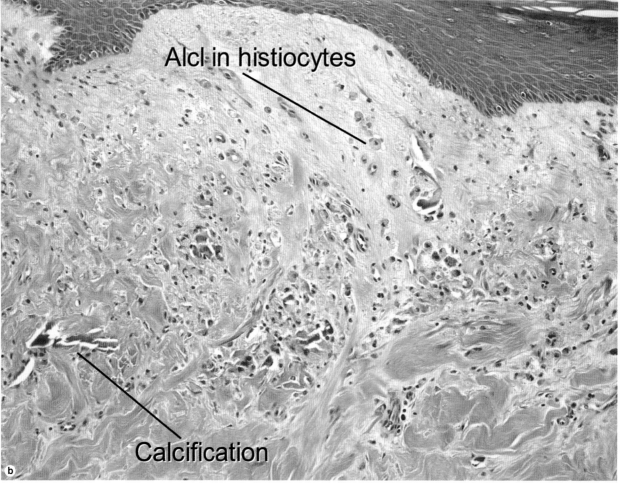

Fig. Ap3.3 (A,B) Aluminum chloride at base of biopsy site

4. Monsel's solution (ferric subsulfate)

- Epidermal effacement and horizontal fibrosis with collagen necrosis and chunky golden, refractile pigment in macrophages
- Perls' iron stain is strongly positive, distinguishing the pigment from melanin

5. Triamcinolone

- Lake of bluish granular to amorphous material, at times surrounded by histiocytic response

Triamcinolone is often seen localized within a keloid or hypertrophic scar where it is iatrogenically injected. It superficially resembles mucin but is negative with mucin stains.

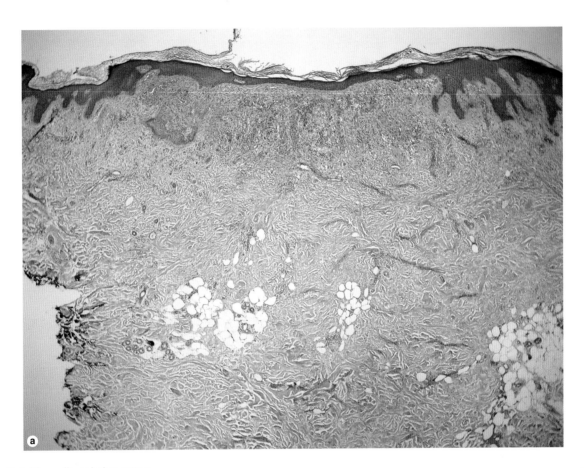

Fig. Ap3.4 Monsel's solution tattoo

continued

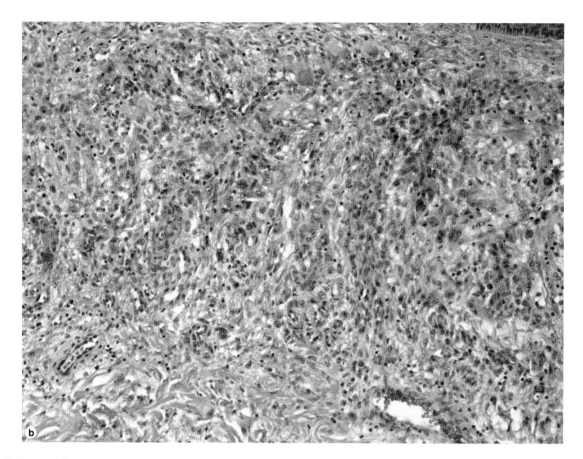

Fig. Ap3.4, cont'd

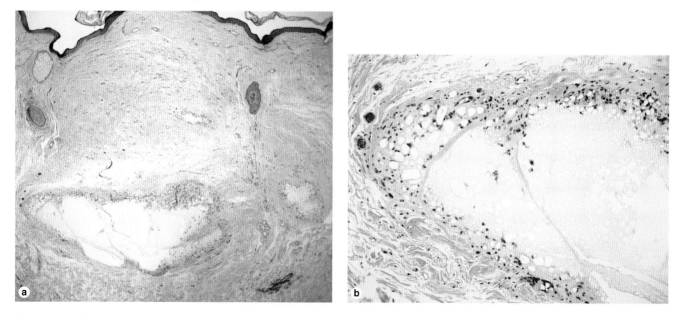

Fig. Ap3.5 (A,B) Triamcinolone in scar

6. Splinter

- Often brown fragment with honeycomb pattern of cell walls.

When plant material is identified in the dermis, it is prudent to perform stains for bacteria and fungi to exclude contaminating organisms.

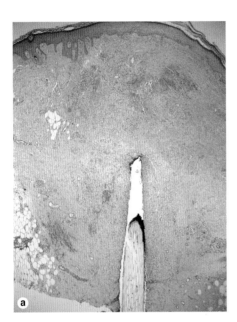

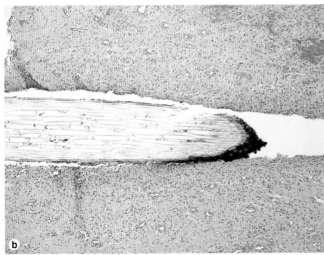

Fig. Ap3.6 Splinter

7. Suture

- Birefringent braided filaments
- Granulomatous foreign–body reaction

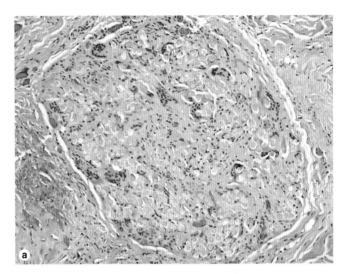

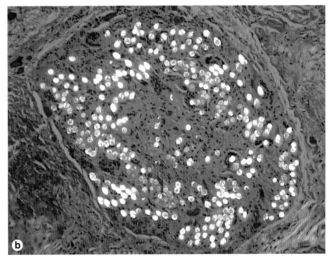

Fig. Ap3.7 (A) Suture. **(B)** Suture (polarized microscopy)

8. Amalgam

- Golden or brown-black fragments and granules free in the dermis or deposited on connective tissue fibers

Amalgam tattoos consist of silver, mercury, and tin and likely occur after accidental implantation during dental procedures. The buccal, gingival, and alveolar mucosa are most commonly affected by these gray-blue macules.

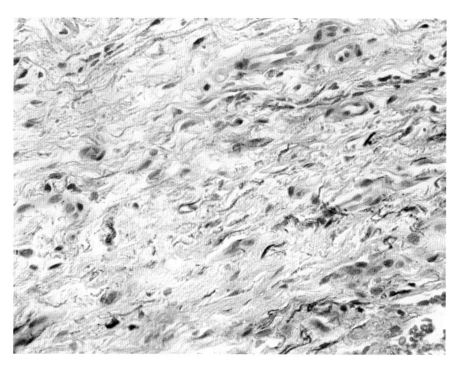

Fig. Ap3.8 Amalgam tattoo

9. Calcium hydroxylapatite

- Nonbirefringent, bluish-gray, round to oval calcific microspheres with variable foreign-body granulomatous reaction

This is a resorbable cosmetic filler that stimulates collagen production. The trade name is Radiesse.

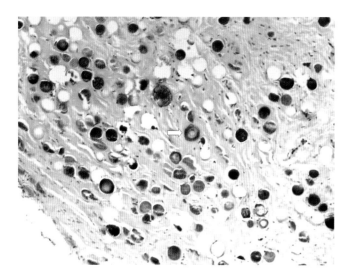

Fig. Ap3.9 Calcium hydroxylapatite filler

10. Hyaluronic acid

- Basophilic material in variable size and shape deposits

This is a resorbable cosmetic filler. Trade names include Restylane, Juvéderm, and Perlane.

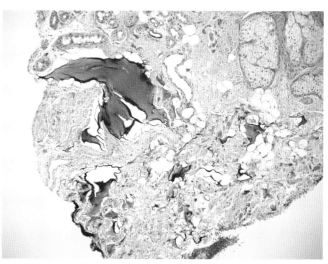

Fig. Ap3.10 Hyaluronic acid filler

11. Poly-L-lactic acid

- Polarizable spiky translucent particles

This is a resorbable cosmetic filler. Trade names include Sculptra and New-Fill.

12. Silicone granuloma

- Empty, variable-sized vacuoles with foreign-body giant cells and fibrosis

Used in soft tissue augmentation. Leakage can occur after trauma to breast implants and occasionally can migrate to distant sites.

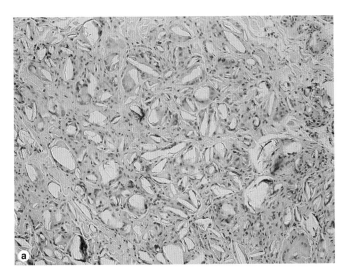

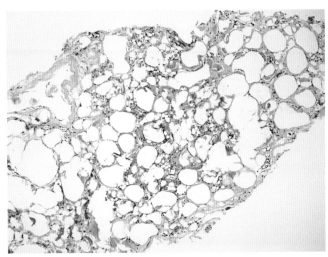

Fig. Ap3.12 Silicone granuloma

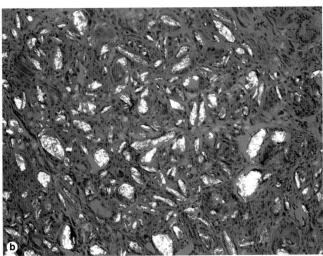

Fig. Ap3.11 (A) Poly-L-lactic acid filler. **(B)** Poly-L-lactic acid filler (polarized microscopy)

13. Argyria

- Minute black granules in the lamina propria of vessels, outlining the basement membrane of sweat glands, and adjacent to elastic fibers

Dietary, medicinal, and industrial exposure to silver-containing compounds results in systemic deposition of silver salts causing a blue-gray pigmentation to the skin, most notable in sun-exposed areas. Localized argyria can occur due to topical application or implantation.

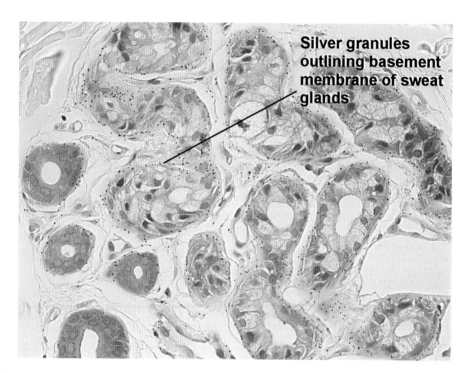

Silver granules outlining basement membrane of sweat glands

Fig. Ap3.13 Argyria

Further reading

Requena L, Cerroni L, Kutzner H. Histopathologic patterns associated with external agents. Dermatol Clin 2012;30(4):731–48.

Requena L, Requena C, Christensen L, et al. Adverse reactions to injectable soft tissue fillers. J Am Acad Dermatol 2011;64(1):1–34.

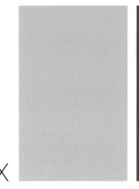

Index

Page numbers followed by "*f*" indicate figures, "*t*" indicate tables, "*b*" indicate boxes, and "*e*" indicate online content.